Praise for *Remed*

"As a work of policy history *Remedy and Reaction* excels.... [Starr] chronicles just how difficult a struggle it has been to make the U. S. healthcare system more equitable and efficient and how far we still have to go."

—Jonathan Oberlander, *Science*

"[A] useful and lucid history of American health reform.... Anyone seeking to understand how difficult it will be to implement President Barack Obama's health care reforms will be enlightened by Starr's readable and engrossing narrative. Highly recommended."   —Jeff Goldsmith, *Health Affairs*

"None of the numerous other histories of US health care policy develops these themes in such an illuminating fashion.... This book provides one of the clearest descriptions and best justifications of the Affordable Care Act published to date.... [An] excellent, cogently argued work."

—Samuel Y. Sessions, *Journal of the American Medical Association*

"[A] remarkable chronicle of the hundred year effort to legislate universal health insurance in the United States.... Nobody with a sense of history—that is, nobody who reads Starr's book—could doubt how sensible and brave was the president's effort to drive the Patient Protection and Affordable Care Act of 2010 through Congress."   —Bernard Avishai, *The Nation*

"Here's the book we've been waiting for—a lucid history of America's struggle over healthcare reform, blending the political, economic, and social pressures that have brought us to where we are, and suggesting where we're headed. With great insight and impeccable writing, Paul Starr explains why that struggle has been particularly bitter and partisan in the United States, why the resulting compromises have left so many people unsatisfied, and why the underlying problems continue to evade us. Brilliant and important."

—Robert B. Reich, Chancellor's Professor of Public Policy,
Goldman School of Public Policy, University of California, Berkeley

"[A] clear, comprehensive, and compelling chronicle of the health care debate.... Starr is at the top of his game."   —Glenn Altschuler, *Huffington Post*

"Remarkable.... There couldn't be a more astute insider to the politics of reform than Starr.... Starr's history of America's battle over whether health care should be a right is an exacting look at politics and policies—and a challenge to Americans to overcome their fear and distrust in order to protect the sick and vulnerable."   —*Publishers Weekly*, starred review

"First, [Starr] objectively draws together the threads of myriad voices and special interests in the century long American health care debate and weaves them into a wholly comprehensible pattern. . . . Second, Starr cogently explains the highlights of the recently passed and highly controversial Affordable Care Act. . . . In sum, this self admitted universal health care advocate and seasoned realist leaves readers questioning, as he does, whether Americans can 'summon the elementary decency toward the sick that characterizes other democracies.'"
—Donna Chavez, *Booklist*, starred review

"The best summary and political analysis of health care reform I've read. . . . Starr nails every nuance while taking the analysis one level deeper than any other treatment I've read."　　　　　—Austin Frakt, *Incidental Economist*

"[I]f I were forced to assign only one book to summarize the historical context, political constraints, and policy dilemmas that shaped the 2010 Patient Protection and Affordable Care Act (PPACA), I would definitely choose this tart and briskly paced 300 page work. I would do the same if I had to recommend one book to a well-informed colleague who obsessively followed the 2009 and 2010 legislative debate leading up to the PPACA. I was surprised by how much I learned reading *Remedy and Reaction*, as I was a close observer and partisan participant in that story."　　　—Harold Pollack, *Public Administration Review*

"Three decades ago Paul Starr wrote the definitive history of American medicine. *Remedy and Reaction* now offers the definitive analysis of American health care reform—its history, nature, and continuing vulnerability."
—Timothy Jost, coeditor, *Transforming American Medicine:
A Twenty Year Retrospective*

"*Remedy and Reaction* is the story of health care in America, told by the man who knows it best. Whether you're a serious scholar or just a serious citizen, you should read this."　　　　　—Jonathan Cohn, senior editor, *New Republic*

"Paul Starr, who gave us a magisterial account of the history of American medicine, now has given us the definitive account of the history of the struggle to enact health reform in America. Starr has done more than just study reform—he was a player in efforts to achieve it. *Remedy and Reaction* is in some ways thus an insider's history, which only enriches the experience of the reader. This book is a lively read, but has depth and insight. From its account of the early experiences in the twentieth century with reform, up through the disappointments in our lifetimes to achieve any comprehensive change, through the enactment of

the Affordable Care Act and the story of its uncertain future, *Remedy and Reaction* is the definitive account of the history of health reform in America."
—Norman Ornstein, coauthor of *The Broken Branch: How Congress Is Failing America and How to Get it Back on Track*

"Few books as important as this one is are as clearly and compellingly written. *Remedy and Reaction* is a brilliant analysis of the political conflicts and compromises that led to the passage of the Affordable Care Act, and a fitting sequel to Paul Starr's masterful book, *The Social Transformation of American Medicine*. The final page came much too soon."
—Shannon Brownlee, author of *Overtreated: Why Too Much Medicine is Making Us Sicker and Poorer*

"A useful contribution as the country moves forward with the implementation of health care reform."
—*Kirkus Reviews*

"[D]elivers an insightful political analysis."
—Kristen Greencher, *Charlotte Observer*

"[An] interesting and engaging account of the many attempts made over the past century to reform care in this country. As daunting, even wonkish, as this may sound, Starr does an excellent job of explaining the different proposals and identifying the reasons why some succeeded where others failed so spectacularly."
—Dennis Rosen, *Boston Globe*

"[C]oncise and beautifully written."
—Michael Gusmano, *Commonweal*

REMEDY AND REACTION

PAUL STARR

Remedy
and
Reaction

THE PECULIAR AMERICAN STRUGGLE

OVER HEALTH CARE REFORM

Revised Edition

Yale UNIVERSITY PRESS

NEW HAVEN & LONDON

Yale University Press books may be purchased in quantity for educational, business, or promotional use. For information, please e-mail
sales.press@yale.edu (U.S. office) or sales@yaleup.co.uk (U.K. office).

Set in Scala type by Westchester Book Group.
Printed in the United States of America.

Library of Congress Control Number: 2013933273
ISBN 978-0-300-17109-9 (cloth : alk. paper)
ISBN 978-0-300-18915-5 (pbk.)

A catalogue record for this book is available from the British Library.

10 9 8 7 6 5 4 3 2 1

To Emanuel and Oren, Marghi, and the next generation

CONTENTS

PREFACE TO THE REVISED EDITION

ISSUES OF HIGH IMPORTANCE IN NATIONAL POLICY are not always subjects of high drama in politics, but for the past two years health-care reform has been both. When the Supreme Court heard oral arguments about the constitutionality of the Affordable Care Act in March 2012, the debate over reform became a theatrical event as well as a critical test of national principles. After a young woman testified in favor of the contraceptive coverage under the law, a radio blowhard heard across the country called her a "slut" and a "prostitute" and helped to re-ignite passions over birth control. When the former governor who had passed the program that led to "Obamacare" ran for president and promised to repeal it, health-care reform was thrust first into the Republican primaries and then into the general election.

Since *Remedy and Reaction* was first published in October 2011, the politics of health-care reform has not wanted for surprise and suspense. No one knew at that time whether the Affordable Care Act would survive the Supreme Court or the 2012 election. At the oral argument in the Court over the individual mandate, I was among those sitting in the audience, stunned by the conservative justices' onslaught against the government's case but uncertain at the end how the Court would rule. Its decision turned out to defy almost all informed predictions. The election posed a stark choice between two different paths in health care, but the political debate turned on symbols and secondary issues rather than the big question facing the country: Do we have an obligation to provide health care for all our citizens?

The re-election of Barack Obama ensured that the Affordable Care Act would go into effect, but it is too early to say whether it will become as firmly established in national policy as Social Security and Medicare have been. If Democrats had enough votes, they would extend the new law, and if Republicans had enough votes, they would undo it. Such stability as it has in 2013 is the result of neither party being able to do as it wants. The real test will come when one of them does.

When I first set out to write *Remedy and Reaction,* I thought I would be writing about how America's long war over health care turned out in the end. But there is no sign even of a lull in the battle, much less a peace settlement or national reconciliation. This is not because health care is intrinsically contentious everywhere; it has for historical reasons become peculiarly contentious in the United States. That, at least, is the thesis of this book, and the national experience since the first edition gives me no reason to revise that judgment.

Paul Starr

January 2013

PREFACE AND ACKNOWLEDGMENTS

DURING THE PAST THREE DECADES, I've written about health care as a historian and sociologist and as an advocate for changes in national policy. In
the 1990s that work led me to become involved in some of the events I
would otherwise have studied at a distance, and it may raise a question in
your mind as to what kind of a book this is.

Remedy and Reaction is a history of the American struggle over health-
care reform, which I hope people on all sides will find useful. The three
parts of the book rest on somewhat different foundations: Part One on
standard historical sources; Part Two on both public sources and my direct
knowledge of events inside the Clinton White House; and Part Three on
the methods of journalism and political analysis. Along the way, especially
in Chapter 8 ("The Affordable Care Act as Public Philosophy"), I offer normative judgments of a kind that historians and social scientists usually
refrain from making. Since I have been a participant as well as an observer
in the recent phases of the national debate about health care, I will not test
your patience by pretending to be neutral about it. Whether my involvement and viewpoint are an advantage or a liability in explaining historical
developments, you will have to judge for yourself.

I want to thank my wife and family for their support during the work on
this book in the past year. I am also grateful to the many people in Washington and elsewhere who shared their knowledge with me; to Princeton
University and my colleagues at both the university and *The American*

Prospect; to Timothy Jost and Jon Kingsdale for corrections on some points of law and policy; to two Princeton students, Hope Glassberg and Trace Feng, who provided research assistance; and to my agent Scott Moyers and the people of Yale University Press who have helped bring this project to fruition.

Paul Starr

April 25, 2011

Introduction

AN UNEASY VICTORY

AMONG THE RICH NATIONS OF THE WORLD, the United States stands out for the virulence of its political battles over health care. Unlike the other capitalist democracies, America has long left a large population without insurance coverage; as of 2010, there were about 50 million uninsured at any one time. The United States also spends far more on health care than other countries do—17.6 percent of its gross domestic product compared with an average of about 9 percent in the other economically advanced societies. These differences grew wider from 1970 to 2010. In 1970, when the uninsured were a considerably smaller fraction of the population, health-care costs in the United States were much closer to the levels in western Europe and Canada. Under President Richard Nixon, the United States also came close to enacting on a bipartisan basis a comprehensive health-insurance plan for its citizens. In the following years, however, as the underlying problems of health coverage and costs became more severe, the attempts to remedy them generated more rancorous partisan divisions. In no other advanced country has public responsibility for health costs provoked such deep and bitter conflict.

The ideological warfare over health care in American politics has its antecedents in the battles over health insurance in the first half of the twentieth century. It was in those years that the United States diverged from the more common path in western democracies, failing to establish a general system for financing health care. And when America finally adopted critical tax and health-financing policies in the two decades after World War II, it ensnared itself in a *policy trap,* devising an increasingly costly and complicated system that has satisfied enough of the public and so enriched the health-care industry as to make change extraordinarily difficult.

Escaping from that policy trap has become a politically treacherous national imperative. Hoping to make it less treacherous—to attract support in the center and to avoid arousing the opposition of the protected public or the health-care industry—recent Democratic plans and legislation have called for the expansion of private insurance, once the core element of Republican proposals. The most ambitious of the Democratic efforts, the plan proposed by President Bill Clinton, came to grief in 1994 without the adoption of any legislation. But the supporters of health-care reform believed that they had finally reached their goals in March 2010, when Congress passed the Patient Protection and Affordable Care Act. Savoring the achievement, President Barack Obama and Democratic congressional leaders compared the law to such historic landmarks as Social Security, civil rights legislation, and Medicare.

It remains to be seen whether those comparisons will prove to be apt. Despite the exhilaration its supporters experienced in the moment, the passage of reform was an uneasy victory—uneasy because it was the victory of one party over a united opposition that threatened to repeal the legislation the first moment it had a chance; uneasy because many of those voting in favor had been obliged to accept compromises that they believed might jeopardize the program's success; uneasy because public opinion at the time was sharply divided; uneasy because Democrats had already suffered an unexpected reverse in an election in Massachusetts in January and were worried (for good reason) about more losses in the fall.

The law's passage was also an uneasy victory because its implementation was left in large measure to governors and state legislatures—some of whom fervently opposed the law and would challenge its constitutionality in court—and because no one could be certain the law would withstand all the attacks on it and lead to a stable and popular outcome. Even some of the strongest advocates of reform (and I am one of them) worried that the United States had become so entangled in the knot of problems it had woven in health-care finance that any politically achievable response was bound to be imperfect and to be condemned for its limitations.

Political leadership requires different sorts of courage. Sometimes it is the physical courage to face down a hostile mob—and Democratic members of the House of Representatives had to show that fortitude as they walked to the decisive vote on March 21 through right-wing protesters who spat on them. Sometimes it is the courage to put a political career at risk for the sake of deeply held principles; many legislators had to do that as well. And sometimes it is the courage to make a decision when the choices are less than ideal and the prospects for success are uncertain. All those who voted for reform had to make that leap too.

This book is about why health care in the United States became so vexed a problem. My aim is to provide an analytical account of the struggle over reform, attentive to both stubborn social realities and the critical choices that political leaders and other individuals have made. Institutional and political constraints are not imaginary, but political leadership often involves testing how strong those chains are—sometimes breaking them, and sometimes falling short.

The Making of a National Impasse

Large-scale innovation in national policy has never been easy in the United States, nor was it intended to be. In a parliamentary democracy, a party that wins a legislative majority thereby controls the executive and usually can carry out its program by a vote of the lower house. But America's constitutional system sets up a series of impediments even for a winning party: the division of Congress into two co-equal houses; the short, two-year intervals between congressional elections; the separation of the executive from the legislature; a Supreme Court with lifetime tenure. Additional institutional obstacles have grown up in the form of powerful congressional committees controlled by senior lawmakers and procedural rules in the Senate that enable a minority of 40 members to prevent legislation from coming to a vote. With so many veto points along the journey to law, supporters of major reforms usually cannot put them into effect by winning only one election.

After gaining power, they often need to retain it through several elections in order to control every point where their program may be blocked.

The American political system does offer ways of working around its impediments. The most important of these is the ability of the states to serve as "laboratories of democracy" for policies blocked at the national level. States also face constraints: federal law often limits their authority, and they cannot let their taxes and regulations get too far out of line with those of other states, lest businesses and jobs go elsewhere. Nonetheless, national reforms have often begun with state programs, and the federal system enables Congress to build in flexibility for states so that they may, for example, set eligibility and benefits for a program above a national minimum, obtain waivers of particular requirements, or opt out of some programs entirely.

In nearly a century of struggle—from 1915 until 2010—the advocates of a public program to provide all Americans access to health care and shield them from the costs of illness tried virtually every course possible in a federal system. At first they sought to pass laws in the states. Later they offered proposals for a federal program that would have been carried out through the states and allowed them to opt out. Still later, they tried purely federal measures. Then while some reformers advocated a federal program, others went back to pushing for action in states where they had the best chance of success. But they were unable to pass and carry out a universal program at either the federal or the state level, at least until they succeeded in Massachusetts in 2006.

The failure of the more ambitious proposals led to the adoption of a series of compromises benefiting particular groups to varying extent. As they had from early in American history, some states and local governments provided support for hospitals and clinics for the poor. Beginning after World War I, Congress established a separate hospital and medical system for veterans. In the 1940s and '50s, the federal government began providing a tax subsidy for those with employer-provided private health insurance. In 1965 Congress enacted a purely federal program for the elderly (Medicare) and a mixed, federal-state program (Medicaid) for specific categories of poor people. Some federal and state programs targeted funds to support treatment for particular types of disease. Nonetheless, many

Americans remained without access to care or financial protection when illness struck.

By the second half of the twentieth century, the United States was the only major advanced society without a system for providing health care for all its citizens. After the enactment of Medicare and Medicaid, roughly 10 to 12 percent of people remained without coverage in the early 1970s. Then, in line with other measures of growing economic inequality and insecurity, the uninsured population began to increase, rising to 16.7 percent of Americans, or 50.7 million people, in 2009.[1] These Census Bureau figures are estimates of the numbers of uninsured at a given time. The number who lose insurance for some period during a year is about 50 percent higher, and according to a Treasury Department study, almost half of the non-elderly population, 48 percent, were uninsured for some time over the decade from 1997 to 2006.[2] Many with insurance also had coverage that proved inadequate in serious illness, particularly if they had a pre-existing condition or their policy had other exclusions. As a result of the various limitations of the insurance system, Americans experienced forms of economic insecurity virtually unknown in the other advanced countries: "medical uninsurability," "medical bankruptcy," and "job lock" (inability to start a business or change jobs for fear of losing health benefits).

During the past 40 years, America also became an outlier in health-care costs. In 1970 the United States spent 7 percent of GDP on health care, the same proportion as Canada, about the same as Sweden (6.8 percent) and Denmark (7.9 percent), more than France (5.3 percent), and considerably more than Britain (4.5 percent). By 2007, in dollar terms, the United States spent two and a half times per capita as much as the average of other rich countries—and more than 50 percent more than the next highest spenders (Norway and Switzerland).[3] Since health expenditures vary directly with national income, the United States would be expected to spend more on health care than other countries did. But by the early 2000s, health spending was 42 percent greater in the United States than its income would predict.[4] Variations in disease rates also do not explain these differences in spending, nor do Americans visit the doctor more often or spend more time in hospitals. The main difference is not volume but price—Americans pay more for drugs, medical equipment, hospital care, and doctors' visits.[5]

High costs and spotty insurance inevitably lead to less access to care: in a 2008 study, 52 percent of Americans with incomes below the median reported that they went without medical treatment or a prescription because of cost, compared with 24 percent of the comparable group in Germany, 18 percent in Canada, and 9 percent in Britain.[6] And despite the excellence of American medicine at its best, the U.S. system did not show up particularly well in international comparisons. A rating of the overall performance of health-care systems by the World Health Organization in 2000 ranked America's thirty-seventh.[7]

With all the many problems of America's health-care system, why has it been so hard to change? Three familiar lines of explanation focus on special interests, national values, and the daunting complexity of the problems of health care and health policy.

The "special interests" that many people have in mind as obstacles to change are the insurance and pharmaceutical companies, hospitals, physicians, and others who make money from health care. The basic equation of health economics remains: health-care costs equal health-care incomes. Since every dollar spent on health care is also a dollar that someone earns from health care, interest groups predictably resist government policies that limit spending. Most businesses do not want regulation by the government or competition from it, and Americans who earn their living from health care are no exception. Physicians, in particular, have historically opposed any intrusion by the state into their professional terrain that would limit their income or autonomy, and during the past century, particularly from 1935 to 1965, "organized medicine" fought repeatedly against a public program for health insurance. As the health-care industry has mushroomed, groups with a stake in the system have also proliferated. When the major European countries created their national insurance systems between the 1880s and early 1900s, health care was a small portion of their economies, probably no more than 3 percent of GDP. In the United States, reforms affect a much larger industry, now more than 17 percent of the economy, and they may threaten more substantial (and more heavily commercialized) interests.

The opposition of physicians and insurers in the first half of the twentieth century was unquestionably a factor in blocking adoption of early proposals for government health insurance programs. But special-interest influence is not as good an explanation as it may initially seem for the persistence of the status quo. In recent decades, the major health-care interest groups have not been uniformly opposed to large-scale reforms, including measures that would cover the uninsured. Faced with political leaders and movements advocating expanded coverage, health-care industry stakeholders have sometimes thrown their support to policies they see as beneficial or at least as less distasteful than other likely alternatives. Economic interests are often hard to calculate. Groups continually face difficult choices about whether to pursue their interests by trying to shape the content of reforms or by blocking them altogether, and even those with shared interests may disagree about what to do because of conflicting political judgments (for example, about the form that legislation is likely to take when it finally emerges from the "sausage-making" in Congress).

The special-interest explanation for the status quo also has another serious deficiency: it seems to imply that if not for special interests, the public would overwhelmingly welcome reform. But one of the legacies of American health policy is that it has split the interests of the public. The government has given generous tax benefits for private health insurance to unionized workers and other employees of businesses that offer health benefits. Veterans have their medical system, the elderly and the disabled have Medicare, and some of the poor qualify for Medicaid. These members of the protected public may still be vulnerable to problems in paying for health care if their status changes, as when insured workers lose their jobs. But they may worry less about those possibilities than about the unknown risks of reforms that could upset arrangements that satisfy them reasonably well. The persistently uninsured are a mostly low-income population with no coherence, organization, or political power, even though the numbers uninsured at any one time have grown to about 50 million. In contrast, the protected public is not only larger but also consists of highly organized and vocal groups.

Moreover, many of those who are reasonably well protected—veterans, the elderly, the families of employees with good benefits—believe that they have earned their coverage, whereas others have not. These moral perceptions contribute to the intense, often vituperative tenor of public debates about health care. If political leaders favoring reform had to worry only about overcoming resistance from interest groups in the health-care industry, reform would certainly not be easy. But it is all the more difficult because the partial measures of the past have attached the protected public to the status quo and given many people a moral argument against doing anything on behalf of the uninsured. Rising health costs and other problems with health care do not necessarily lead members of the protected public to accept the need for change; on the contrary, they may cling to the protections they have all the more tightly and insist that they not be taxed to pay for anyone else.

Like the special-interest account, the national-values explanation for the failure to change the system has an immediate attraction. Americans, according to this argument, are more devoted to individual liberty than are people in other countries that have adopted universal health insurance. Not only are Americans individualistic; they are particularly suspicious of the federal government. There is no question that suspicion of government does run deep in the United States, though it is the anti-government attitude on the right that particularly distinguishes American political culture. American conservatives have been far more anti-statist than European conservatives, who have often played a central role in expanding the welfare state.

Yet an explanation based on national values alone runs into difficulties. If the commitment to individual liberty shaped all of our institutions, many things would be different in the United States. For example, laws and social practices might protect privacy in America more strongly than elsewhere. But, in fact, protections of the privacy of personal data are stronger in Europe than in the United States, and American courts have also significantly downgraded rights to privacy under the Fourth Amendment. Where privacy rights have come into conflict with concerns about national security, privacy has lost out. Despite these developments, privacy advocates have had great difficulty mobilizing public support for their cause. Their appeals to liberty—to the vision of "negative liberty," freedom from government—have been to little avail despite American individualism.

Or consider education. Why isn't the phrase "socialized education" part of the American political vocabulary? Public schools paid for through taxes became established in the nineteenth century when Americans were concerned, among other things, about Americanizing immigrants. The legacy of those past choices shapes thinking about education today. Parents who want to send their children to a private school still have to pay taxes, however much they may resent it, to support a system of universal public education. To be sure, if Americans had to design an educational system from scratch in the current ideological climate, public schools might not be the result. But that is the point: institutional legacies shape how people apply their values to specific spheres.

American values also did not prevent the establishment of Social Security, Medicare, and many other programs that demand just as great a departure as universal health insurance from traditions of self-reliance. Americans have found ingenious ways to reconcile those programs with their values. Even as many say they favor self-reliance, they accept Social Security and Medicare and, in fact, would be outraged if those were taken away. Moral values are complicated. Americans are egalitarian as well as individualist, but in health care as in many other areas, their values often point in opposite directions. People do not resolve their ambivalence simply through quiet self-reflection. Political groups attempt to mobilize widely shared values on behalf of their positions, and especially when an issue festers for decades, political conflict often turns differences in moral values into well-worn scripts of warring ideologies.

This is precisely what has happened in health policy: During the early and mid-twentieth century, the organized medical profession and the insurance industry shaped a script for thinking about health care that elevated their cause from mere self-interest to larger concerns about freedom and the American way. That interpretation had special resonance especially during the long American conflicts with Germany and the Soviet Union, each of which could be successively identified with "socialized medicine." These battles have left a legacy in the ideas and language that American conservatives summon when they oppose proposals for government financing of health insurance. In the other rich, capitalist democracies, conservative parties generally do not question the basic proposition, resolved long ago in those countries, that the costs of health care should be primarily a public obligation. Only in the United States is public responsibility for health-care costs equated with a loss of freedom. With equal passion, those who support broader government responsibility insist that leaving millions of people unable to afford health care is a grievous moral and political failure. With more than one-sixth of the economy at stake, health care is bound to provoke sharp conflict. But because Americans have raised the choices about health care to a high ideological plane, the difficulties in negotiating change have become even greater.

The sheer complexity of the American health-care system also sets it apart from the health systems of other countries. Not all countries with universal health coverage have a single, governmental plan, but even those with multiple insurance funds typically have standardized rules regulating payment and other matters. In contrast, Americans pay for health care through a myriad of different private insurance plans and public programs, each with its own rules and paperwork. The resulting complexity has an economic dimension: the administrative costs of American health care are far greater than the costs of other systems with more unified or standardized organization. The system's complexity also has a psychological dimension: to many of the sick and their families health insurance is mystifying. And complexity has a political dimension. The intricacies of health care finance and policy are hard for most people to follow. Some advocates of reform would like to sweep away all the many different private plans and public programs and institute a single, simple, government system, but that approach threatens to provoke interest-group resistance, ideological opposition, and the anxieties of the protected public all at once. Seeking to avoid those provocations, liberal reformers in recent decades have tried instead to build on and modify existing law and institutions. But that approach necessarily makes their proposals complicated too, opening them up to misunderstanding and misrepresentation, even to the suspicion that they have insidious provisions secretly buried deep inside them.

Some features of the health-care system make it especially difficult for Americans to understand their own interests clearly. If every family had to pay a lump-sum bill every month for health insurance, the system's costs would probably not have grown to their present proportions. But most of the employed do not make such a payment. The costs of health insurance are typically divided between an employee and employer share, and even the employee share is deducted in advance from paychecks. Economists generally agree that the employees also ultimately bear all or nearly all of the company's share as well as their own, but most people do not experience health costs that way. They think the company is paying for most of their health insurance and often have no idea how much the total bill is. Nor do they recognize that their insurance is substantially subsidized by the government because the employer's share is excluded from taxable income. Every aspect of this financing system serves to obscure its true costs. So when people who have good health benefits evaluate reforms, they do so from a standpoint shielded from the full realities of the problem.

To make matters worse, the discussion of health care takes place in a political environment low in trust. The complexities of health policy would not pose as great a problem for reform if the American public had confidence in American institutions. But confidence has been low for decades, and suspicions of malevolent intent are pervasive.[8] While the advocates of reform play on distrust of private insurers, the opponents play on distrust of government and politicians. Low trust has usually been more of a problem for the advocates of reform, however, because cynicism undermines the belief in public remedy that is essential to any popular movement for large-scale change.

Each of the impediments to change that I have mentioned has been formidable in its own right, but they have been devastating in combination. American political institutions make innovation difficult, but the barriers are especially large when reform has the potential to provoke so many different sources of interest-group, ideological, and popular opposition. Not only did the institutional arrangements enrich the health-care industry; they substantially protected large and well-organized groups in society, obscured how much the system was costing them, and encouraged them to believe they earned their protection and therefore deserved it, while others did not. This is the policy trap the United States worked itself into through the twentieth century, a deeply dysfunctional system that the country could not readily bring itself to change. To escape from that trap would require artful and determined leadership seizing opportunities created by a shift in underlying conditions.

A Window for Reform

When Democrats won control of both the presidency and Congress in 2008, they saw a chance of breaking through the national impasse on health care, as they had tried to do after winning the 1992 election. But if the reform effort had failed again as it had 16 years earlier, there would have been no shortage of persuasive explanations for the outcome. After all, defeat would have been consistent with a long historical pattern in health-care reform, and most of the obstacles that previously stood in the way of action had not vanished.

The institutional and ideological obstacles had certainly not lessened. The Senate was still the graveyard of legislation. The Republicans' use of the filibuster had become so routine that Democrats could not pass bills of any significance, unless related to the budget, without at least 60 votes. A sharper ideological cleavage between the parties also made reaching those 60 votes more difficult. As of the early 1990s, Senate Republicans still included a significant number of moderates, but their numbers had dwindled sharply. By 2009, every Republican in the Senate had a voting record to the right of the most conservative Democrat.[9]

The divide in the Senate reflected a broader pattern of polarization in American politics that guaranteed that health-care reform would again be the subject of ideological warfare. With the rise of Fox News, conservative Republicans had acquired a powerful means of shaping opinion that the party had lacked in the early 1990s. And with a large share of the protected public still satisfied with the status quo, public opinion would be just as divided in 2009 as it had been 16 years earlier. Fiscal constraints had certainly not eased. Coming into office in January 2009 amid a severe economic crisis and widening budget deficits, a new Democratic president could have declared that the recession required putting off health-care legislation.

Nonetheless, the new makeup of Congress and the maturation of a long-run shift in the position of health-care interest groups made it a reasonable gamble for Obama and congressional Democrats to press for health-care reform. The 2008 election put the party in the strongest position it had been in Congress in more than 30 years, giving Democrats a margin of 256 to 178 in the House and bringing them in striking distance of 60 votes in the Senate. As of January 2009, they had 56 senators as well as two independents who caucused with them. Then in March one Republican (Arlen Specter) switched parties, and in July a Democrat (Al Franken) was finally seated after recounts and appeals of a close race in Minnesota. The resulting 60 votes, if they could hold together, were the Democrats' first filibuster-proof majority since 1978, and though it lasted less than half a year, that ephemeral majority was more liberal than the earlier one because it included fewer conservatives from the South, none in leadership positions. This was crucial: the leadership of both chambers and the control of key committees would be in the hands of Democrats who were committed to passing health-care reform. President Obama and the chair of the Senate Finance Committee, Max Baucus, would try to win some Republican support. But while the polarization between the parties made it hard to pass health-care legislation on a bipartisan basis, it increased the ability of the Democrats to act on their own.

In addition to this new political majority, another condition favoring legislative action was a rapprochement between health-care interest groups and the reform elements in the Democratic Party. That process had already begun by 1993, when Clinton proposed a plan for universal health coverage that relied on competition among private insurance plans, but Clinton had also sought cost controls and market reforms that the industry refused to accept, and the marriage was never consummated.

By 2009, after several years of private meetings, the representatives of the drug companies, hospitals, doctors, and even some of the insurers were ready to throw in their lot with Democratic reformers if the stakeholder groups could avoid provisions they regarded as deal-breakers. They had come around to the view that the current framework of insurance was unsustainable. From 2000 to 2006, premiums for family health coverage had increased 87 percent, compared with cumulative inflation of 18 percent and cumulative average wage growth of 20 percent.[10] That figure for average wage growth, however, chiefly reflected growth in earnings at the top of the scale; real median household income had declined 3 percent since 2000.[11] Health-care inflation was driving the price of insurance to so high a level, particularly for people who bought coverage individually or through small businesses, that there was a danger of those markets going into a death spiral. As higher premiums led younger and healthier people to stop buying coverage, the population continuing to insure would get older and sicker and the cost of insurance would become prohibitive.

For the health-care and health-insurance industry, reform offered a viable alternative to the dismal scenarios for the status quo. In rough outline, the "grand bargain" that most of the industry was prepared to accept would require the insurance companies to cover any applicant regardless of pre-existing conditions at rates not based on an individual's health status, provided the government require everyone to be covered, subsidize those with low incomes, and refrain from imposing regulatory controls that the industry opposed. Although the insurance lobby in the end did not endorse the legislation (and the "Big Five" for-profit insurers actively fought it), the other major health-care interest groups were satisfied with the framework of reform and, in some cases, struck explicit deals with the White House and Senate to limit how much they would be asked to give up in cost containment.

While bridging differences with interest groups, Democratic leaders were reaching a consensus among themselves about the architecture of reform. The breakthrough in Massachusetts in 2006 had helped to crystallize views about how to proceed. The acceptance of the Massachusetts model was reflected in the health-care proposals of the major candidates for the 2008 Democratic presidential nomination and in congressional discussions between the election and the inauguration. Observers would make much of the fact that unlike Clinton, Obama left it to Congress to write health-care legislation. But in 2009, unlike 1993, congressional Democrats already agreed on the direction they were going to take, and it was the same direction that Obama favored. He didn't need to jump-start or guide the legislative process by drawing up his own bill and sending it to Congress (though the Obama White House secretly did draw up a bill internally that it never found necessary to release).

Like Clinton, Obama came to see the government's own fiscal interests as a reason to undertake reform, not a reason to postpone it. Long-term control of the deficit would be impossible without instituting general means for controlling health costs. Huge increases in Medicare and Medicaid were already built into federal budget projections. By shaving even a small percentage off future growth in existing programs, Democrats could generate savings that would finance much of the cost of covering the uninsured. And by adopting changes in tax and spending provisions that would have their biggest effects in the "out years," they could improve the long-term budget outlook. Although Clinton also saw health-care reform the same way, Obama and congressional Democrats in 2009 were more successful in devising a plan that the Congressional Budget Office would ratify as contributing to deficit reduction.

Perhaps the crucial difference between the Clinton and Obama efforts was that in 2009 all parties knew how the story had ended in 1994: Congress did nothing and the Democrats suffered a historic defeat at the mid-term elections. In 2009, Republicans were looking to reenact the past and Democrats to avoid repeating it. Rather than enter into negotiations or offer a serious alternative, the Republican congressional leadership sought only to block the Democrats. For fear of another electoral defeat, some Democrats wanted to proceed with modest steps in health care or to emphasize other issues entirely. But the predominant response in their party was to press ahead and correct what they now saw as earlier failings. On the left flank of the party, many believed that Democrats had failed in 1993 because of the absence of grass-roots organizing for health-care reform. This time, rather than wait for the opposition to mobilize, unions and other liberal groups took early steps to create an extensive field operation to build popular support for the struggle ahead. In the Senate, the leaders of the two committees that would take up legislation established a collaborative relationship to avoid the wrangling that helped to derail legislation in 1994. In the House, Speaker Nancy Pelosi assumed a central role in coordinating the work of the three committees with jurisdiction over health care and eventually took direct control of the final negotiations. The seeming lessons of 1994 were also not lost on the right flank of the party. The conservative or "Blue Dog" Democrats knew that when health-care reform failed the previous time, their counterparts suffered major losses at the mid-term elections. This time they did not split their party's ranks by lining up behind an alternative bill as they had 16 years earlier, and enough of them voted for the legislation to enable it to squeak through. If the Health Security Act had not failed in 1994—and if Democrats had not interpreted its failure as a reason for their losses that year—the Affordable Care Act probably could not have passed in 2010.

One reason that the memory of 1994 loomed so large under Obama is that nearly all of the central players in Congress and the administration were veterans of the earlier battle over health care. The major exception was the most important player of all, Barack Obama. But the Clinton experience also affected Obama because of an accident of political history. He ran into Hillary Clinton on his way to the Democratic presidential nomination, and the race between them, rather than being settled quickly, was drawn out for months, forcing Obama to debate Clinton 21 times. The debates usually turned to health care, a subject that Clinton knew thoroughly from her role in the reform effort of the early 1990s. At first, Obama's efforts to discuss health care were vague and vacuous, but Clinton's formidable knowledge and debating skills forced him to master health policy. In the primary campaign, Obama's primary disagreement with Clinton concerned the individual mandate—the requirement that people carry health insurance—which Obama opposed, except in regard to children. By the time he wrapped up the nomination, Obama had told one campaign aide, Neera Tanden, who asked him about the mandate, "I kind of think Hillary was right."[12] And when he entered the White House, not only could Obama hold his own on health policy with the experts; he was also far more committed to health-care reform than anyone had had a reason to expect when he first became a candidate.

The influence that the fight for the nomination had on the new president's attention and commitment to health-care reform was only one of many contingencies that factored into the outcome. No weighing of all the social, economic, and political conditions—some favoring the passage of reform, others militating against it—can explain why Obama and Congress finally broke the legislative impasse on health care. At several points, the reform effort was pronounced dead, and it might well have died if President Obama, House Speaker Nancy Pelosi, and Senate Majority Leader Harry Reid had not brought it back to life. Leadership mattered. But that is not to say that political institutions, interests, and ideological forces were irrelevant to the legislation that Congress passed.

The conditions in 2010 created a window for reform, but it was not a big one. To squeeze legislation through that window, Democrats had to work around the many constraints that might otherwise have doomed their chances for passing a bill. And working around those constraints helped to shape the central choices they made, including the choices that left the law vulnerable to counterattack.

Choices and Vulnerabilities

In the abstract, nations have a wide array of options to choose from in health-care finance and organization, but at any particular historical moment the alternatives that receive serious political consideration are far more limited. After Obama's election the constraints were especially tight because the new administration and Democrats in Congress committed themselves to build on existing arrangements and to use health-care re- form to bring about long-term deficit reduction. The effort to provide all Americans access to medical care and protect them from economic ruin had a liberal inspiration. But the Democrats were trying to accomplish that goal through means that were centrist, if not conservative.

The political constraints accepted by President Obama and Congress influenced two of the most consequential choices in health-care reform: the general framework for expanding coverage and the timetable for insti- tuting that expansion. Of course, within the general design and timetable, there were many other important choices: what services to cover (the most difficult issue would be abortion), whom to cover (the most controversial group would be immigrants), how much to subsidize coverage (a key deci- sion would be how far above the poverty line subsidies would reach), and how to pay for the expansion of coverage and control costs (the toughest problem would be a so-called "Cadillac" tax on high-cost health plans).

But the general architecture and timetable of reform were especially important because more than anything else, they defined the political terrain on which new struggles would be fought. Instead of building on Medicare—the program Democrats had earlier hoped to be the foundation of a universal system—the Affordable Care Act built on Medicaid and pri- vate insurance, two institutions that many reformers had long expected to supersede. And instead of carrying out the change expeditiously, Congress and the president put off implementation of the main provisions of the law until January 2014, nearly four years after its passage.

Consider the range of models for health care finance and organization already existing in the United States that, at least in theory, might have served as bases for extending health coverage. At one end of the spectrum are systems with government-owned and -operated facilities staffed by personnel paid by the government. This is "socialized medicine" or "government health care" in the true sense of those terms. The largest American example is the veterans' health-care system; Great Britain has its National Health Service, available to all as a matter of right. But in the United States none of the leading proposals for universal coverage has ever called for a national health service on British lines.

In recent decades, the three major systems that reformers have considered as potential models or bases for expanded coverage have instead been Medicare, Medicaid, and private insurance. Like the veterans' system, Medicare is financed primarily with federal taxes, but it pays for the services of private doctors and hospitals chosen by the beneficiaries. With its roots in Social Security, Medicare covers virtually the entire population over age 65, not just those in need. Proponents of universal coverage long hoped to replace private health insurance with a single federal insurance plan along the lines of Medicare, as it was traditionally organized (that is, without the private plans introduced mainly by Republicans since the 1990s). By 2010, however, leading Democrats no longer supported a "Medicare for all" or "single-payer" plan, though this approach still had support on the left.

Rather, the Democratic proposals now focused on extending Medicaid for the poor and making private insurance affordable for others without insurance. Unlike Medicare, Medicaid serves only people who are determined to be in need, and the responsibility for running the program rests with the states, which split the expense with the federal government. To keep down their own costs, many states have restricted eligibility to only a fraction of the poor and kept fees for doctors and other health-care providers so low that many of them refuse to accept Medicaid patients. The long-standing aim of liberals was to bring Medicaid beneficiaries into the mainstream through a system of national health insurance based on Medicare or by integrating the poor into private insurance (as the 1993 Clinton health plan would have done). But, in the absence of comprehensive health reform, Congress had incrementally extended federally mandated Medicaid coverage to increasing numbers of the poor, especially children. Defending Medicaid in 1995 and 1996 against a Republican attack, Democrats became more convinced of the program's value. Then in 1997 Congress added another federally subsidized, state-run program, the Children's Health Insurance Plan, for children in near-poor families. By 2008 a consensus had gradually formed among Democrats that instead of abolishing Medicaid and CHIP, health-care reform should try to remedy their defects and extend them to cover all of the poor and near-poor.

The consensus view also held that private health insurance would serve as the base for extending coverage to people who are not poor but have nonetheless been unable to afford or obtain coverage or have simply taken the risk of going uninsured. But extending private insurance would require overcoming the existing market's severe limitations.

Access to health insurance in the United States depends on employment. Large companies generally offer broad health coverage at relatively good rates, subsidized by the federal government through the exclusion of employer contributions from taxable income. Large companies also generally shield their employees from the most pernicious insurance practices, such as rescissions of coverage after the filing of claims. But the system has worked much less well for employees of small firms, the self-employed, part-time workers, and people without a regular job. Small businesses have paid high rates for limited coverage, and at the low-wage end of the labor market, employer-provided health insurance has been scarce. Individuals who buy insurance on their own have had the worst deal of all—high prices for coverage with numerous restrictions.

These disparities have arisen for systematic reasons, not simply as a historical accident, as some suppose. If the government leaves the health-insurance market to voluntary choice, the costs of administering coverage are sure to be higher for small groups and individuals than for big employers. Individual consumers and small businesses also lack the knowledge and purchasing leverage at the disposal of a large firm. Not unreasonably, insurers worry that in individual and small-group markets, those who sign up for insurance are likely to be at risk of high health costs (a problem known as "adverse selection"). In a voluntary market, insurers have every incentive to avoid covering the sick and instead to cherry-pick the healthy from among the individuals and small groups that apply for coverage. But if they do so, millions of people will remain uninsured.

From the 1940s to the early 2000s, proposals to extend health coverage by building on private insurance came in a variety of forms. Republicans usually favored additional tax subsidies for private insurance. In 1971, President Nixon broke with Republican orthodoxy when he proposed a near-universal program that required employers to pay for private coverage for their workers and dependents and created a voluntary federal program for everyone else. Liberals at that point generally opposed any program using private insurers. But beginning in 1979, Democrats led by Senator Edward M. Kennedy abandoned their earlier commitment to a single federal insurance system and supported a system of competing private insurers, though Kennedy would have made both employer contributions and individual participation mandatory. In the late 1980s, Democratic proposals, while requiring employers to pay for coverage, offered them a choice between private insurance and a government plan. Another approach, taken by the 1993 Clinton health plan, required employers to pay into a regional purchasing alliance that would offer a choice of private plans to nearly the entire population below age 65. In 1993, the main Republican moderate alternative, introduced by Senator John Chafee of Rhode Island, rejected an employer mandate but relied instead on vouchers for low-income people and a requirement that individuals carry coverage.

By the early 2000s, the dominant view among those supporting universal health insurance was that merely providing subsidies in a voluntary market would do too little, while removing health insurance from the employment relationship would be too disruptive. Democrats favored some minimum requirement for large employers, if only to prevent them from dropping coverage. The focus of reform, however, would be on the individual and small-group insurance markets, where the problems were concentrated. A key step would be the creation of insurance exchanges—similar to the Clinton plan's alliances but more limited in scope—to enable individuals and small businesses to shop for coverage among standardized plans. There also needed to be new rules for the market, requiring insurers to offer coverage to any eligible individual and prohibiting them from denying it for pre-existing conditions. But if reform did that alone, healthy people would rationally wait to insure until they got sick, and no insurance system can work unless the healthy as well as the sick pay into it. So there had to be some means to prevent people from opportunistically paying for insurance only when ill. The individual mandate—a measure identified with moderate Republicans in the early 1990s—became the preferred solution to that problem.

The individual mandate was not an essential requirement for the legislation—there were other solutions to the problem that the mandate answered. But perhaps because prominent Republicans had endorsed the idea, Democrats underestimated the problems it would cause. Polls later showed it to be the most unpopular provision of the Affordable Care Act, and it became the focal point of legal challenges to the law's constitutionality. But during the congressional deliberations, neither conservative Democrats nor Republicans focused much attention on the mandate, and neither the White House nor congressional leaders showed interest in alternatives.[13]

How quickly could the health-insurance system move to these new rules? The direct precedent was Massachusetts, which began instituting its new system in six months and began enforcing the individual mandate about a year after Governor Mitt Romney signed the law. The biggest federal insurance program, Medicare, went into effect on July 1, 1966, not quite one year after Congress created the program. In late 2008, between Obama's election and his inauguration, his transition team had MIT economist Jonathan Gruber develop cost estimates for health reform with January 1, 2012, as the effective start date, leaving nearly two years to prepare the way.[14]

But fiscal concerns immediately began causing second thoughts in the administration about a two-year start-up. The effects of cost-containment measures would likely be small at the beginning, though they would grow with time. Expanding coverage quickly would therefore have the biggest net cost in the early years. And because of budgetary conventions, the program's cost would be estimated over its first 10 years. If coverage could be postponed, the estimate of its cost would be lower.

An additional issue arose because of the pressure in the Senate to leave the establishment of the insurance exchanges and other aspects of implementation to the states. Assigning that role to the states necessarily meant allowing more time for states to pass complementary legislation and to start up insurance exchanges.

These considerations militated in favor of pushing back the start date from January 1, 2012, at least to January 1, 2013. That date would still have likely made health-care reform a fait accompli if a Republican president took office on January 20, 2013. But a January 2013 start for coverage would mean that open enrollment in health plans would take place around the time of the November 2012 elections. At a closed meeting, Senator Robert Menendez of New Jersey indicated his opposition: if something went wrong then, it could jeopardize the chances of Democrats who would be running for election that year. The Medicare prescription drug program, enacted in 2003, had severe problems when its main provisions went into effect in 2006, and Democrats were worried about a repeat of that experience.

Congress considered two other startup proposals. The bill that initially came out of the Senate Health, Education, Labor, and Pensions (HELP) Committee called for a rolling start, allowing states to start their exchanges as they were ready, beginning in 2012. Another idea was to start up the program on July 1, 2013. But the Treasury Department objected that because the insurance subsidies were in the form of federal tax credits, it would be difficult for people in some states but not others to be eligible for the credits, or to have tax credits for insurance for just half a year.

If Obama or congressional leaders had felt strongly about the startup date, these objections to a January or July 2013 start, or to a rolling start, could have been overcome. But the White House made no effort to have the program go into effect at an early enough date to prevent a possible successor in 2013 from undoing the program. According to congressional staff, the senators and representatives involved in the legislation also never focused much attention on the startup date. They were preoccupied with other aspects of the legislation.

The White House solution to the slow startup was to focus instead on some short-term reforms, such as changes in health insurance regulations, as well as a small "high-risk pool" for the medically uninsurable, which could take effect more quickly. Ironically, the administration itself had already excoriated high-risk pools as an inadequate policy, and the Affordable Care Act funded the pools at so low a level that they would likely help few people before 2014.[15] The postponement of reform until that time did help keep down the cost of the program. It just did so by exposing the entire program to the risk of being overturned by a new administration before it could be carried out. And the inclusion of an individual mandate exposed the program to the risk of being overturned by the Supreme Court—a fate from which it was ultimately saved by an act of clemency by the chief justice.

This, then, was the general architecture of reform that became the basis of the Affordable Care Act of 2010: a two-pronged expansion of coverage through Medicaid and private health insurance, all on a slow timetable that stretched beyond the next two elections. If the bill that originally passed the House of Representatives had prevailed, the federal government would have run a national insurance exchange, and that exchange would have offered a new government insurance plan (the "public option"). But the main legislation came instead from the Senate, which turned the exchanges over to the states and excluded any new federal insurance plan. Nonetheless, conservatives denounced the Affordable Care Act as "socialized medicine" and a "government takeover" as if it nationalized the health-care industry. None of the compromises made by Democrats softened Republican opposition in the slightest. Just before the Senate began debate on the legislation, Senator Orrin Hatch said, "It's going to be a holy war."[16]

Rather than settling the long conflict over health insurance, the Affordable Care Act launched the struggle into a new phase. States with conservative leadership immediately went to court to challenge the constitutionality of the individual mandate and other provisions of the law. After Republicans won back control of the House of Representatives in the 2010 election, they voted to repeal the Affordable Care Act and sought to use every means at their disposal to block it from being carried out. Republican victories in state elections also brought to power governors and legislators determined to thwart the federal reform. In June 2012, however, the Supreme Court upheld nearly the entire law, and the following November the voters re-elected President Obama and a Democratic Senate, making it impossible for Republicans to carry out their promise to repeal the Affordable Care Act before its main provisions went into effect in 2014. But at the state level Republican governors and legislators continued to refuse to co-operate in carrying out key aspects of the law.

When Congress passed Medicare and Medicaid in 1965, the legislation seemed to lay to rest philosophical opposition to government responsibility for health-care costs. But what was settled in those years became unsettled again. Americans are still at odds over the most basic question about health care: whether it is a requirement for a free life that the community has an obligation to provide or a good that needs to be earned (and if you can't earn it, too bad for you). This conflict was not written into the American charac-ter or national tradition. It was not inevitable that Americans would work themselves into so deep a tangle of problems in health care as they have. Only history can help us make sense of a health-care system that, from the perspective of its results, makes very little sense at all.

PART I

THE GENEALOGY OF HEALTH-CARE REFORM

CHAPTER 1

Evolution through Defeat

FOR AMERICAN LIBERALS IN THE TWENTIETH CENTURY, health insurance for all was a persistent dream and a perennial disappointment, often on the horizon but always seemingly just beyond reach. After the death of one veteran advocate, Congressman Claude Pepper, in 1989, Democrats ruefully told one another that when Pepper arrived in heaven, he asked, "Will America ever have national health insurance?" and the Lord said, "Yes, but not in my lifetime." Before World War I, the reformers of the Progressive era had won the enactment of food and drug regulation, antitrust law, labor legislation, national parks, the Federal Reserve, and workers' compensation—but met defeat on health insurance. During the 1930s and '40s, the New Deal and its successor, the Fair Deal, definitively established federal responsibility for the overall stability and growth of the economy and led to the passage of Social Security, collective bargaining laws, financial regulation, a minimum wage, and the GI Bill—but not health insurance. The era of liberal reform in the 1960s and '70s added civil rights legislation, antipoverty programs, regulation of occupational safety and consumer products, environmental protection, Medicare for the elderly, and Medicaid for some of the poor—but not universal health insurance.

If Americans came to know one thing about the history of battles over health insurance, it was that a government program to make health care a right of citizenship had always been defeated. The specter of failure loomed so heavily over the national memory in health policy that public figures and the news media even attributed defeats to presidents who had never attempted to pass universal health care.

Yet this is not the story of an unchanging movement with an unchanging result. Health-care reform in the United States has been an evolving political project. While there have been historical continuities from one era to another, the objectives of reform have shifted as American politics and the economics of health care have changed. As a result, the enterprise of reform has undergone a complete transformation.

Health insurance first emerged as a public issue during the Progressive era, particularly during the years between 1915 and 1919, when reformers proposed health insurance as a program at the state level, primarily intending to provide income support for industrial workers during spells of illness. During a second period, beginning in 1935, reformers sought an expansionary health insurance program with national scope to finance medical care for the entire population. The pursuit of national health insurance continued until 1950, when liberal policy experts decided to downsize their aims to a hospital insurance program for the elderly, later to be known as Medicare. Along with favored tax status for employment-based insurance (definitively established in 1954), the enactment of an expanded version of Medicare in 1965 provided significant protection against the financial risks of illness to a majority of the public and channeled an increasing flow of the nation's income into health care. As a result, when efforts to pass national health insurance resumed in the late 1960s, the political environment of the movement had changed. Proposals for universal coverage had to deal with the skyrocketing costs of both public and private insurance. Instead of proposing an explicitly expansionary program, reformers increasingly sought changes in both the organization and the finance of health care to contain costs as well as to extend coverage and improve services. Gradually, the definition of the aim changed from "national health insurance" to "comprehensive health-care reform."

The substance and context of reform have changed so drastically over the past century that no single cause can possibly account for the outcome. From one phase to the next, the dominant paradigms for policy have changed. So have the political alliances in favor of and against reform. Neither political parties nor key interest groups have held to the same positions. Early defeats and limited successes have complicated the fulfillment of the aim of universal coverage, as large parts of the public secured protection. Vast financial interests have developed that would not exist if earlier struggles had turned out differently. In short, the fate of health-care reform cannot be explained without examining the critical decision points along the distinctive historical path that policy and institutions have followed in the United States.[1]

Progressive Health Insurance, 1915–1919

The earliest proposals for government-sponsored health insurance in the United States took their cue from programs enacted earlier in Europe. Before their governments intervened, many European workers were insured through sickness funds established by mutual societies, unions, and employers, which provided cash benefits to make up for lost wages as well as payment of doctors' services. When governments first began subsidizing voluntary funds or made participation in sickness insurance compulsory, they did so as part of a series of measures to limit the threat of impoverishment from four major types of risks: workplace accidents, sickness and disability, old age, and unemployment. Germany led the way, enacting sickness insurance in 1883, and Britain adopted national insurance in 1911. The early focus of social insurance on workers—the programs typically applied first to industrial workers and only later to their dependents and others—reflected a mixture of economic and political objectives. By relieving economic insecurity among wage earners, political leaders such as Germany's Iron Chancellor, Otto von Bismarck, and Britain's Liberal leader, David Lloyd George, were trying to deny socialist parties their appeal and to integrate the working class into the existing political order. Sickness insurance was also expected to increase the wealth and power of a nation through the improved health and efficiency of its labor force and army.

As government health insurance programs continued to spread in Europe, the idea at first drew little interest in the United States, though many states did adopt workers' compensation programs (industrial accident insurance). The Socialist Party in the United States, far weaker than its European counterparts, endorsed compulsory health insurance in 1904, but it had little impact. Although economic regulation was gaining ground by then, laissez-faire ideas still permeated public policy, especially judicial thought. In that era's classic test of economic regulation, *Lochner v. New York* (1905), the Supreme Court struck down a statutory limit on the working day on the grounds that the law interfered with freedom of contract. The federal government still had only a peripheral role in public health and no role in financing medical services, except for merchant seamen. State and local governments were increasingly involved in public health measures but generally kept out of the provision and financing of medical services, except through public hospitals and clinics for the poor. Even in the private sector, protection against the costs of illness was limited. Commercial health insurance had hardly developed, and although many fraternal lodges, some unions, and a few employers provided sick pay and medical benefits, these ways of spreading the costs of illness were less common in the United States than they had been in Britain and Germany prior to government intervention.

The first significant reference to health insurance in American politics came in 1912—the year after Britain passed its National Insurance Act—when Progressive Republicans bolted from the GOP to form the Progressive Party, nominated Theodore Roosevelt for president, and had a line in their platform supporting social insurance, including protection against the costs of sickness. After succeeding William McKinley, Roosevelt had served as president from 1901 to 1909. The notion that health insurance is "something that Washington has been talking about since Teddy Roosevelt was president" (as President Obama put it in 2010 in one of many references) is a misunderstanding.[2] During his years in the White House, Roosevelt had never addressed health insurance, and his speeches during the 1912 campaign did not discuss it.[3] This silence is understandable because at that time no one had yet formulated any specific proposals for health insurance, and the general understanding was that all such issues were properly the responsibilities of the states, not the federal government, if for no other reason than the certainty that the Supreme Court would have overturned any federal legislation of that kind. The real significance of Roosevelt's presence on the ticket of a party that endorsed compulsory health insurance is that he was representative of a faction of Republicans favorably disposed toward the idea, and if that faction had been stronger, it might have been able, together with Democrats, to enact health insurance at the state level. Such an alliance did come very close to success in one state.

It was just after the 1912 election that a small, primarily academic group of reformers, the American Association for Labor Legislation, convened a meeting to discuss social insurance and decided to focus on developing a health insurance program. The group's proposal, published in 1915, called for sick pay at two-thirds of wages for up to 26 weeks, payment of medical bills, a maternity benefit for both insured women and the wives of insured men, and a small benefit at death to cover burial costs. On the premise that middle- and upper-income people could take care of their own expenses, the program applied only to workers (and their dependents) making less than $1,200 a year, except for domestic and casual employees. The group estimated that the benefits would cost 4 percent of wages and proposed that those costs be divided among workers and employers, each to pay two-fifths, and the government, to pay the remaining fifth. In the advocates' view, health insurance had to be compulsory because low-income workers could not afford it unless contributions from employers and government were required along with their own.[4]

The reformers of the Progressive era presented compulsory health insurance not as a special interest of labor or the poor, but as a general interest of an enlightened society. Citing data from charities and other sources indicating that illness was a primary cause of poverty, they argued that spreading the costs of sickness would reduce the prevalence of destitution and dependency. By paying for effective medical care and giving employers and government incentives for preventive and public health measures, compulsory health insurance would also reduce the social burden of disease. The labor-law reformers had made similar arguments in promoting workers' compensation (also a form of compulsory insurance), and their success in gaining the adoption of that program gave them confidence about the prospects for passing health insurance. The campaign for workers' compensation had enjoyed the support of many employers, such as those represented in another moderate reform group, the National Civic Federation, which brought together corporate and labor union leaders. But employers had a clearer interest in workers' compensation than in health insurance. Jury verdicts against companies in workplace accident cases were rising, and many employers preferred the predictability of a compulsory insurance program to the uncertain costs of litigation. Regarding health insurance, business representatives came to a different conclusion. They objected to the provision for sick pay because it might increase malingering, and although they had been forced to accept some liability for workplace injuries, they refused to accept responsibility for the costs of all illnesses of their employees, much less for the medical costs of their employees' dependents.[5]

While employers were hostile, labor leaders had a mixed response to the reformers' health insurance proposal. At that time the American Federation of Labor generally opposed public social programs, including a minimum wage, on the grounds that workers should look to unions for protection, not to the government. Based on his own experience as a leader of the cigar workers, the president of the AFL, Samuel Gompers, saw health benefits as a way for unions to build their membership. But some of the state labor federations and individual unions did support compulsory health insurance, and the AFL would eventually reverse its opposition in the 1930s.[6]

Another potential source of support, women's groups, also faced divisions in their ranks in response to the AALL's insurance proposal. The leader of the National Consumers League, Florence Kelley, opposed the maternity benefit because, in her view, single, working women would be taxed for a benefit that was of no use to them. But other women leaders in both the labor and suffrage movement vigorously supported the AALL's proposal for health insurance, including the maternity benefit.[7]

Though unable to secure unified labor and women's support, the labor-law reformers at first enjoyed the cooperation of the American Medical Association in the drive for government-sponsored health insurance. The AMA had been the ally of social reformers in passing other public health and regulatory legislation and attacking medical quackery. In the view of many doctors, including prominent leaders of the profession, compulsory health insurance would benefit physicians as well as their patients by financing medical care for many people who otherwise could not afford it. But discontent percolated up from the county medical societies, typically dominated by an inner fraternity of successful specialists. These physicians worried that government would follow the pattern of fraternal lodges, unions, and employers in driving down physicians' incomes by forcing them to compete for contracts to care for groups on a per capita (or "capitation") basis. The doctors' concerns were not fanciful. Some of the reformers, having learned from European experience that paying physicians by fee for service could create budgetary problems, hoped to use capitation payment. An AMA leader, Alexander Lambert, Theodore Roosevelt's personal physician, proposed as a compromise that doctors be paid fee-for-service but out of local funds with a fixed budget. Another reformer of the time, Michael M. Davis, after visiting the Mayo Clinic, suggested that health insurance could help promote group practice. Because physicians objected to all such ideas, reformers quickly abandoned them, but the concessions were futile. Physicians' groups—at the county, the state, and eventually the national level—turned against compulsory health insurance and played a central role in its defeat.[8]

From the beginning of the Progressive campaign, the most implacable opponent of a government program was the insurance industry, even though it had no stake at that point in health insurance. By offering a funeral benefit, however, the AALL's model bill struck at one of the most profitable lines of business for companies such as Prudential and Metropolitan Life—the door-to-door sale of "industrial insurance" by an army of insurance agents, who collected 25 cents or so a week from working-class families for policies that provided a death benefit to cover the costs of a final illness and burial. Reformers argued that because the insurers' high marketing costs absorbed a large share of the money spent on the burial policies, a government program would better serve workers. But by threatening insurers through the inclusion of a funeral benefit, reformers stirred them to oppose the health insurance program in its entirety, which the companies saw as a dangerous precedent for a wider government assault on the whole enterprise of private insurance.[9]

At first, from 1915 to 1917, momentum seemed to be gathering in favor of a government insurance program. A half-dozen states established commissions to study the issue and make recommendations, but the Progressive movement had already peaked and was beginning to falter. In the 1916 election, the Progressive Party broke up, and after the United States entered

World War I in April 1917, the war effort absorbed much of the energy that had previously gone into domestic reform. Amid intense anti-German war propaganda, moreover, the opponents of compulsory health insurance emphasized that the idea had originated in Germany and attacked it as un-American. It was in this atmosphere that health insurance went down to defeat in a state referendum in California.[10]

The one state where compulsory health insurance came close to passage was New York, where both labor and feminist organizations provided strong support for the legislation in the face of opposition from an alliance of physicians, insurers, and employers. In March 1919, nine Progressive Republicans joined with the Democrats in the New York State Senate to pass a health-insurance bill that had the support of the recently elected Democratic governor, Al Smith. In the Assembly, however, the powerful Republican speaker Thaddeus Sweet, an upstate manufacturer, succeeded in keeping the legislation from reaching a vote. And when women's groups, now empowered with the franchise, failed to turn Sweet out of office in the 1920 election, the Progressive campaign for health insurance was over.[11]

If New York had adopted a health insurance program in 1919, it might have had national ramifications. The unemployment insurance program that Wisconsin adopted in 1932 helped pave the way for federal legislation in 1935. In Canada, the health insurance plan adopted in Saskatchewan in 1946 played a comparable role as a stepping stone toward a national program. If a state health insurance program had developed in New York, private insurers might have established a new and profitable business selling supplementary policies and relaxed their opposition to a government program as long as it was limited in eligibility and benefits. A New York program would have received national attention when Governor Smith became the Democratic presidential candidate in 1928 and might have influenced Smith's successor as governor of New York, Franklin Delano Roosevelt, who might then have made different choices when he became president in 1933.

But the opponents defeated a government health insurance program in every state where the idea was introduced, a perfect record that testifies to the underlying structural impediments in the Progressive era. Compulsory health insurance did not have the same level of political sponsorship in America as in Europe. The primary impetus came from neither of the two major parties but instead from third parties and reformers outside government. And those reformers never had substantial organized support because the political dynamic that had been at work in Europe had no counterpart in the United States.

The American labor movement was comparatively weak and never represented a serious challenge to the established parties, much less to the state itself. National elites were therefore not looking for new ways to integrate workers into the political order. Under those circumstances, the more narrow and immediate interests of employers, insurers, and physicians could dominate the political process. But although this underlying pattern heavily biased the outcome of the first battles over health insurance, things might have been different in the 1930s, when the next historical phase began.

The New Deal and National Health Insurance, 1935–1950

Proposals for publicly sponsored health insurance changed by the time the idea was revived during the New Deal. During the four decades beginning in 1935, reformers made a series of efforts to introduce or expand health coverage, all of them sharing certain assumptions about the purposes of reform. While the more universal programs failed, several partial measures passed, and as a result, America's health insurance system took a path unlike that of any other country.

No period in the twentieth century provided more favorable general political conditions than the New Deal for passing a universal health program. The forces unleashed during the Depression of the 1930s opened the way for social legislation on a national scale by bringing to power a president, a congressional majority, and ultimately a majority on the Supreme Court who broke decisively with the premises of laissez-faire. Industrial workers unionized, and the new leadership of the labor movement supported public social programs. Although President Roosevelt consistently upheld an affirmative view of government's responsibilities, he did not follow a single-minded program through his 12 years in office. Rather, he tested different approaches, responded to interest-group pressures, and adjusted to shifting political demands. And those pressures and demands, as he interpreted them, led him to back off twice from embracing proposals for health insurance that many in his party supported.

During the 1930s, the dominant objectives of health insurance proponents changed in critical respects. The replacement of lost wages during sickness and the provision of paid maternity leave and a funeral benefit receded from priority or disappeared entirely. Reformers sought health insurance as a means of protection against the costs of health care, and instead of merely covering medical costs, they sought to expand access to services for what were increasingly seen as legitimate and universal medical needs. No longer focusing only on workers, they offered proposals that would apply to the middle class as well. And rather than calling for action solely by the states, they wanted the federal government to provide health insurance, at first via state programs and later directly to the public.

These shifts reflected new economic realities and political assumptions. Since the Progressive era, medical costs had grown larger than wages lost to illness and now represented a problem not just for workers, but for many in the middle class as well. By focusing on medical costs alone, reformers also hoped to avoid the political opposition that other provisions, particularly the funeral benefit, had stirred up in the Progressive era. The rise in medical costs was the result of two developments long in the making, each in some way due to the response of American society to changes in science. In the late nineteenth and early twentieth centuries, legislatures enacted progressively stricter licensing laws for doctors, raising requirements for medical education; the effect of those laws was to close many medical schools and reduce the supply of physicians at a time when demand for their services was growing. Under these conditions, doctors were able to increase their fees and incomes (which was one reason why organized professional support for government health programs diminished). The second factor in higher medical costs was the growth and transformation of hospitals. During the nineteenth century, hospitals had been conducted on a largely charitable basis mainly for the poor, but antiseptic surgery and other scientific advances had turned the hospital into a medical workshop for doctors treating patients from all classes. Although the change had already begun by the Progressive era, a federal survey in 1918 in Columbus, Ohio, still put hospital expenses at only 7.6 percent of average family medical bills, which amounted to less than $50 a year, half of which went to physicians.[12] By 1929 a foundation-funded national commission, the Committee on the Costs of Medical Care, estimated hospital costs at 13 percent of a total family medical bill averaging $108.[13] For patients, however, the problem was not just the growing average expense, but the increasing variance of costs due to high hospital bills in a small number of serious illnesses. This new situation was responsible for the rising concern about medical costs among people of "moderate means." The Depression further magnified those concerns.

When middle-class families began having trouble paying for hospital care, hospitals had a financing problem too, and in the late 1920s and early 1930s individual hospitals and hospital associations in Texas, California, and other states created the first plans for groups of employees to buy insurance for hospital expenses. These plans, which evolved into the Blue Cross system, were run on a nonprofit basis and at first covered only a small number of people, leaving the general problem of financial insecurity in illness unresolved.[14]

Reformers saw public and nonprofit health insurance as a response to growing medical needs as well as rising medical costs. Beginning with the report of the Committee on the Costs of Medical Care in 1927, the standard argument of reformers was that as a result of advances in science, all Americans, even the affluent, needed more medical care than they were receiving. Health insurance became a way not merely of distributing the financial risks of illness, but of budgeting larger expenditures for medical care.

In European social insurance legislation, health insurance had typically followed workers' compensation, and that was the sequence that Progressive reformers had expected to follow in 1915. But the Great Depression altered political priorities. With millions out of work and a grass-roots movement among the elderly demanding help from the government, unemployment relief and old-age pensions became more urgent than health insurance. Legislative activity in the states had already registered the shift in focus by the time Roosevelt took office in 1933. Wisconsin provided a model for unemployment insurance, and five states had adopted old-age pension laws since 1929. So it is not surprising that when Roosevelt established the Committee on Economic Security in 1934 to prepare social

insurance proposals, he indicated he was especially interested in unemployment and old-age insurance, though health insurance also fell within the
committee's charge.[15]

From the beginning, though, the prevailing view on the committee,
chaired by Secretary of Labor Frances Perkins and made up entirely of administration officials, was that health insurance would have to be delayed
because the AMA's opposition might sink the entire bill. When the committee made its report in January 1935, it offered specific proposals for unemployment and old-age insurance but only general principles for dealing
with health-care costs. Roosevelt gave the committee three more months to
study health insurance, but he buried that report when he received it. In its
set of principles, the committee made every effort to mollify physicians: it
said they would remain in private practice, their participation in insurance
would be voluntary, and they could choose their method of reimbursement.
Nonetheless, the AMA went into high gear to oppose any action, and key
congressional leaders made it clear health insurance would get no consideration. When the Social Security Act passed Congress in August 1935, it included only some secondary provisions related to health care.

Roosevelt returned to health insurance two more times. Perhaps his
best opportunity to pass legislation came in the two years after his landslide reelection in 1936, when the Democratic caucus enjoyed lopsided
margins in both houses of Congress (347 to 88 in the House, 79 to 17 in
the Senate). In 1937 the president authorized another internal administration group to work on a proposal for a national health program, which
he received the following February. Besides urging federal aid for maternal
and child health care, hospital construction, and the disabled, the proposal called for two kinds of grants to states: the first for medical care of
the poor and the second for health insurance for the general public. An
administration-organized public conference on the national health program in June 1938 seemed to build momentum for the initiative, but
events then followed the same course as three years earlier. The AMA
mobilized in opposition, congressional leaders signaled they would block
any bill, and Roosevelt decided to put health insurance off to another day.
Stymied repeatedly by conservative Democrats in Congress, the president tried to purge them in the 1938 midterm elections, but the outcome

instead was a conservative coalition of Republicans and southern Democrats who from that point on blocked major New Deal initiatives. Although Senator Robert F. Wagner of New York introduced a bill in 1939
incorporating watered-down recommendations from the 1938 health program, the proposal died for lack of support even from the administration.
A much broader bill, first introduced in 1943 by Senator Wagner, Senator
James Murray of Montana, and Representative John Dingell of Michigan,
would have expanded Social Security to include comprehensive health
insurance, disability benefits, and more generous support in old age, all
to be financed by mandatory employer and employee contributions. But
the Wagner-Murray-Dingell bill, though developed by officials inside the
Roosevelt administration, never reached the floor of either house of Congress.[16]

As he looked ahead to peacetime during the war, Roosevelt began one
final effort to press for health insurance. In his State of the Union address
in January 1944, he called for an "economic bill of rights" to fulfill the
hopes for security Americans were fighting for in the war. Among those
rights were a "right to adequate medical care" and a "right to adequate protection from the economic fears" of sickness. But Roosevelt was never able
to follow through. His close adviser Samuel Rosenman was preparing a
health insurance program and an accompanying speech for Roosevelt
when the president died on April 12, 1945.[17]

What explains the omission of health insurance from the New Deal?
The explanation cannot be "individualism" in general. Other policies adopted in those years required no less a departure from individualism than
a health insurance program did. One recent history says that health insurance simply did not "grab" Roosevelt.[18] But he took up the issue three times,
and rational political calculations based on the conditions of the times
adequately explain his decision not to move ahead in 1935 and 1938 (death
seems a pretty good excuse in 1945). The Depression shaped the priorities
of reform, subordinating health insurance to other goals. The interest-
group power of physicians helped to tip the political balance against health
insurance, particularly in 1935, when AMA's opposition to the Social Security
Act could well have endangered its passage. At the start of his second term,
when Roosevelt might have passed health insurance, he made a series of

major blunders—including the failed effort to "pack" the Supreme Court and the decision to cut deficit spending, which plunged the economy back into the Depression—thereby squandering a political opportunity he would never have again. Underneath Roosevelt's calculations were the institutional realities of American politics. A party in a parliamentary system that won an election on the scale of the Democratic victories in 1932 and 1936 would have been able to pass a health insurance program. But the bastions of conservative resistance in Congress, particularly in the Senate Finance and House Ways and Means Committee, limited the power of a president, even one elected in a landslide.

After Roosevelt's death, Harry Truman took up the cause his predecessor had never fully embraced and, in a message to Congress in November 1945, became the first president to call for national health insurance. Modeled on Social Security, the program was to be federally run, compulsory, and nearly universal in its reach. The president denied, however, that it was "socialized medicine," insisting that "our people would continue to get medical and hospital services just as they do now."[19] If Truman had succeeded in enacting health insurance, it would have been consistent with the pattern at that time in western Europe, where many governments were expanding rights to social welfare, including health care. It was in 1946 that Britain established its National Health Service, which unlike the previous national insurance system provided treatment through state-financed hospitals and doctors at no charge to patients. But in the United States, the political conditions for universal health care were much less favorable than in Europe. In 1946 Republicans gained control of Congress, and although Democrats took it back when Truman won the presidency in his own right two years later, health insurance legislation still faced steep institutional, interest-group, and ideological barriers.

The 1949 battle over Truman's program may have been the closest the United States has ever come to adopting a unified national health insurance system with no separate provision for the poor. But even so, the struggle was not close. Within Congress, opponents of a government program chaired key committees, and in the country at large the AMA dominated the public debate, lining up support from hundreds of organizations and financing a massive advertising campaign against "socialized medicine."

The AMA played on the ideological climate of the early Cold War. As the AMA's public relations agency framed the issue, defeating national health insurance was a struggle to preserve the "American way" against insidious and subversive forces attempting to foist socialism and communism on an unsuspecting public. Truman himself never followed up his call for national health insurance with a specific plan. Although he said he supported the Wagner-Murray-Dingell bill in principle, he never actually endorsed it, nor did he present an official administration bill. Neither house of Congress acted on the issue during his presidency.[20]

The failure of Truman's program was one of the great dividing points in the history of health-care reform. While rejecting national health insurance, Congress approved programs that Truman proposed for aid for hospital construction and medical research, which substantially increased investment in technologically intensive medical services. Other Western democracies created insurance programs for low-income workers before they built modern medical facilities; public policy in the United States followed the reverse sequence, raising the level of capital investment in health care before extending insurance. In 1950 Congress also enacted a small program of federal aid partially reimbursing the states for the medical costs of welfare recipients; this was the germ of Medicaid. And in what would prove to be a fateful turn, a study commission created within the Truman administration in 1951 responded to the president's crushing defeat on national health insurance by introducing a proposal for just 60 days of hospital coverage for the elderly on Social Security. Though nothing came of it at first, this idea was the germ of Medicare.

The Growth of the Protected Public, 1950–1965

The United States took the critical steps in the formation of its health-care financing system in the two post–World War II decades, when it turned decisively toward private employer-based insurance and created separate federal programs for the elderly and for the poor. These were the years when the United States ensnared itself in a policy trap—a costly, extraordinarily complicated system which nonetheless protected enough of the public to make the system resistant to change.

Before the 1930s, commercial insurers had been slow to offer health coverage out of concern that only individuals with high costs would sign up (adverse selection) and that the administrative costs of marketing policies, evaluating applicants, collecting premiums, and paying claims would make the coverage too expensive to sell. The early Blue Cross plans demonstrated, however, that basing health insurance on employee groups made it a viable enterprise because the employer's regular payments cut overhead and risk and the employed are relatively healthy. Employer-based health insurance then spread during World War II, when federal authorities allowed companies to add health insurance despite wage-and-price controls, and coverage soared after the war when millions of unionized workers received health benefits through collective-bargaining agreements.[21]

Federal policy reinforced this system after the election of Dwight Eisenhower as president in 1952. As employer-provided insurance had grown, federal law had been unclear as to whether the employer payments counted as taxable income. In 1953, the Internal Revenue Service ruled that a contribution to an individual health insurance policy was taxable even though a contribution to a group policy was not. To resolve the ambiguity, the Eisenhower administration proposed a blanket exclusion for all employer contributions, plus an expanded medical-expense deduction. When one senator at a hearing asked how much the exclusion would cost, a representative of the administration admitted, "We haven't any figures at all on that."[22] No one else seemed interested either, though the exclusion proved to be one of the most costly federal health policies ever adopted. Neither was there much concern about the policy's distributive impact. Yet excluding employer contributions from taxable income favored people with higher incomes for three separate reasons. The higher an employee's income, (1) the more likely he or she was to receive health insurance; (2) the more generous those benefits were likely to be; and (3) the more valuable any exclusion or exemption would be, especially with the high marginal tax rates of the 1950s. Health-care interest groups and conservative journals argued for the tax exclusion partly on the grounds that it would help thwart a government program. And even labor leaders backed the exclusion, oblivious to its distributive inequities or its likely long-term political effects in weakening the movement for national health insurance.

As the health insurance market expanded in the post–World War II era, it also became more competitive, though not in a way that benefited the sick. The Blue Cross plans originally offered coverage at a "community rate"—the same price for all employee groups in an area. But when commercial insurers entered the market, they went cherry-picking, selling coverage to employers with younger and healthier workers at a cheaper "experience rate." That form of competition left Blue Cross with a more costly population and ultimately no choice but to adjust to its competitors' pricing practices, which meant higher rates for individuals and groups with higher costs.[23] The opponents of Truman's program had argued that voluntary insurance could eventually cover all Americans except the poor, but they had failed to take into account the dynamics of the market, which made it difficult even for nonprofit insurers to cover high-cost groups such as the elderly and the disabled.

Meanwhile, as a result of the establishment of Social Security, the federal government and its officials became more concerned with the problems of the elderly. Unlike European countries, the United States had established old-age insurance before acting on health insurance. And by so doing, the federal government created a corps of policy experts and program executives whose vision for health care reflected their experience in initiating and building Social Security. Some of these experts—such as Wilbur Cohen, who became the go-to expert in the field during the middle decades of the twentieth century—served almost continuously in government from the New Deal through the 1960s. Members of Congress as well as the executive branch relied on Cohen and his colleagues for ideas, technical work, and the drafting of legislation.[24] After national health insurance was defeated under Truman, it was the Social Security policy experts who proposed a limited program of hospital insurance for the elderly. Even when the political winds shifted in a more liberal direction in the 1960s, they continued to call for hospital insurance for the elderly as an incremental step that they hoped would eventually lead to a system of universal coverage on the same public-financing principles as Social Security. They would be disappointed in that larger aim, however, partly because of the compromises struck in taking what they thought would be the first steps.

No other country has created separate health insurance financing for the elderly; it is a peculiar American invention, established without a full appreciation of the political consequences of singling out the elderly for special treatment. To be sure, once employer-based insurance had taken root, a separate program for seniors had a definite rationale. The elderly didn't fit into an employer-based model, and most couldn't afford to buy coverage on their own, especially as the insurance market moved away from community rating. In the early post–World War II decades, seniors continued to be a relatively needy group, with a higher poverty rate than the working-age population had. The supporters of a hospital insurance program for seniors believed that integrating it into Social Security would give it immediate legitimacy. As the elderly had a right to their Social Security benefits earned by contributions during their working years, so they could now be understood to have earned a right to hospital insurance.

During the Eisenhower administration, the Social Security program experts and liberals in Congress concerned about social welfare initially focused on adding disability coverage to the old-age insurance system. Disability insurance did not face the political obstacles of health insurance—the AMA and other health-care interests were not opposed—and it passed in 1956. Almost immediately thereafter, liberal attention shifted back to health insurance and to the idea of adding 60 days of hospital coverage for Social Security beneficiaries. The first effort to pass such a program in Congress began with the introduction of a bill by a Rhode Island congressman, Aimee Forand, in 1957.

Recognizing the appeal of adding hospital insurance to Social Security, the opponents in Congress tried to preempt it in 1960 by enacting a program targeted to the elderly poor and run by the states. Known as Kerr-Mills for its two sponsors, both Democrats—Senator Robert Kerr of Oklahoma and Representative Wilbur Mills of Arkansas, the powerful chairman of the House Ways and Means Committee—the program extended to the medically indigent elderly the earlier program of federal aid to the states for welfare recipients' medical care. Under the program, the federal government paid 50 percent to 80 percent of a state's costs for medically impoverished seniors. The lower a state's per capita income, the higher the share of its spending the federal government reimbursed. Nonetheless, many southern and other states with large low-income (and, not incidentally, minority) populations restricted eligibility and covered only very limited services or did not participate in Kerr-Mills. In fact, 90 percent of the money spent under Kerr-Mills went to five states with 32 percent of the nation's population—California, New York, Massachusetts, Michigan, and Pennsylvania.[25] In other words, a bill supported by moderate to conservative representatives from the South and the West yielded a program that distributed funds mainly to the more liberal states.

Kerr-Mills, however, did not stop the political movement for what became popularly known as Medicare (though "Hospicare" would have originally been a more appropriate name). The hospital insurance proposal was a prominent issue for John F. Kennedy in his 1960 campaign, and public opinion polls indicated wide support for the idea. Despite the limited nature of the proposal, the opposition from organized medicine and conservative Republicans was just as fierce as it had been to national health insurance. A good example is a speech that Ronald Reagan, at that time an actor and spokesman for General Electric, recorded in 1961 for use in Operation Coffee Cup, a campaign against the bill by the women's auxiliary of the AMA. The Medicare bill, Reagan explained, was part of a larger plot to bring socialism to America, all the more dangerous because of its seeming humanitarian rationale. Soon the government would be telling doctors where to practice. If Americans didn't rise up against "socialized medicine" and the Medicare bill, Reagan warned, "one of these days you and I are going to spend our sunset years telling our children, and our children's children, what it once was like in America when men were free."[26]

While Kennedy was alive, a coalition of Republicans and southern Democrats blocked Medicare and other liberal initiatives. As chairman of Ways and Means in the House, Mills was the single most formidable congressional obstacle to the hospital-insurance measure, though support for it was growing in his committee as Democrats were added in the early 1960s. The Medicare legislation finally began to advance after Lyndon B. Johnson became president in the wake of Kennedy's assassination in November 1963. In 1964, the original proposal for limited hospital insurance was tacked on to a Social Security bill and passed the Senate 49 to 44 (filibusters were rare in those days, except on civil rights). As taped White

House telephone conversations show, Johnson talked with Mills in June about expanding Medicare in the House to cover physicians' services, which the president referred to as an addition with "sex appeal." Although Johnson courted Mills relentlessly, insisting the congressman would get all the credit and the glory ("It will be the biggest thing you have ever done for your country"), Mills backed off and blocked the hospital insurance program from becoming law. But when Johnson won a landslide victory over Barry Goldwater that November, the huge Democratic congressional majorities he brought with him made it virtually certain that Medicare would pass the next year.[27]

Indeed, rather than just enacting the limited hospital insurance measure, Congress ended up passing a broadened Medicare program, much as Johnson had discussed with Mills the previous year. The expansion, however, came about in a surprising way that made it appear to be a concession to conservatives, which in some ways it was. As 1965 began, the AMA and Republicans were criticizing the Democrats' Medicare proposal not only because it established a form of compulsory insurance, but also on the grounds that it covered only hospital costs. Now, for the first time, Republicans offered a serious alternative: a federally subsidized, voluntary insurance program that would cover physicians' bills as well. Mills took them up on the idea and, in what came off as a grand synthesis, combined three elements: the Democrats' compulsory hospital insurance program, which became Part A of Medicare; the Republican voluntary program to cover physicians' bills, which became Medicare Part B; and an expansion of the Kerr-Mills program (no longer restricting it to the elderly poor), the approach favored by the AMA, which became Medicaid. This "three-layered cake" was the basis of the legislation that both houses of Congress adopted in 1965.[28]

Mills' maneuver has generally been regarded as a brilliant legislative coup and a liberal victory. It was a brilliant coup, but it was not exactly a liberal one. Medicare and Medicaid did bring health care to millions of people who otherwise would not have received it, and those services resulted in significant improvements in health and well-being.[29] But the 1965 legislation was also a source of the persistent inequalities and high costs of the American health-care system.

By creating separate and unequal programs for the elderly and the poor—one piggy-backed on the shoulders of Social Security, the other shackled to public assistance ("welfare")—the 1965 legislation institutionalized two tiers of public financing for health services. The benefits that the elderly receive in the upper tier have been understood as an earned right, even though seniors have never paid enough in payroll taxes to earn their insurance coverage (in fact, the first wave of beneficiaries didn't pay anything). That moral claim has nonetheless given Medicare political security, making it unthinkable (at least until recently) to rescind the program, cap it, or cut it in a recession. In contrast, the recipients of Medicaid, like welfare, are not regarded as having earned any right, and that lack of a moral claim has made Medicaid politically insecure and more vulnerable to cutbacks.

The legal provisions for the two programs reflect this difference in their moral underpinnings. While Congress established Medicare on a national basis, it left Medicaid to the vagaries of the states; Medicare provided the same benefits to the elderly wherever they lived, but Medicaid did not do the same for the poor. States did not have to participate in Medicaid (Arizona did not establish a Medicaid program until 1982), and they had wide discretion about eligibility criteria, the scope of covered services, and payments to health-care providers. According to a formula favoring the poorer states, the federal government paid between 50 percent and 77 percent of a state's Medicaid expenditures, but as under Kerr-Mills, the states in the South and Southwest bearing the smallest share of costs nonetheless restricted eligibility the most severely. The federal law originally linked eligibility for Medicaid to eligibility for welfare, thereby limiting the program to the poor who fit into the eligible categories: the aged, blind, disabled, and families with dependent children. If a state agreed to run a Medicaid program, it had to cover all welfare recipients, though it could also receive federal funds for covering the poor with incomes up to 133 percent of the state's cut-off for welfare as long as they fell into the eligible categories. But because states varied in their criteria for welfare and their willingness to cover others among the poor, many of the poor who could qualify for Medicaid in, say, New York could not qualify in Mississippi. The more liberal states were also more liberal in the range of services they covered. Even in those states, however, the lower moral standing of Medicaid was reflected in payment rates to doctors that were so low that many refused to take Medicaid patients.[30]

Though Medicare did not carry the stigma of Medicaid, the Medicare benefit package was not generous. To pass Medicare in the Senate, the Johnson administration and party leaders fought off efforts by liberals to add coverage of prescription drugs and catastrophic medical costs— omissions that would come back to haunt them. But Medicare's financing provisions for the services it did cover were all too generous and created another kind of structural problem for health care. Spooked by the long opposition of the AMA to a federal program and anxious to have the full cooperation of doctors and other health-care interests in implementing Medicare, the Johnson administration and Congress failed to impose any cost restraint on health-care providers. The Medicare legislation explicitly denied the government any power to set rates: "nothing in this title shall be construed to authorize any federal officer . . . to exercise any supervision or control over the . . . compensation of any institution . . . or person providing health services."[31] Following the practice of Blue Cross (which the hospitals had originally established), Medicare Part A and Medicaid paid hospitals according to their costs. The higher a hospital's costs, the more it would be paid—a surer way of promoting health-care inflation could not have been devised. Any hospital that cut its cost would be reimbursed less. Medicare Part B paid doctors their "customary" fees, assuming them to be in line with "prevailing" rates in their area or to be "reasonable." But the legislation set no standard for reasonableness, and it required the government to outsource claims payment to the insurance industry. Acting as "carriers," merely passing along the costs to the government, the private insurers had no incentive to exert any control. Like hospital costs, doctors' fees surged immediately after Medicare went into effect in 1966. Fulfilling a promise to the AMA, Mills even insisted that hospital-based specialists such as pathologists, radiologists, and anesthesiologists, who were typically paid by salary at the time, instead be paid fee-for-service under Medicare Part B—a provision that led to the vast enrichment of those specialties in years to come. As a result of all these decisions, Medicare's costs proved to be much higher than the Johnson administration projected.[32]

Nonetheless, the implementation of Medicare has strangely been considered a success. The startup one year later, on July 1, 1966, went off without a hitch: The doctors and hospitals cooperated, and there were no waiting lines for care, as some had feared. Moreover, the ideological as well as interest-group opposition disappeared, partly because the doctors discovered how much money they could make out of the programs and no longer had any interest in rousing popular opposition to "socialized medicine." The final compromises struck by Mills also lent the legislation a bipartisan air. Although only ten Republicans in the House voted for the bill on the critical motion, many more joined in on the final roll call, and it passed 313 to 115.[33]

But while Mills' three-layered cake helped to achieve ideological reconciliation, it added a tremendous amount of complexity to health-care finance. Not only was Medicare divided into two parts working on different principles, but many of the elderly also bought private supplemental insurance to make up for the program's limitations, and if they were poor enough or spent down their assets and ended up in a nursing home, they might also be covered by Medicaid. Medicare's administrative costs were considerably lower than those of private insurance because the government didn't do any marketing or take any of the countermeasures to avoid costly enrollees that added so much to private insurers' overhead. But together with the myriad private insurance plans, the multiple government payment systems required hospitals, doctors, and other providers to hire legions of administrative personnel. Critics of a single, federal insurance plan had said it would be a bureaucratic nightmare, but the more unified or standardized systems in other advanced countries have much less bureaucracy. It was political compromise in America that made health care in the United States bureaucratically complex.

Compromise also led to other perverse effects. In a universal system, people do not have to be poor enough to qualify for health care, but that is how Medicaid worked, and its original link to welfare created a problem analogous to job lock. Just as many people found themselves unable to quit a job because they would lose health benefits, so many of those on welfare faced the loss of health coverage if they took the kind of job typically available to them—low-wage work without health insurance. So if Medicaid recipients suffered from chronic health problems or had a sick child, they had a strong incentive to stay on welfare. The Medicaid-welfare link may have increased the welfare rolls by about one-fourth.[34]

The Americans who remained without any health coverage were dispro-portionately the working poor—low-wage workers and their families, with access neither to employment-based insurance nor to a public program—as well as individuals whom private insurers deemed "uninsurable" be-cause of their medical history. Thanks to Medicare and Medicaid, the uninsured population was low enough in 1970, probably between 10 and 12 percent of the population, that the goal of universal coverage seemed within reach.[35] Thanks also in part to the two programs, sharply rising health care costs helped to trigger widespread criticism and rethinking of health care. That shift in thinking opened a new era in the pursuit of a rational and just health-care system.

CHAPTER 2

Stumbling toward Comprehensive Reform

AFTER CONGRESS PASSED MEDICARE IN 1965, many liberals expected to pursue the strategy of incremental enlargement that they had followed with Social Security since 1935: start out with limited benefits for a limited population, then gradually raise the standards and add new groups until the program provided a decent level of universal protection. That might have been the subsequent history if Medicare had not had economic and political consequences that made it difficult to extend. Yet even after the election in 1968 of a Republican president, Richard Nixon, the great question about national health insurance was not *whether* it would be achieved, but in *what form*. Worried about the costs, many conservative and centrist Democrats preferred a new federal program that would cover only the biggest medical bills, an approach known as "catastrophic insurance." Republicans who supported universal coverage generally preferred to build on private insurance for the employed and on Medicaid for the poor.

By this time, the rhetoric that Ronald Reagan and other conservatives had used in fighting the passage of Medicare seemed over the top. The elderly had not been ruined by giving them health insurance. Doctors did not have to practice where the government ordered them. The sun had not set on freedom. Even though its costs outstripped predictions, Medicare proved so popular no national politician dared suggest repealing it. But while the old ideological battle died down for a while, it did not disappear. The conflict over whether to have government-financed health insurance at all turned into a conflict over how much America should rely on government or the market in carrying out a new program.

Yet those were not the only possibilities. Besides employing government or the market with conviction, policy-makers could do a little of each without doing anything effectively. On universal coverage the two sides could fight one another to a draw, which is, in fact, what they did. This is not to say that the policies of the 1970s and '80s made no difference. Without exactly intending to do so, they transformed private insurance into managed care. Yet national policy didn't succeed in either controlling costs or providing secure coverage to all. The idea that reform had to be "comprehensive" grew out of years of policy-making that often had unintended and unhappy consequences when it was not deadlocked or ineffectual.

Political Deadlock, 1969–1980

Around 1970 health care in America went through a drastic public reassessment that initially favored efforts to achieve universal coverage. Instead of deferring to the judgment of health-care professionals, the press and political leaders began to subject health care to more critical scrutiny. Perhaps the organization of the health-care system failed to serve the interests of either efficiency or fairness; perhaps fee-for-service payment for doctors and cost-based reimbursement for hospitals were not the best ways to finance medical care. Perhaps the system was no system at all and needed more deliberate planning. The rate of growth in medical costs more than doubled, from 3.2 percent in the seven years before 1965 to 7.9 percent in the five years after. From 1965 to 1970, state and federal health expenditures rose at an annual rate of 20.8 percent. Deprivation co-existed with excess: while many Americans remained without access to services, studies identified patterns of excessive hospitalization, unnecessary surgery, and other inefficiencies. Suddenly, people on all sides were saying there was a "crisis" in health care. "We face a massive crisis in this area," President Nixon said in July 1969. "Unless action is taken within the next two or three years . . . we will have a breakdown in our medical system." Public opinion polls also registered wide agreement with the statement, "There is a crisis in health care in the United States."[1]

To liberals, the crisis demonstrated the need for a system of national health insurance with built-in spending constraints. In 1968, labor leaders had spearheaded the organization of a new Committee for National Health Insurance, and the following year Senator Edward M. Kennedy of Massachusetts toured the country to do hearings on the crisis. A bill Kennedy co-sponsored with Representative Martha W. Griffiths of Michigan provided for a single, comprehensive, federally administered system of national health insurance to replace existing private plans and government programs. The coverage would begin at the "first dollar" and make health care free at the point of service. While doctors would continue in private practice and hospitals would remain under their existing ownership, the federal government would set a national budget, and health-care providers would have to stay within prescribed spending limits.[2]

As the next presidential election approached, Nixon became convinced that he needed his own health insurance proposal to compete with Kennedy's. Health care was attracting increased attention from the media; for example, the June 7, 1971, issue of *Time* magazine featured a cover story on health care, and on June 8, according to taped conversations in the Oval Office, the president told his aides, "If the media can make the environment an issue, then they sure as hell will make health an issue—with the help of Teddy Kennedy. . . . So what we're playing in the health game is really a defensive maneuver. In addition, of course[,] to trying to deal with the real problem . . . effectively."[3]

Nixon's effort to compete with Kennedy on liberal terrain was entirely in keeping with his general pattern as president. Politically, Nixon and liberal Democrats detested and distrusted each other, but substantively they were closer than their mutual hostility suggested. Throughout Nixon's presidency, liberal assumptions dominated national debate and the Democrats continued to control Congress, but Nixon often sought to defeat them by offering alternative policies in an effort to co-opt their supporters. Despite cuts in antipoverty programs, for example, Nixon proposed a minimum guaranteed income. He presided over increases in Social Security, introduced affirmative action, adopted wage-price controls, embraced Keynesian economic policy, and agreed to the establishment of new regulatory agencies for environmental protection and occupational health and safety—all violations of traditional Republican orthodoxy. Nixon's Tory reformism came out nowhere more clearly than in health care. In fact, he was the first president of either party to send a specific plan for near-universal health coverage to Congress.

Nixon's 1971 national health strategy—the first of two major plans he offered as president—sought, first of all, to fill in the gaps in the insurance system. The core of the proposal was an employer mandate: employers would be required to pay three-fourths of the premiums for health insurance for their workers and dependents, though the minimum required coverage could have significant deductibles and co-payments and a $50,000 annual limit. A proposed Family Health Insurance Plan, with less generous benefits, would cover the unemployed and the poor at no charge to the poorest and on a sliding-scale subsidy for families with incomes up to $5,000 (121 percent of the 1971 federal poverty level for a family of four). In response to congressional Republicans who were unhappy about the employer mandate, the administration agreed to exempt small businesses with fewer than 10 workers. But Nixon defended the mandate forthrightly in a March 1972 message to Congress, citing "precedents of long-standing under which personal security—and thus national economic progress—has been enhanced by requiring employers to provide minimum wages and disability and retirement benefits and to observe occupational health and safety standards." Nixon also called for the federal government to finance 100 percent of Part B of Medicare, eliminating the premiums paid by the elderly.[4]

The second part of Nixon's 1971 health strategy aimed at restraining medical costs and introduced a new term, "health maintenance organization," for an old idea: payment of health-care providers for comprehensive services per person (capitation payment) rather than by individual fee for service. Beginning in the 1930s, a small number of nonprofit health plans had developed on a prepaid basis in conjunction with physician group practices. These prepaid group practice plans started out with a left-wing reputation due mainly to opposition from the AMA, which denounced them as socialized medicine and tried to put them out of business. A campaign by the medical association to blacklist doctors who worked for the plans led to a 1943 Supreme Court decision holding that the AMA had violated the antitrust laws. The most successful prepaid group practice plan, Kaiser

Permanente, became the largest health-care system in California and thus well known to Nixon, who came from the state. Policy advisers to the Nixon administration—including Paul Ellwood, the Minneapolis physician who coined the term "health maintenance organization" in 1970—presented the idea as a way to create incentives for preventive health care and efficient services and a more competitive health-care market. In a stunning reversal, what conservatives had once denounced as socialized medicine they now hailed as a capitalist solution for health care.[5]

The early 1970s saw a profusion of proposals both to expand health coverage and to control costs, and in 1972 Congress did extend Medicare to two groups below age 65: end-stage renal disease patients (who faced a life-or-death need for kidney dialysis) and people with disabilities who had qualified for Social Security disability insurance for two years. In another incremental step, when Congress created a new minimum national cash benefit for the aged, blind, and disabled poor (Supplemental Security Income), it required states to cover the beneficiaries in their Medicaid programs. The same legislation sought to limit unnecessary medical services by authorizing the establishment of panels of physicians to review treatment under federal health programs, but like several other regulatory and planning measures of the 1970s, the review system failed to control costs.[6]

With the 1972 election on the horizon, Congress and the Nixon administration were unable to reach an agreement on universal coverage. At the beginning of his second term, however, Nixon made a comprehensive insurance plan a top priority, assigning responsibility for developing the proposal to Caspar Weinberger, his new Secretary of Health, Education, and Welfare. By that time, the Watergate scandal had already become a central preoccupation for the president, and as the cover-up unraveled that year, Nixon became increasingly desperate to win back public favor. A bold health care proposal offered him that possibility. In addition, because the scandal forced out the president's top advisers in the White House, Weinberger and his staff had a free hand to formulate health policy. In a memo to Nixon in November 1973, Weinberger argued that a "broad and comprehensive [health] plan" would "demonstrate that the administration has a positive and effective position in health care and that the government is not paralyzed." Despite opposition from other members of his cabinet,

Nixon went ahead with the plan, though he modified some aspects of it. Weinberger had recommended financing the plan by treating employer contributions to health insurance as taxable income, but Nixon rejected that proposal.[7]

Like his 1971 plan, Nixon's new Comprehensive Health Insurance Plan relied on an employer mandate to cover workers and their dependents and a public program for everyone not otherwise insured. But this time the employer mandate required generous benefits and limited cost-sharing, and the government program was also broad in scope and open to anyone who couldn't obtain private insurance, with no income limits on eligibility. Speaking on the radio on February 5, 1974, the day before he sent his health program to Congress, Nixon referred to comprehensive health insurance as "an idea whose time has come."[8]

Its time might very well have come that year if the Watergate scandal had only wounded Nixon instead of destroying him. Until August 1974, when Nixon resigned, moves were afoot to find common ground on health care. Beginning in mid-1972, Kennedy had reached out to Wilbur Mills and met privately with him to work out joint legislation. The Kennedy-Mills bill that emerged from those discussions in April 1974 called for two departures from Kennedy's earlier proposal: it included some cost-sharing by patients and gave private insurers a role as fiscal intermediaries. Even though the bill still called for a universal, tax-financed, comprehensive, federal insurance program, Kennedy's long-time allies in unions refused to go along, insisting on first-dollar coverage as a matter of principle. Kennedy was not deterred. "There is a ball game going on up there, and I'm going to be a part of that ball game," he declared at a meeting in downtown Washington of the Health Security Action Coalition. Some in the audience called him a "sellout."[9]

Meanwhile, Senator Russell Long, chairman of the Senate Finance Committee, had built up a majority on his committee for a bill creating a federal program to cover catastrophic health costs. Coverage would begin after 60 days of hospital care and after $2,000 in doctors' bills. The 1973 version of Long's bill, co-sponsored by Senator Abraham Ribicoff, Democrat of Connecticut, also called for replacing Medicaid with a new program to cover the medical costs of low-income people regardless of their employment, family status, or eligibility for welfare. A third part of the plan required the standardization of private insurance policies that covered the costs that the federal catastrophic-insurance program left out.[10]

Both Democrats and Republicans signaled interest in a compromise. Although Democrats had long promoted the issue, the Republican leaders in the House and Senate wrote to Nixon in April that it was "imperative" that Congress "enact a bill to lift the burden" of high health costs. In talks encouraged by the president, aides to Nixon and Mills met to discuss a synthesis of the president's proposal and Kennedy-Mills. That June, Kennedy announced, "A new spirit of compromise is in the air," and suggested a bill could reach the president's desk by the fall.[11]

To be sure, key differences remained. While Kennedy-Mills relied on a payroll tax, Nixon's financing relied on an employer mandate, which allowed him to say that his plan involved no new taxes. Nixon's plan also did not require individuals who could afford coverage to purchase it, which meant that, unlike Kennedy-Mills, it would not cover everyone. During their careers, however, Mills, Nixon, and Kennedy all enjoyed success playing against type—Mills by reversing himself on Medicare; Nixon by embracing policies identified with his opponents, most spectacularly in his diplomatic opening to China; and Kennedy, by leading the early efforts at deregulation. The key players, in short, had enough flexibility to have struck a deal. But Nixon's resignation on August 6, 1974, prevented any final negotiation. In the ensuing two weeks, while Gerald Ford, Nixon's successor, was still promising to sign health insurance legislation, Mills tried to achieve a grand synthesis by stitching together a bill with elements of Nixon's proposal, Kennedy-Mills, and Long-Ribicoff. But Mills was able to win only a bare majority, 16 to 15, on the Ways and Means Committee. The opposition came from Mills' fellow southern Democrats and most of the Republicans; the committee's liberals backed the chairman despite their reservations about his plan. Deciding that he lacked enough support to bring the compromise measure to the floor, Mills declared a "hopeless deadlock," signaling an end to the effort, even though Long was still interested in pursuing a deal.[12] Many Republicans had never been enthusiastic about Nixon's proposal in the first place, while labor-oriented progressives anticipated major gains in the 1976 election and therefore saw no reason to settle for a compromise. Speaking for the Committee for National Health Insurance, labor leader Leonard Woodcock said his group preferred no legislation to any compromise. In what would be the final straw, the political career of the traditionally staid Mills came to a dismal end that fall after the Washington, D.C., police found him driving drunk at night with his headlights off, accompanied by a strip-tease dancer with whom he was having an affair. Mills' alcoholism and private troubles may have prevented him from negotiating the kind of deal on national health insurance that he had struck nine years earlier on Medicare.

It may seem unsatisfactory to say that the fate of national health insurance hinged on the peculiar circumstances of the Watergate affair and the private lives and political fortunes of individual leaders. But if political leadership fails when the window for reform is open, the moment may pass and the window may close. And so it did. Because of larger changes in political economy that would alter the entire political landscape, the possibilities for a bipartisan agreement on health insurance were about to disappear. The era of national health insurance, as liberals had conceived it, was over, and a new phase in health reform was about to begin.

In 1975 President Ford did not resubmit Nixon's health insurance plan to Congress on the grounds that it would exacerbate inflation. At first it seemed that the movement for national health insurance had only paused. But the slow growth and high inflation of the mid-1970s—"stagflation," people called it—proved to be a major turning point for American society and politics.

In retrospect, the mid-1970s marked the end of a liberal era of shared prosperity. Since the 1940s, economic growth had been strong, income inequalities had fallen and remained low, and the middle class had expanded. Under those conditions, the public had supported rising expenditures for education, health care, and other public programs, and those programs contributed to the wide diffusion of gains from economic growth. But beginning in the mid-1970s, economic inequalities increased sharply, many Americans saw real declines in their incomes, and conservative anti-government and anti-tax sentiment spread. Much of the hostility focused on welfare, but the discontent affected general attitudes toward government, and in several states, notably California in 1978, voters passed referenda capping or rolling back taxes.

In this changed climate, the primary focus of concern about health care shifted from coverage to costs. Under the wage-price controls that Nixon imposed in August 1971, the growth in health-care costs was relatively subdued, but it surged when price controls expired for the health-care sector in May 1974. A change in the tenor of thinking about medical costs took place in the same period. When the 1970s began, the press and political leaders were questioning whether medical care was efficiently organized. By the middle of the decade, some influential critics had moved on to raise more fundamental doubts about whether medical care was effective in reducing mortality and improving health. This wave of criticism echoed an old tradition of "therapeutic nihilism" that doubted medical treatment to be of any use. The idea that public improvement is hopeless—the "futility" thesis, as Albert O. Hirschman calls it—is a recurrent theme of conservative thought, and during the 1970s a variety of services such as the schools and prison rehabilitation came under attack along the same lines. Perhaps all the increased spending for health, education, and other social programs was a waste of money. In fact, the evidence on medical care showed that it did improve health and well-being, but the new therapeutic nihilism nonetheless undercut the movement for equal access. After all, what point would there be to equalizing access to something that did little or no good?[13]

The slowing economy, rising government deficits, and attacks on the value of medical care forced the supporters of health-care reform to put more emphasis than ever on cost containment. A rift opened up, however, between those who believed that national health insurance could itself be a way of controlling costs and those who insisted that cost containment had to precede the extension of coverage.

The labor leaders who in the spring and summer of 1974 had refused to accept the Kennedy-Mills compromise, much less Nixon's plan, were right that the post-Watergate elections would bring a bumper crop of Democrats to Washington. But they were wrong that those Democrats would press for immediate action on national health insurance, much less for a plan with first-dollar coverage. The Democrat who was elected president in 1976, former Georgia Governor Jimmy Carter, vaguely endorsed national health insurance at a point in his campaign when he needed labor support, but once in office he balked at taking any action. Carter had other priorities in domestic policy, though he proved ineffectual in making progress on any of them. His main concern about health care was cost control, and in April 1977 he submitted legislation—never passed by Congress—to limit the rate of increase in revenue that hospitals received from all sources, public and private. Although Carter told Kennedy and labor leaders that he would submit a national health insurance bill, he kept putting it off. Carter's economic advisers opposed a bill, and Carter's own thinking about health care, according to one of his aides, emphasized "volunteerism and Christian noblesse oblige. . . . He did not see health care as every citizen's right, nor did he think government has an obligation to provide it" but instead "preferred to talk movingly of his deep compassion and genuine empathy for those who suffered for lack of health care."[14]

The dispute among Democrats over health insurance came to a head in July 1978, when Carter informed Kennedy that rather than endorsing a comprehensive plan, he would support phasing in expanded coverage over a period of years, with each additional step being contingent on meeting targets for cost control and requiring new action by Congress. Viewing this approach as politically hopeless, Kennedy announced: "We intend to proceed now, on our own—with the Administration if possible, without the Administration if necessary."[15]

The following year, Kennedy introduced a new proposal for universal coverage, but as so often happens, the politics overshadowed the substance of a policy proposal. Preconceptions about Kennedy and liberalism also prevented journalists at the time (and some historians since then) from appreciating the significance of the shift in liberal thinking that Kennedy's plan represented. As Kennedy writes in his final memoir, he had "negotiated long and hard" with the leadership of the AFL-CIO and United Auto Workers to give up on a single, federal insurance system and instead to support a proposal based on competing private insurance plans.[16] Kennedy was still calling for universal, mandatory coverage, but now with choice of private insurers. Consumers would get a card entitling them to insurance, which they could use to obtain coverage from Blue Cross, a commercial insurer, an HMO, or an independent practice association (a form of prepaid plan using independent doctors). How much consumers would pay for a card would depend on their income and employment. Employers would pay 65 percent of the cost for their workers and dependents, while government would pay for the poor. Because the card would not identify the source of payment, the poor would not bear the stigma of Medicaid. To discourage cherry-picking, the payment received by insurers would be adjusted to reflect the actuarial risk of their enrollees, and if consumers chose plans that operated more efficiently, they would get rebates or extra benefits. The entire system would run under budget limits.[17] This proposal, though it failed at the time, is the origin of the plan that Bill Clinton would propose in 1993 and, to a lesser extent, the law that Barack Obama would sign in 2010.

When Carter finally issued his own plan in June 1979, it turned out to be an echo of Nixon's, though a rather faint echo at that. Like Nixon, Carter called for employers to insure their workers and dependents and a public program for everyone else. But while Nixon's plan featured comprehensive benefits, Carter proposed to start off only with catastrophic health insurance, with further steps depending on cost containment. The proposal, however, was quickly forgotten. The next month, Carter gave a speech to the nation declaring that it suffered from a crisis of confidence. Then he asked for the resignation of his cabinet, firing five of them and bringing on a crisis of confidence in his own leadership from which he never recovered. Broad economic and social trends were only partly responsible for the turn to the right that culminated in the election of Ronald Reagan in 1980. Carter himself deserves a lot of the credit.

The split between Kennedy and Carter on health insurance was not only a matter of political rivalry. It also reflected a basic divergence between liberal and centrist Democrats in their understanding of health-care reform. Kennedy saw universal health insurance as an opportunity to restructure health-care finance with new incentives and comprehensive budget limits. Carter saw universal coverage as a burden that the government could bear only if it first controlled costs. But Carter's hospital cost-containment bill would have only superimposed a layer of regulation on hospitals while leaving in place all the incentives that were driving costs; health-care providers could have evaded the controls by shifting inpatient procedures to ambulatory settings (as, in fact, new technology would increasingly allow them to do). Moreover, by providing catastrophic coverage alone without covering primary or preventive care, the first phase of Carter's insurance program would have reinforced American medicine's bias toward high-cost, high-tech services. Carter and his economic advisers were trying to be prudent by taking small steps, but the steps were too small to have remedied the problems and their vision was too cramped to win public support. When the House of Representatives defeated the hospital cost-containment legislation in November 1979, the whole basis of Carter's health insurance strategy collapsed. For the time being, Democrats were at an impasse.

Yet while the battles over national health insurance in the 1970s failed to yield any action, something significant had changed by the end of the decade: the cause itself had been redefined as comprehensive health-care reform. Any serious proposal for universal coverage also had to be a plan for cost containment. Previously, "comprehensive" as a modifier of reform referred to the scope of coverage; now it meant addressing the problems of the health system in all their dimensions—access, cost, and quality of care. The change was reflected on both sides of the ideological spectrum. Earlier conservative proposals mainly echoed trade-association views reinforcing the status quo, but by the late 1970s, market-oriented health-policy analysts were arguing that the health-care industry needed substantial change. Stronger antitrust enforcement was one theme of this critique. More support for HMOs and other alternatives to traditional fee-for-service medicine was another. The Stanford economist Alain Enthoven brought many of these threads together in a proposal for universal health insurance that called for consumers to choose among competing integrated health plans in their community. Under Enthoven's approach, the government would also change the tax treatment of insurance so that people had to use after-tax dollars to pay any extra amount above the lowest-cost plan.[18] While Enthoven was proposing a market model for universal coverage, Kennedy was abandoning a single governmental system and incorporating elements of competition into his approach. Under different political conditions, these developments might have signaled a promising ideological convergence.

But Reagan's election foreclosed that possibility by knocking universal coverage entirely off the national agenda.

Political Reversals, 1981–1990

The 1980 election was the first of three national elections in 30 years bringing to power Republicans promising to reverse the expansion of government. Unlike the Republicans elected in 1994 and 2010, President Reagan did not initially make federal health-care programs a central focus of attention, though in his first budget he sought to cut Medicaid and other federal health programs rather than expand them. The "Reagan revolution" was also expected to usher in a general shift of emphasis in health policy from government to the market. Even before 1981, the health-care industry was already becoming more of a field for corporate enterprise primarily because of the profitable opportunities created by the absence of effective cost controls in either private insurance or government programs.[19] It might be easy, therefore, to imagine that the 1980s saw a coherent shift from regulation to the market as the driving force for change.

But during the 1980s, health policy followed an unexpected course. In the end, instead of being cut, Medicaid was expanded. In his last year in office, Reagan signed an expansion of Medicare that was quickly repealed. And in the single most important reversal, instead of relying more on market mechanisms, the Reagan administration sought and received stronger regulatory authority to control the prices that Medicare paid hospitals. The 1980s continued a pattern that had already emerged in the Carter years— a greater emphasis on costs than on coverage. But instead of a general program to contain overall health costs, the main impetus for change came from cost-control measures taken separately by the payers, public and private. Medicare was the most important payer of all, and when the federal government changed how Medicare paid hospitals in 1983, it set in motion developments that transformed the health-care system and ultimately the national debate about reform.

As an opponent of Medicare before its enactment, Reagan had warned that it would bring government control over health care. In reality, the original Medicare program had brought no control even over the prices paid to hospitals and doctors for treating the elderly. So it was a supreme irony that the government would finally begin to set those prices through a policy that Reagan himself would sign into law.

What finally broke the grip of the hospitals (and later the doctors) on the methods of Medicare payment was the acute fiscal crisis that developed after Reagan cut taxes and increased military spending in 1981 and the economy then plunged into the worst recession in decades. Falling revenues intensified pressures on the Social Security Trust Fund, which made up for an imminent shortfall by borrowing money from the Medicare Hospital Trust Fund even though that fund faced its own difficulties because of soaring hospital costs. Under Carter, the hospital industry had organized a voluntary effort to restrain inflation, but once Congress defeated Carter's hospital cost-containment bill, all restraint collapsed. With hospital costs rising 18 percent in 1981, the congressional leaders who had backed the industry against Carter were ready to support tougher policies.[20]

Crises create opportunities for change, but the political use of a crisis depends on the remedies at hand and the leadership in power at the moment. During the late 1970s, several states had obtained federal approval to experiment with rate-setting for hospital care of Medicare beneficiaries as well as other patients. Under a system introduced in 1980 in New Jersey under a Democratic governor, hospitals began receiving a flat payment per admission adjusted for the patient's diagnosis, a method developed by researchers at Yale University. This system of prospective payment by "diagnosis-related groups" (DRGs) aimed to give hospitals an incentive to control costs, in contrast to Medicare, which reimbursed hospitals retrospectively on the basis of the costs they incurred. Early reports about the new system were encouraging, and Reagan's Secretary of Health and Human Services, former Pennsylvania Senator Richard Schweiker, was familiar with the New Jersey experiment from his connections with the state and his work on the Senate Finance Committee. Overruling staff who favored other approaches, Schweiker made the DRG system the administration's policy even though it meant that the government, not the market, would set prices. "[F]iscal necessity overwhelmed political ideology," Rick Mayes and Robert Berenson write in a history of the policy.[21] The new payment system, which proved to be the biggest change in Medicare since its enactment, was rushed through Congress early in 1983 with virtually no public debate as part of bipartisan legislation bailing out Social Security.

Phased in during the mid-1980s, prospective payment put hospitals at financial risk for the first time. If the cost of a patient's treatment exceeded the DRG payment, a hospital would lose money, but if the cost was lower, it could turn a profit. In the first years of the new system, hospitals did very well indeed because Medicare started out paying them at levels that reflected the industry's historic costs, which allowed plenty of room for savings. So while the system slowed the growth in Medicare's hospital costs, hospital profit margins hit new highs. The belief that prospective hospital payment was a success led Congress to introduce a comparable reform in the payment of physicians. Adopted in 1989 and carried out three years later, the new system replaced the payment of "reasonable" charges with a fee schedule based on an analysis of the resources required for different services (a "resource-based relative value scale," or RBRVS).

From the beginning, Congress adjusted prospective hospital payment for various purposes, providing higher rates to teaching hospitals to support medical education and research and continuing to reimburse capital expenditures of all hospitals on a cost basis. Additional payments were also targeted to institutions caring for a "disproportionate share" of the poor and uninsured. In short, rather than just being a program for the elderly, Medicare became a means of carrying out health policy for the broader society, including indirectly some coverage of the uninsured. The decision to pay for capital costs was particularly important. Because Medicare beneficiaries represented roughly 40 percent of hospital revenue, Medicare continued to defray 40 percent of the cost of any new hospital investment. The federal government did not cover 40 percent of a new school building that a local district wanted to build, but it did pay for 40 percent of a new wing built by the local hospital, no questions asked. The contrast in the physical plant and technological resources of hospitals and schools in the United States is partly the result of this difference in policy.

By the late 1980s, Congress responded to the hospitals' high profit margins under the new system by ratcheting down annual payment increases. The resulting savings had obvious appeal to legislators for use in reducing the deficit or funding other programs. But as Congress pressed down on Medicare rates, it led hospitals to shift costs to privately insured patients, driving up health insurance premiums and focusing the attention of employers and insurers on how they could reduce their own costs. Instead of providing full coverage, many employers began requiring workers to pay increased deductibles and co-payments. But the most important development was the "managed care revolution."

The growth of HMOs had been relatively slow even though Congress in 1973 had adopted legislation to promote them. As they were originally conceived, HMOs required substantial commitments of capital as well as the development of new managerial capacities and new ways of thinking among both doctors and patients. In the classic "staff" or "group" organizational models, the doctors are salaried or form partnerships that contract with the health plan; in looser models, independently practicing physicians enter into contracts to serve as the plan's exclusive providers. In the mid-1980s, the pace of change began to pick up as insurers created a broader set of alternatives to conventional fee-for-service insurance. "Managed care" came to refer to any form of health coverage that did one of two things (or more likely both): regulating treatment decisions and contracting selectively with health-care providers. To regulate critical decisions, insurers often required pre-authorization for hospital admissions and expensive tests and procedures. In "gatekeeper" plans, patients had to obtain referrals from a primary-care physician before seeing specialists. Selective contracting enabled insurers to demand discounts from providers, who might lose large numbers of their patients if they refused to make concessions. Under a new hybrid managed-care plan, the "preferred provider organization" (PPO), patients were not locked into a plan's network. Instead, insurers offered enrollees more complete coverage if they used in-network than out-of-network providers.

These new insurance plans transformed the character and image as well as the structure of "alternative delivery systems." Aiming to provide high-quality, coordinated care, the original, nonprofit HMOs had experienced lower costs as a side effect, mainly because their members spent less time in the hospital. The new, mostly for-profit managed-care plans were set up to make money by demanding discounts from providers and requiring checks at critical decision points in a course of treatment. The more aggressively the insurers pursued that course, the more they created adversarial relationships with both physicians and patients and raised suspicions that they were refusing to cover necessary care. But despite those suspicions, the new managed-care plans could be established more quickly and cheaply than the classic HMOs, and their enrollment began to grow rapidly as premiums for fee-for-service insurance increased. In 1978, 95 percent of employees with health benefits still had traditional fee-for-service insurance. By 1988 that proportion dropped to 71 percent, as managed care gained an increasingly wide foothold.[22]

Another change in the private market that gained momentum in the 1980s was the spread of self-insured employee health plans that effectively operated free of all regulation. In 1946, under the McCarran-Ferguson Act, the federal government left insurance regulation largely to the states. But in 1974, Congress passed the Employment Retirement Income Security Act (ERISA), preempting state laws that regulated benefit plans established by employers and unions, if the plans were self-funded and bore insurance risk. At the time the legislation was passed, the debate about it focused on pension plans; few employers had self-insured health plans, and hardly anyone realized ERISA would apply to health benefits. But as health costs rose, increasing numbers of firms used the law to escape from state insurance regulations. ERISA effectively undermined the capacity of states to curb abusive insurance practices and to create a pool for community-rated policies that included the employees of large firms. Despite preempting state law, the federal government also did not step in to set standards. One exception came in 1986, when Congress extended to workers a right to buy group health coverage for up to 18 months after being laid off. Known as "COBRA coverage" because it passed as part of the Consolidated Omnibus Budget Reconciliation Act, it did not include any assistance in paying for insurance. After all, helping the unemployed pay for coverage might have required a tax increase.

The Emergency Medical Treatment and Active Medical Labor Act, another measure adopted by Congress as part of the 1986 omnibus budget legislation, also expanded access to medical care without any increase in taxes. Adopted in response to widespread reports of hospitals "dumping" uninsured patients in desperate need of care, the law gave individuals an explicit right to emergency medical treatment by hospitals that participate in Medicare. Once again, Congress was using Medicare indirectly as a basis for serving wider social purposes.[23]

Although national health insurance was off the agenda, the late 1980s did see two major federal efforts to extend health insurance coverage. One of these involved an expansion of Medicare and proved a resounding failure, while the other involved an expansion of Medicaid and proved a quiet success. Both illustrated the problems of trying to increase coverage without raising taxes to pay for it.

At first, the resounding failure appeared to be a story of constructive bipartisanship. In 1988 President Reagan signed the Medicare Catastrophic Coverage Act, which passed the House by a final vote of 328 to 72 and the Senate by a vote of 86 to 11. Public opinion polls at the time showed overwhelming support for the legislation. But the next year Congress repealed nearly the entire law, and "Medicare Catastrophic" became a cautionary tale about the political perils of health-care reform.

The origins of the program partly explain its fate. Although the proposal to add Medicare coverage for catastrophic medical expenses emerged from the Reagan administration, the idea never had its full backing. The impetus came entirely from Otis Bowen, a doctor and former Republican governor of Indiana who became secretary of Health and Human Services in 1985. During his wife's long battle with cancer, Bowen had become concerned about the limits of Medicare coverage for hospital and physician services. Many of the elderly bought private supplemental insurance to pay those bills, but Bowen thought those "Medigap" policies were a bad deal because up to 40 cents of every premium dollar went for administrative costs and profits, compared with Medicare's administrative overhead of 3 percent. So Bowen proposed to extend Medicare's hospital and physician coverage through a flat premium of $4.92 a month to be paid by all beneficiaries. Within the administration, conservatives were appalled by a proposal that would effectively substitute a government monopoly for a private market, but Bowen steamrolled over internal opposition and released his proposal on November 20, 1986, without White House approval.[24]

By this time, amid the Iran-Contra scandal, Reagan's popularity had declined and Republicans had just lost control of the Senate as well as the

House. Congressional Democrats eagerly seized on Bowen's initiative as an opening for more substantial legislation. With the support of a bipartisan coalition that included virtually the entire leadership of both parties, the final bill added coverage for prescription drugs, expanded coverage for such services as skilled nursing facilities, and provided protections against spousal impoverishment from catastrophic health costs.

Reagan had insisted that he would not sign the bill if it included a tax increase, and to comply with that demand and avoid adding to the deficit, the Medicare Catastrophic Coverage Act required seniors to pay its entire cost through two kinds of premiums. A flat monthly premium of $4 to be paid by all seniors would pay for one-third of the program's cost, while the remainder would be covered by an additional, income-related premium due from seniors who paid income taxes of at least $150. These premiums would take the form of a surtax of 15 percent on their tax liability in 1989, up to a maximum of $800 for individuals and $1,600 for couples; in 1993 the surtax would rise to 28 percent, capped at $1,050 for individuals and $2,100 for couples. Even though this surely looked like a tax to those who would have to pay it, Reagan signed the bill.[25]

The financing provisions of Medicare Catastrophic reflected a changed view of the elderly among national elites. By a variety of measures, the economic position of seniors had improved substantially since the enactment of Medicare, and many Democrats and Republicans in Congress were persuaded that it was no longer justifiable to tax the working-age population to support the retired. As a result, Medicare Catastrophic was the first social-insurance program ever adopted with elderly-only financing. The premise of Social Security and Medicare was, and remains, that workers contribute during their working years to be able to enjoy benefits during retirement, and the original architects of both programs were careful to limit the financial burdens they placed on the affluent to minimize potential opposition and try to ensure that the programs were a good deal for all, rich and poor. Medicare Catastrophic broke from that tradition.

Supporters were nonetheless convinced that the program would be well received. After all, the majority of the elderly would benefit from it, the American Association for Retired Persons supported the law, and 91 percent of seniors backed it, according to an AARP poll in May 1988, just before the law passed. But within months seniors turned sharply against the program. Supporters of the law blamed the shift on hostile and misleading direct-mail campaigns, particularly by a group called the National Committee to Preserve Social Security and Medicare. And it does appear that many low-income seniors were misled into believing that they would pay the surtax. But surveys also indicate that the more informed seniors were, the less they approved of the law. Before the law was passed, the print media paid little attention to the financing provisions, and television news paid no attention at all. The AARP polls before the law was passed had also not made clear to respondents how much they would have to pay. In fact, the program was the first social-insurance legislation to make a substantial number of its beneficiaries— probably about 30 percent—financially worse off because they would pay more in premiums than they would receive in benefits. In addition, about 20 percent of seniors—generally the more affluent ones, who were being asked to pay the most—were retirees whose former employers paid part or all of the premiums of their Medigap policies.[26] The legislation required them to pay for a program that benefited them not at all. It didn't help that soon after the legislation passed, the government raised its estimates of the cost, and by the following year, George H. W. Bush had succeeded Reagan and had no stake in defending the program. In one of the most dramatic reversals in national policy, a bill that had passed Congress overwhelmingly in 1988 was just as overwhelmingly repealed in 1989.

The surprising and little-noticed counterpoint to the failure to expand Medicare was the expansion of Medicaid during the 1980s. In his first year, Reagan called for ending the individual entitlement of the poor to medical care under the Medicaid program and turning it into a block grant to the states. Reagan also wanted to convert a wide range of public health programs into block grants, which meant that the disabled, mentally ill, and other groups weakly represented in many state legislatures would lose protections they enjoyed under federal law. Still holding a majority in the House, Democrats succeeded in maintaining the Medicaid entitlement and other key policies but agreed to budget cuts. As a result, federal spending on Medicaid was held flat during a recession when expenditures would ordinarily have risen because many laid-off workers lost their health insurance. The resulting crisis in health care for the poor during the early 1980s boomeranged against Republicans, however, strengthening support for Medicaid. In 1984, largely through the work of Rep. Henry Waxman, chairman of the health subcommittee of Energy and Commerce, Congress began extending Medicaid coverage for low-income pregnant women and children. Year by year for the rest of the decade, Congress extended coverage a little further, typically first as an option for the states and then as a mandate. The biggest steps came in 1989 and 1990 when Congress mandated that states phase in Medicaid coverage of all children in families whose incomes fell beneath the federal poverty line and all children up to age five in families with incomes up to 33 percent above the poverty line. Millions of children would gain health coverage as a result of these low-profile measures. In addition, when Medicare Catastrophic was repealed, Congress left in place the provisions of the law relating to Medicaid, which required state Medicaid programs to cover the cost of Medicare deductibles, co-payments, and other expenses for the elderly poor. These "dual eligibles" would come to represent a growing financial obligation for the states.[27]

Like the financing arrangements for Medicare Catastrophic, the Medicaid mandates were another way for Congress to circumvent the need to raise federal taxes to pay for health coverage. The mandates gradually made Medicaid a more consistent national program, especially in the coverage of low-income children. Expanding coverage for poor children responded to a pattern that was the inverse of what had been happening among the elderly. While poverty had fallen among seniors, it had risen among families with children. Nonetheless, the nation's governors were increasingly irate about the burdens of unfunded mandates. Congress, Arkansas Governor Bill Clinton complained, was trying to achieve "universal coverage using the states' credit cards as the financing mechanism."[28] Clinton wasn't against universal coverage; he just thought there needed to be a better way to do it.

Medicare prospective payment and the rise of managed care brought substantial change to health care but no slowdown in the overall rate of growth in costs during the 1980s. The evidence on each of the policies made it seem as though they were effective. Medicare's new system for paying hospitals slowed the program's hospital costs, and managed-care plans extracted discounts from providers and reduced costs for inpatient care. But providers figured out how to adapt to Medicare's new rules, moving services out of the hospital and shifting costs to other payers. The classic HMOs showed significant savings, but the new forms of managed care had a modest impact.

Although prospective payment was a more rational way to pay health-care providers than cost-based reimbursement had been, the new system mainly displaced costs from Medicare to the privately insured. By 1990, many employers had come around to the view that reform had to be comprehensive—comprehensive in the sense that it had to apply to both the public and private sectors, lest government just make things worse for business.

The United States, moreover, was now reaping the consequences of its earlier decisions. For decades public policy and the health-care financing system had promoted investment in hospitals and other costly facilities and encouraged the training of medical specialists rather than primary practitioners. No doubt much good came out of these investments, particularly in medical research. But these long-standing policies created an internal dynamic that fed on itself, generating continued growth in health expenditures that the half-way cost-containment measures of the 1980s were incapable of checking. Health costs in the United States continued to outpace economic growth. Between 1980 and 1992, health costs grew so much faster than the economy as a whole that the health-care sector jumped from 9.3 percent to 13.6 percent of GDP—an additional 1 percent of GDP every 34 months, far beyond what health care in other countries cost.[29] Higher costs put health insurance out of reach for more people. So even though universal coverage had dropped off the national agenda in the 1980s, the underlying forces were about to bring it back—not as national health insurance, but as comprehensive reform.

The American Path in Health Insurance

How had the United States ended up in 1990 with the most expensive health care system in the world and a rising proportion of people without health insurance?

Many people have tried to find one explanation for the absence of universal health insurance in the United States, but from a historical standpoint, it is better to divide the problem into two parts. The first part concerns the period before job-based private insurance was established and reformers began pursuing a separate program for the elderly: Why in the first half of the twentieth century did the United States fail to adopt a government health insurance system that originally would have been aimed, as in Europe, at industrial workers? The history after Medicare raises a different question: Why after adopting a program for the elderly did the United States fail to extend it—or to use some mixture of public and private insurance—to make coverage universal? The two periods raise different questions because employment-based insurance and Medicare drastically altered political conditions. It is one thing to establish a government program in a field where private institutions are absent or weak. It is another thing entirely where private institutions are well established and not only the majority but the most vocal groups enjoy significant protection. The explanation for the persistence of a social pattern (in this case, the absence of universal coverage) is often entirely different from the explanation of its origins.

In Europe, as I suggested in the previous chapter, governments created health insurance programs for workers in the late nineteenth and early twentieth centuries as part of a larger effort to co-opt the appeal of socialists and integrate workers into the established political order. The relative weakness of unions and socialists in the United States meant there was no corresponding political basis for a government health insurance program when reformers first tried to pass it in the Progressive era. Consequently, the more narrow interests of employers, insurers, and (eventually) doctors were able to prevail. In the 1930s, the overall political conditions shifted in support of government social programs, but political priorities changed too, and Roosevelt opted for unemployment and old-age insurance rather than health insurance, with the opposition of organized medicine helping to tip the political calculus. The AMA then served as the central organization inspiring and coordinating opposition to Truman's call for national health insurance in the late 1940s, when Democrats no longer held congressional majorities of the kind they had at the height of the New Deal. In each of these periods, interest groups opposed to health insurance fanned broader ideological opposition, identifying a government health insurance program with the enemy regimes of Germany and the Soviet Union. Their framing of the question left a legacy in American conservative thought identifying "socialized medicine" as an evil of a deeply insidious kind.

The failure of national reform in the 1940s allowed the consolidation of employment-based, private insurance and led the earlier advocates of national health insurance to focus instead on hospital insurance for the elderly on Social Security. Here the sequence of development of American social policy was crucial. Unlike other countries, the United States introduced old-age insurance before health insurance, and the success of Social Security then laid the basis for framing a health-care program around the elderly. Moreover, the steady, incremental expansion of Social Security encouraged a misleading analogy that gave false comfort to the visionaries of Medicare who expected it to be the first step on the road to national health insurance.

Social Security was well suited to incremental expansion. The generation that initially entered the program—many of whom had lost their savings during the Depression—received an especially good deal in retirement income, and every time Congress extended the program to cover additional workers, contributors increased faster than recipients, improving the program's finances. Social Security was also entirely compatible with private employer pensions; the program provided a base retirement income, which pensions and individual savings could supplement. This experience suggested health insurance could also follow an incremental path.

But the 1965 legislation establishing Medicare did not create the same favorable conditions for program expansion. Instead of serving as a foundation for national health insurance, Medicare functioned more like a prophylactic against it. The failure to build in cost controls at the inception of the program led many people to conclude that a universal program on Medicare's principles would be fiscally irresponsible. By establishing Medicaid as a separate program, Congress complicated efforts to create a unified financing system. Medicare brought the elderly into the protected public along with those who had employer-provided insurance; the program encouraged seniors to see themselves as having separate group interests that are morally superior to those of the poor on Medicaid. Although the passage of Medicare was not the result of a well-organized lobby for the elderly, it helped to create one. Bringing the privately insured into Medicare would have also posed enormous problems. Most employees who received health insurance as a fringe benefit believed they were getting it virtually for free, and many unionized workers as of the 1960s and 1970s had first-dollar coverage, which Medicare did not provide. Liberals could not pass the taxes for a government program that would have given the privately insured as good a deal as they thought they had. And as Kennedy discovered in 1974, labor leaders resisted a government plan that would give them less than they had won through collective bargaining. Once employment-based insurance and Medicare were established, a large bloc of voters saw little for themselves in a program to cover the remaining uninsured—except for higher taxes. As the repeal of Medicare Catastrophic showed, it even became difficult to raise the floor in Medicare for the elderly.

In short, federal policy toward health insurance exhibited a pattern that was the reverse of Social Security. The incremental health policy measures adopted after World War II—tax benefits for the employed and Medicare for the elderly—blocked a universal public system. When Kennedy and other liberals finally decided in the late 1970s to accept private insurance as a means of achieving universal coverage, it was too late: they were unable to get consensus in the Democratic Party, much less find a negotiating partner among the Republicans.

National health insurance had no route forward except to become a program of comprehensive reform, aiming to control costs as well as to expand coverage. This new phase in thinking, however, created its own distinct tensions. To make universal health insurance into an instrument of cost containment threatened its popular appeal. Health insurance might come to seem less like a moral cause than an argument about economic management. Like some of its advocates, the idea of health care for all had passed from an idealistic youth to a grim maturity.

Still, new opportunities for change might arise. New windows for reform might open. A universal insurance program had actually never had the full commitment and highest priority of presidential leadership. In a best-selling book published in 2009, *The Healing of America,* the journalist T. R. Reid writes, "From Theodore Roosevelt to Barack Obama, half a dozen U.S. presidents have come to office promising 'health care reform' and 'universal coverage' "; Reid then refers to "the Roosevelt, Wilson, Truman, and Nixon reform plans."[30] But this picture is wrong. Teddy Roosevelt never addressed the problem when he was president, and there never was a Roosevelt plan. Wilson never supported health insurance in any form, and there never was a Wilson plan. Harry Truman called for national health insurance in principle but never submitted or endorsed legislation. Nixon was the first to submit legislation, but as a defensive maneuver in 1971 in preparation for his reelection campaign the following year, and then as a desperate move in 1974 when he was trying to save his presidency during Watergate. Carter also only submitted a plan late in his term, in his case to ward off a challenge from Kennedy in the Democratic primaries.

What president was the first to "come to office promising 'health-care reform' " and to propose legislation for "universal coverage"? That would actually be Bill Clinton in 1993.

PART II

FRUSTRATED AMBITIONS, LIBERAL AND CONSERVATIVE

CHAPTER 3

The Shaping of the Clinton Health Plan,
1991–1993

AFTER A DECADE IN THE POLITICAL WILDERNESS, universal health insurance returned to the national agenda in November 1991, just in time to influence the next year's presidential race. The triggering event was a special election for a U.S. Senate seat in Pennsylvania, where the Democratic candidate, Harris Wofford, called for making health care a right and came from 40 points behind to win an upset victory. At the time the country was mired in a recession, and the combination of high unemployment and double-digit increases in health-care costs aggravated worries about health insurance, which Wofford's advisers had argued was becoming a concern even for the middle class. Polls confirmed the potency of the health-care issue, and in the week after he won, the media settled on that explanation for his victory.[1] So began a new season of political opportunity for health-care reform.

The underlying reason for the heightened attention to health insurance was the pressure from rising health-care costs, amplified by the federal clampdown on Medicare payment that led hospitals to shift costs to the privately insured. From 1987 to 1993, private insurance premiums jumped 90 percent, while wages increased only 28 percent, with the result that fewer Americans could afford health coverage.[2] Despite the limited expansion of Medicaid eligibility, the uninsured population rose to 38.6 million in 1992, an increase of 5.2 million from 1989.[3] In response to higher costs, employers cut back health benefits, shifting a larger share of the premium to their workers, reducing the scope of coverage, and introducing more tightly controlled managed-care plans. Neither companies nor workers were happy about the trends: surveys of both business executives and the public at large showed that by wide majorities, they thought that the health-care system needed to be fundamentally reformed or completely rebuilt.[4]

The political reverberations of Wofford's victory and the ensuing media coverage were evident even among long-time opponents of national health insurance. Looking ahead to his reelection campaign, President George H. W. Bush endorsed tax credits to extend coverage. In the Senate, a group of 20 Republicans co-sponsored a bill introduced by John Chafee of Rhode Island that established a right to coverage and made it universal through vouchers for low-income people and an individual mandate—a requirement for individuals to carry insurance. In a striking departure, both the American Medical Association and the Health Insurance Association of America endorsed employer-funded universal coverage. Several other influential groups, including the American Hospital Association, introduced their own proposals for universal coverage. To many observers, health-care reform didn't only seem possible; it had an "aura of inevitability," as George D. Lundberg, the editor of the AMA's *Journal,* put it. In May 1991, all ten of the AMA's scientific journals were devoted to the crisis of health care costs and access, and in a lead editorial Lundberg wrote: "If the Iron Curtain can be lifted, the Warsaw Pact dissolved, and East and West Germany politically reunited, all quite rapidly, because it was the right thing to do and the time had come—surely we in this rich and successful country can manage to provide basic medical care because it too is the right thing to do, and the time has come." Similar sentiments came from the lips of countless public figures at the time.[5]

But as of the early 1990s, the support for reform was missing one critical element: an agreed-upon remedy. While there was a negative consensus that something was wrong with the health-care system, there was no positive consensus about how to fix it.[6] The plethora of proposals signaled wide interest in reform, but not necessarily a readiness to make sacrifices to reach common ground. Even Democrats were a long way from settling on a policy; the disagreements among them were just as great as they had been during the clash between Carter and Kennedy a decade earlier. A substantial faction on the left wing of the party favored a Canadian-style, government-run insurance system (a solution that in the late 1980s had come to be known as "single-payer"), while moderate and conservative Democrats supported cautious, incremental, market-oriented reforms. Between these two groups were many liberals, including leading Senate Democrats, who endorsed a plan called "pay-or-play," which sought to achieve universal coverage through a requirement that employers cover their workers by either "playing" (providing insurance directly) or paying a tax into a public program.

Health care was a prominent but by no means the top issue in the Democratic primaries. The candidate who emerged with the nomination, Bill Clinton, emphasized the economy and talked at least as much about reforming welfare as about reforming health care. During the primaries, he had gathered a group of health policy advisers from Democratic circles in Washington that favored pay-or-play. But during the general election, a second group of advisers gained influence and Clinton decided to shift to a new approach that they favored—a plan for universal coverage based on consumer choice among competing private health plans, operating under a cap on total spending (an approach known, in the shorthand of health policy, as "managed competition within a budget"). Although the media did not recognize its significance at the time, a speech that Clinton gave in September announced his support for a system of universal coverage based on "competition within a budget," and this approach became the framework for the plan that he submitted to Congress the next year.[7]

How that plan took shape has been widely misunderstood. On January 25, 1993, five days after his inauguration, Clinton named his wife to chair a newly established President's Task Force on National Health Care Reform. From that moment, the public had the impression that the president had delegated responsibility for the administration's reform plan to Hillary Clinton and the health care task force. This belief became so firmly established at the time and was so frequently repeated in subsequent years that it is probably impossible to change, but it is not what happened.

Bill Clinton decided on the general design of his health proposal before Hillary became involved, and he never gave up control of the policy-making process in the White House. As a governor and a presidential candidate,

Clinton had developed a detailed knowledge of health policy and firm beliefs about what ought to be done. He saw health-care reform through the prism of economic policy, believed that curbing the long-term growth in health costs was a national imperative, and insisted that even while making coverage universal, health-care reform had to bring down future costs below current projections for both the government and the private economy. Among Clinton's close advisers, Ira Magaziner championed the view that these aims were achievable. When Clinton named Hillary the chair and Magaziner the director of the health-reform effort, their job was not to choose a policy, but to develop the one that the president had already adopted.

Despite all the attention it received, however, the President's Task Force—consisting of members of the cabinet and several other senior officials—proved to be useless for reaching decisions and drafting the plan. It immediately became the subject of litigation and dissolved at the end of May without making any recommendations. The work of developing the plan fell to a small team of advisers and analysts who worked under Magaziner, meeting frequently with both the president and First Lady. Beginning in March and continuing in a stop-and-go fashion until September, the decision meetings about the plan took place outside the structure of the task force, usually in the Roosevelt Room of the White House. Bill Clinton ran these meetings himself; Hillary was present, but there was no question who was in charge. The decisions about the plan were the president's.

My knowledge of this process is first-hand. After advising Wofford during his Senate campaign, I worked briefly with Senator Bob Kerrey of Nebraska, one of Clinton's rivals for the presidential nomination. Magaziner first brought me into the internal discussions of health policy in the Clinton campaign after reading the manuscript of a book I had written, *The Logic of Health-Care Reform*, which developed a plan for universal coverage based on managed competition within a budget. As a senior White House health-policy adviser, I took part in the decision meetings with the president, helped to draft the health plan, and at various times represented the White House in discussions with cabinet departments, members of Congress, and groups outside the government.[8] In the fall of 1993, while remaining a consultant on contract to the White House, I returned to teaching at Princeton, where I revised the paperback edition of *The Logic of*

Health-Care Reform to make it a defense of what had now evolved into the Clinton plan.

So much attention has focused on why reform failed under Clinton that many people fail to ask the prior questions: What led Clinton to make health-care reform a central goal from the first days of his presidency? Why did he turn to a new approach that was unfamiliar to Congress as well as the public? And why did he and so many others, including his opponents, ever think he could succeed?

A New Framework

Wofford's victory and the 1992 presidential race set off intense discussions in political circles and the press about the approach to health-care reform that a new administration and Congress might take. In early 1992 the news media typically presented a menu for reform that had three main alternatives: a Canadian-style, single-payer system, pay-or-play, and the tax-credit approach proposed by President Bush. If a fourth possibility, "managed competition," received attention, it was often confused with conservative, free-market ideas (*managed* competition is, by definition, not a free market). A universal health insurance plan that combined managed competition and a budget cap on health spending was not on the menu at all.

The single-payer model—a unified government insurance plan, at either the federal or the state level—was the latest incarnation of the social-insurance framework that had been the basis of the Wagner-Murray-Dingell bill of the 1940s, Medicare in its original form, and Senator Edward M. Kennedy's Health Security Act circa 1970. The traditional base of support for a government program to replace private insurance had waned: Kennedy and the unions had given up on that approach in 1979 and by the early 1990s were supporting pay-or-play. But single-payer had new support from other progressives, particularly because of the attention given to Canada's health insurance system.

To many people, the experiences of Canada and the United States over the two previous decades seemed like a natural experiment. As of 1970, both countries devoted 7 percent of GDP to health care. Then, in 1971, Canada established a single-payer system (operated separately by each of its provinces), while the United States did not enact any program for universal coverage. By 1990, though the United States left 38 million uninsured, it was spending more on health care than Canada—11.9 percent of GDP compared with 9 percent. A study showing administrative costs to be sharply higher in the United States than in Canada had a particularly telling impact. According to one estimate, Canada's lower costs were due in roughly equal proportions to reduced bureaucratic overhead, lower physician fees, and lower hospital costs. The Canadian system imposed "global budgets" on hospitals and physicians, forcing them to keep their spending and fees within annual budget caps. Single-payer advocates argued that these caps enabled Canada to avoid regulating individual doctors' decisions; as one metaphor had it, while America tried to put a leash on every cow in the pasture, Canada just put up a fence. Single-payer advocates also pointed out that Canadians retained free choice of doctors, whereas many Americans in managed-care plans did not.[9]

Democratic leaders in Congress were unwilling, however, to go back to a position that had been decisively defeated before. Single-payer faced the unified opposition of all the major health-care interest groups, and it required a steep increase in taxes to pay for the health care of everyone under age 65, not just the uninsured. To be sure, the taxes would replace private insurance premiums, but most insured Americans did not see the share of premiums paid by their employers. Single-payer supporters could argue that the overall costs of health care would be cheaper, but to those with employer-provided insurance, it would not appear that way. Many employer health plans also had benefits that were broader than Medicare or Medicaid, the two government health programs Americans could look to as examples. From the standpoint of the protected public, therefore, single-payer could appear to threaten higher taxes for worse coverage. And, not without reason, many Americans were skeptical that the government could run one-seventh of the economy.

The second option, pay-or-play, attempted to circumvent the opposition to single-payer by giving employers and unions the option of keeping the private insurance they had established or negotiated. But pay-or-play posed difficulties of its own. Individual consumers would have no choice about whether to enroll in the government program or a private plan; under pay-

or-play, that decision belonged to employers, potentially raising fears among many of the privately insured that their employers would dump them into an inferior public program like Medicaid. In fact, there was reason to be concerned. While firms with relatively healthy workers and higher wages would buy private insurance directly, the government program would attract employers with older and less healthy workers and lower wages. Burdened with the most expensive people to insure, the public program would appear to be costly and inefficient and, like Medicaid, face pressures to keep down its expenses, perhaps paying doctors so little as to make it difficult for enroll-ees to find a physician. According to estimates at the time, employers par-ticipating in the public program would have to pay a tax of 7 percent to 9 percent of wages. For many congressional Democrats, that provision alone was a deal-breaker.

The third option, introduced by the Bush administration as the presi-dent's reelection campaign got under way, called for a new program of tax credits for low-income individuals and families to buy private insurance. The administration proposed overriding all state requirements for specific benefits in health insurance and called upon the states to develop a "basic" package to be purchased with the tax credits. The program did not take on the larger problem of health-care costs. And to avoid endorsing a tax in-crease in an election year, the administration did not propose any way to finance the new tax credits.[10]

Among Democrats, the objections to each of these alternatives opened the door to a different strategy. In an influential pair of articles with Rich-ard Kronick, Alain Enthoven had reworked the consumer-choice, managed-competition proposal that he had developed originally as an option for national health insurance in the late 1970s, and as the 1992 election ap-proached, Enthoven was collaborating with a group based in Jackson Hole, Wyoming, on a revised proposal for managed competition.[11] The central thrust of these ideas was to create a system of universal coverage in which consumers would make informed, cost-conscious choices among alter-native health plans with population-based budgets. Although presented as a way to stimulate market forces, managed competition required a great deal of new regulation. The proposals called for an employer mandate, though of a particular kind: the required employer contributions could be excluded from taxable income only up to the premium of the lowest-cost plan in a region. With the employer share set at a flat, fixed-dollar amount, consumers would have to use their own after-tax dollars to pay the extra cost if they preferred a more expensive plan.

Many people misinterpreted "managed competition" to mean "competition among managed-care plans." But managed competition describes a framework of choice among health plans, not all of which need be managed care. As a modifier of "competition," "managed" refers to a way of structuring the market for insurance so as to discourage insurers from trying to exclude people likely to need care. Insurers would be required to offer open enrollment and standardized benefit packages and to set premiums without respect to an applicant's health or claims experience. The total premium payments that the plans received, however, would be risk-adjusted—that is, they would receive more money for a higher-risk population and less for a healthier one. A "sponsor"—a large employer, a public agency, or a "health insurance purchasing cooperative" acting on behalf of small and medium-size firms—would do the managing of the competition. The sponsor, not individual insurers, would enroll consumers in plans and provide comparative information about costs and quality of care. Regular measurement of consumer satisfaction and health outcomes would help people make informed choices during open-enrollment season. The Jackson Hole proposal introduced the term "accountable health partnership" to describe an integrated medical system that agreed to be held accountable for its performance on the basis of regular monitoring of its service.

The managed-competition approach had some clear advantages as a strategy for introducing restraint on health-care spending. Other efforts to confront consumers with the costs of their decisions, such as increased patient cost-sharing, typically focused on decisions at the point of treatment, when people are often in no condition to compare the quality and price of different doctors and hospitals (information that, in any case, is usually unavailable). Managed competition focused instead on decisions at the point of enrollment, when consumers can evaluate alternatives. Moreover, the approach recognized that the critical decisions affecting costs are in the hands of physicians and other providers. The real aim of managed competition was to force the providers to work together in integrated health plans to deliver "value for money." Many people worried that HMOs and other managed-care plans had an incentive to deny necessary care. The purpose of regular monitoring of the quality of care and consumer satisfaction was to counteract that incentive and provide feedback to both consumers and professionals about how well the plans were performing.

Nonetheless, managed competition had some serious limitations. The integrated health plans that were central to the vision did not exist in many parts of the United States. Although the plans could be developed in metropolitan areas, it would take years to build them, and it was unrealistic to expect competing, integrated health plans to emerge in rural areas and small towns. The competitive vision could also not readily be applied to low-income communities that had few providers. Holding plans accountable for performance was an attractive idea, but the measures of accountability were also still to be developed. And though HMOs had demonstrated savings, managed competition was still a theory. The approach required changes in the tax code and many other laws and had not yet been put to a test in the United States or anywhere else. Whether managed competition would control health costs in practice was therefore still open to debate.

But perhaps it was not necessary to rely entirely on the competitive mechanism to control costs. Other western democracies set budgets for health spending, an idea adopted by single-payer proposals in the United States. The concept of a budget limit, however, did not require that there be only a single payer. Kennedy's 1979 proposal for universal coverage with private health insurance included a budget limit for the plans. In 1991 Senator Bob Kerrey of Nebraska introduced a plan for universal coverage that had an overall budget for health spending and gave consumers a choice between a government insurance program (the direct antecedent of what later came to be called the "public option") and private alternatives. The Catholic Health Association also had a proposal for competing private insurance plans under an overall government limit on spending. All these proposals, however, allowed for competition only on quality, not on price.

In February 1992, just as the 1992 presidential race was heating up, California's insurance commissioner, John Garamendi, introduced a proposal that had elements of both single-payer and managed competition. Under the Garamendi proposal—developed largely by his deputy Walter

Zelman—consumers would obtain insurance not through their employers, but through a regional "health insurance purchasing corporation" set up by the state. (Because it was a state proposal, the Garamendi plan did not cover people eligible for Medicare, Medicaid, or other federal programs.) The HIPC would contract with HMOs and other managed-care plans as well as one traditional fee-for-service plan and would manage the competition among them, ensuring open enrollment, standardized benefit packages, no discrimination against people with pre-existing conditions, and risk-adjusted payment to the plans. Garamendi proposed to finance coverage with a state payroll tax, which would pay the full premium for the two lowest-cost plans, leaving consumers to pay the difference for plans with higher premiums. The Garamendi plan resembled single-payer in that the revenue for health insurance came primarily from a payroll tax and all of it would go into one pot; the pooling of risk would therefore be community wide. But because the proposal would offer consumers a menu of private plans at different prices, it would force the plans and providers to worry about losing subscribers to more appealing alternatives. And because all the funds for insurance passed through the HIPC, it could serve as a means of regulating total spending for health coverage.[12]

The Garamendi plan helped to crystallize the idea that there might be practical and political advantages from combining elements of models for reform usually thought to be incompatible. While a regional purchasing cooperative serving all consumers was a "sponsor" of managed competition, it was also, in effect, a single payer of plans and therefore potentially had other means of controlling costs. With its enormous buying power, a regional purchasing cooperative could exert countervailing power in bargaining with health plans over their premiums. It could "cap through capitation"—control health spending by limiting the per capita payments to plans. Global budgeting in other countries typically involves separate budgets for hospitals and physicians; the HIPC's payments to health plans could, in effect, set a more comprehensive budget, giving health plans flexibility to shift resources between inpatient and ambulatory care. The HIPC also had the advantage of breaking the linkage of health insurance to employment. Under the existing system, most consumers were limited to the plan or plans offered by their employer instead of being able to choose among the full range of alternatives in their area. The HIPC could give them more choices, and it would enable employees of small companies and those who bought insurance individually to get the benefits of large-scale purchasing enjoyed by the employees of large firms.[13]

The concept of a budget cap is different from "all-payer rate regulation," that is, setting uniform prices for each of the services performed by doctors, hospitals, and other providers. A budget cap sets a ceiling on expenditures rather than trying to specify prices for all the individual services paid for under that ceiling. The cap could be conceived in different ways. In the Garamendi plan, the payroll-tax revenue that paid the premiums of the two lowest-cost plans was one kind of budget cap. A statewide purchasing cooperative could also set an allowable rate of increase for the average premium of all plans and deny rate increases that would break that cap. In short, depending on how it was conceived, the budget cap could be more or less stringent.

Out of these ideas emerged the outlines of a national proposal for universal coverage based on managed competition within a budget. Consumers would choose among private health plans offered through a regional purchasing cooperative. All the plans would offer standard benefit packages at community rates (along with separately priced supplemental policies). Money would flow into the cooperatives from employers and employees, from other people according to their ability to pay, and from government. Money would flow out to the health plans according to the numbers who enrolled and the actuarial risk they represented. Employers would contribute a fixed amount, say, 75 percent or 80 percent of the lowest- or next-to-lowest-cost plan, with the federal government subsidizing contributions from small employers so as to limit their costs to a fixed percentage of payroll. The government would also subsidize low-income people, limiting their premiums and out-of-pocket costs.

The federal government would establish a right to affordable health care, provide much of the financing, and set a limit to the rate of growth of expenditures through the purchasing cooperatives. The budget cap would serve as a fail-safe mechanism in case other restraints on spending proved inadequate. The states could carry out the program in substantially different ways. The price-and-quality competition envisioned by Enthoven might be sufficient to contain costs in metropolitan areas with numerous health plans. In other areas where competition was limited, the purchasing cooperative could hold down costs by using its countervailing power. In rural states, the most effective policy might be for the cooperative to act as a single-payer. Such decisions could be left to the states. A series of papers in 1992 tried to work through the countless issues this hybrid approach raised.[14]

Clinton's Decisions

Political observers often dismiss the positions that candidates take during campaigns as mere posturing, but the 1992 presidential campaign had a critical influence on the policies the winner followed once in office. Before the New Hampshire primary in February, Clinton issued a white paper setting out an ambitious agenda for health reform: universal coverage with a guaranteed benefit package, employment-based financing, cost containment in part through global budgeting, the use of health networks as an option for providing services, an emphasis on preventive and primary care, and expanded support of long-term care emphasizing care in the home. All these elements would be incorporated into the legislation Clinton proposed to Congress in 1993. The white paper, however, said employers would have a play-or-pay choice to cover their workers or pay into a public program, and that proposal did not survive.[15]

Once Clinton turned to the general election, his early support of pay-or-play became a source of concern to his political advisers, who worried that Republicans were going to attack him for endorsing a plan with a 9 percent payroll tax that could be a back door to a government-controlled health system. Some on Clinton's campaign staff argued that he didn't need to discuss health policy in any greater detail. Polls indicated that voters overwhelmingly preferred him to Bush on health care and trusted Democrats more than Republicans on the issue. Clinton nonetheless authorized Ira Magaziner, who had worked on Clinton's campaign manifesto, *Putting People First,* to explore whether a managed-competition approach could serve as an alternative to pay-or-play, and in August a meeting in Washington brought together Clinton's original health policy advisers with a group assembled by Magaziner to support managed competition under a budget. The second approach appeared to have two distinct political advantages: The financing could rely on employer-paid premiums rather than a payroll tax, and managed competition was a better fit with Clinton's general appeal as a New Democrat willing to break with liberal orthodoxy. A reform plan that combined the security of universal, comprehensive coverage with consumer choice and competition in the delivery of services was, in a sense, the logical byproduct of Clinton's efforts to create a political coalition that could span the ideological differences within the Democratic Party.

A fragile consensus in favor of a half-turn toward managed competition emerged from the August meeting. The next month, a small delegation presented that option to Clinton on the campaign trail in East Lansing, Michigan, and on September 24, in a speech in New Jersey and an accompanying press release from Little Rock, Clinton called for universal health coverage "privately provided, publicly guaranteed" under a system of "competition within a budget."[16]

Clinton's embrace of competition may not have had any effect on the election; most reporters didn't register that he had made a shift, and Bush's campaign never aired television spots that it prepared on health care, apparently concluding that they would only highlight an issue on which Bush did not enjoy public trust. Yet Clinton's September turn did matter a great deal after the election because it guided work on the proposal to Congress that he introduced almost exactly one year later.

Clinton's adoption of a framework for reform did not resolve whether he would make health care a top priority and, if he did, how he might go about it. As president-elect, he revised his priorities in light of higher deficit forecasts that fall, the vote for third-party presidential candidate Ross Perot (whose campaign focused on the deficit), and the counsel he received from his economic advisers. Retrenching on an economic stimulus and eventually abandoning his promise of a middle-class tax cut, Clinton opted for deficit reduction in the hope that it would lead to lower interest rates and stronger growth. Another Democratic president cut in Carter's mold might at that point have also walked back his campaign promises of health-care reform. But the higher deficit forecasts highlighted how critical it was to control the cost of health care. If health costs kept gobbling up revenue, they would make long-term deficit reduction impossible and sharply circumscribe what the new administration could accomplish in other areas. Comprehensive health-care reform therefore held more than one attraction. If reform contained health costs, it would contribute to the success of Clinton's economic program. And at a time when he was downgrading other progressive commitments, a high-profile commitment to universal health insurance could bolster his popular support, particularly among Democrats.

A remark that Clinton made at the beginning of an internal White House meeting some months later may shed light on his thinking. In 1936, Clinton ruminated, the Depression had not ended, but Franklin D. Roosevelt won reelection because he had passed Social Security and other measures. Perhaps health security could do the same for him in 1996 even if his economic program did not bring results by then. He referred to both health-care reform and his economic programs as "gambles" but said he was comfortable with the odds on both of them, and he could win if either one paid off. As it happened, he was right, though it wasn't his gamble on health care that proved to be the winner.

In his first days in office, Clinton had good reason to make health-care reform an immediate goal of his presidency and to keep direct control over the reform effort. There appeared to be exceptional political forces aligned in support of reform and strong pressures to move quickly, and those considerations argued for an accelerated timetable. Originally, the president asked for a reform plan to be ready within the first 100 days.

Yet the kind of reform that Clinton believed necessary was alien to the Washington health bureaucracy and unfamiliar to members of his own cabinet. Ironically, the same concern that would motivate so much of the opposition—distrust of the federal bureaucracy—probably also influenced the president's decisions to locate policy development in the White House and to put his wife and Magaziner, an old and trusted friend, in charge. Internal conflicts over the health plan, particularly with top officials at Health and Human Services and the Treasury, would become a consuming preoccupation inside the White House. It was partly these tensions that led to persistent and damaging leaks and the appearance of disarray in the reform effort and to the countervailing efforts to maintain confidentiality and discipline that the critics of Hillary Clinton mistakenly attributed to her allegedly controlling and rigid personality.

Hillary's appointment underscored the president's personal commitment. Although she made no claim at that time to being a health policy expert, she had successfully led a similar effort to develop educational policy in Arkansas, and her gifts complemented Magaziner's. Besides her quick intelligence, she had the personal tact and ease in communicating with the public that would make her an ideal ambassador for the initiative, while Magaziner had the organizational skills, command of detail, and imaginative boldness necessary for mastering an ambitious and complex reform.

The overall direction of policy was not Hillary's choice. She had not been present at the key meetings during the campaign when Clinton had discussed health policy with his advisers, and in the first days in the White House, she was just familiarizing herself with "my husband's plan" (as she referred to it in a meeting I had with her about a week after the inauguration). Whether she fully agreed with that approach wasn't clear. But if she had her reservations, she put them aside and, believing strongly in the aims of reform, worked hard to achieve them. Even though her husband had defined the broad outline of the plan, hundreds of important questions still had to be resolved to turn it into legislation.

But the troubles of the President's Task Force began immediately. Before making the announcement, the White House had not thought to check with legal counsel about the implications of formally designating a "task force," and soon it was facing lawsuits challenging the First Lady's role and demanding that the meetings be public. Under the task force, Magaziner organized some 30 "working groups" concerned with such issues as the design of the purchasing cooperatives. The membership of the working groups quickly rose to more than 500—mostly federal employees, many of them added at the request of their departments, as well as some independent experts, congressional staff (Democrats only), and state health-care officials (Republican as well as Democrat). Their function was only to gather information and to set out options, and they dispersed early in the spring before the plan was written. But the media thought they were actually drafting the president's proposal, and the decision by the White House to exclude the press as well as health-care interest groups created a storm of indignation that the task force was meeting secretly behind closed doors. Normally, presidents consult advisers in private without incurring any criticism. No one would have complained about secrecy if the White House had simply prepared a bill the usual way—entirely behind closed doors, without any formal external participation. The irony was that the very effort to include so many people produced a sense of exclusion among those left out. But the real mistake was creating the task force and working groups in the first place and putting them in the vortex of publicity that the First Lady's appointment guaranteed.

Critics would later say that the task force was so unwieldy that it couldn't meet its deadlines, that the White House should never have developed a proposal but rather left it to Congress, and that it was a mistake to turn over the development of the health proposal to policy wonks instead of politically experienced advisers.

The task force was certainly a public relations fiasco, but the delay in finalizing the White House plan resulted from developments in Congress that were beyond the administration's control. The main impetus for trying to draft the plan in 100 days was to allow it to be incorporated into the budget reconciliation bill, which under Senate rules can pass with a bare majority, not the 60 votes otherwise necessary to shut off debate. But the Senate's Byrd rule limits reconciliation to budget-relevant matters, and when Senator Robert Byrd himself, the guardian of Senate tradition, said in March that the health plan was too far-reaching to be incorporated into reconciliation, the White House had no choice but to delay submission of its health legislation until after the budget passed. During the spring, the president suspended even the internal White House decision-making about the health plan, lest leaks disturb congressional budget negotiations. Winning the budget battle proved more difficult and took far longer than anyone expected. The reconciliation bill was finally adopted on August 6 without a single Republican vote, passing the Senate only because of Vice President Al Gore's tie-breaker. Clinton addressed Congress about the health plan the next month.

The decision to write a bill in the White House was also a response to congressional realities. During the previous two years, neither the House nor the Senate had been able to make progress on a health reform bill, even one that would merely have drawn a veto from President Bush and served as an election issue. While George Mitchell, the Senate Majority Leader, had supported pay-or-play, he was unable to get any proposal with an employer mandate through the Senate Finance Committee. In the House, Speaker Tom Foley had little power over his caucus, and each committee was a fiefdom all its own. Dan Rostenkowski, chair of Ways and Means, told Clinton that the White House had to come up with a health bill to get Congress to act.[17]

The notion that Clinton made a mistake in delegating responsibility for his health plan to policy wonks might be correct if he had actually delegated responsibility. But the president worked through the policy step by step in Roosevelt Room meetings often lasting two hours or more, and Magaziner was continually in touch with both of the Clintons to decide important issues. The political thinking behind the decisions did not work out, but that is not to say the president made the policy with no eye to politics in the first place.

Clinton's original decision to embrace managed competition was an effort to skirt the political problems of pay-or-play, especially a steep payroll tax, and he continued to be determined that his health plan avoid any general tax increase, though it did include a 75-cent-a-pack hike in cigarette taxes. Yet for political as much as policy reasons he was also determined that health-care reform reduce the deficit over the long term. It would be no easy feat to achieve universal coverage while reducing the deficit without any general tax increase. The president's various decisions about the health plan stemmed from an effort to achieve all three of these seemingly contrary political objectives and from a recognition that he would have to adjust the balance among them as he moved from building public support to getting legislation through Congress.

Some aspects of the Clinton plan were assumed from the start and never seriously in doubt. The plan would create an entitlement to a standard level of health insurance for all citizens and legal residents, but not for unlawful immigrants. Consumers would acquire that insurance through purchasing cooperatives, soon renamed "regional health alliances" at the instigation of political advisers who thought that the term "cooperative" sounded too leftist. The alliances would be required to offer at least three kinds of options—traditional, fee-for-service insurance as well as health maintenance organizations and preferred provider plans. (Because fee-for-service was being killed in the market by adverse selection, it would have actually been more likely to survive as a result of the risk-adjustment process in the alliances.) Benefits, co-pays, and other features would be standardized so as to make it easier for consumers to compare prices. Health plans would have to offer coverage to everyone without exclusions of pre-existing conditions, and they would be paid according to the actuarial risk of the population they enrolled. The poor, including those currently receiving acute-care services under Medicaid, would receive subsidies for mainstream coverage through the alliances. Medicare, however, would remain a separate program, and the elderly would receive prescription-drug coverage through Medicare for the first time. States would have the option of creating a single-payer system for the population below age 65.

At the first decision meeting in the Roosevelt Room, Clinton made it clear that, as a former governor, he wanted the states to carry out the reforms. The federal government would set the overall rules, but the states would set up the regional alliances and decide how they would be governed. The decision to give the states control of the alliances meant that reform could not move forward until the states enacted complementary laws and set up the alliances. As a result, the plan would take several years to implement, with a projected phase-in between 1996 and 1998.

The most divisive issues within the White House had to do with the scale of the program and its financing. Health insurance plans range from minimal, barebones insurance to inclusive, first-dollar coverage. Some economic advisers, particularly Robert Rubin, the chair of the National Economic Council, leaned toward a less generous, catastrophic package, while the health-policy team favored a more comprehensive one. The argument for the more comprehensive approach was both political and policy-minded. It would be nearly impossible to rally support for a barebones package; people with good insurance would see it as a threat to the coverage they had, even if it was intended as a floor. The barebones approach would also leave much of the inequality in access to care that health-care reform was supposed to overcome. Those who could afford supplementary coverage would buy it (as many Medicare beneficiaries did) to reduce or eliminate cost-sharing, increasing their use of services and raising the costs of the basic package. Managed competition was aimed at controlling costs a different way; it called for a broad, uniform benefit package and sought to generate price competition among health plans in delivering that package. These arguments implied broad, though not all-inclusive, benefits, and in its final form, the Clinton plan called for a standard benefit package that fell just above the median—slightly more generous than average, but not as generous as the package typically provided by large employers. Moreover, much of the cost of the proposals under consideration lay in the benefits for the elderly and disabled, including a new long-term care program as well as Medicare prescription-drug coverage. Cutting the benefits for the population under age 65 didn't actually have as much impact on projected public spending as many of the economic advisers originally thought.[18]

The president also had to resolve a series of difficult questions about the financing of those benefits. Despite his rejection of a payroll tax during the campaign, that option emerged again within the White House as one of several alternatives. A payroll tax had the advantage of clarity and simplicity; it could be set at a level that would raise enough funds to pay for a low-cost plan, leaving consumers to pay any extra amount for more expensive options. The alternative was a "capped premium," an option that business representatives preferred in negotiations with the White House, though the battle over "payroll versus premium" dragged out for months.[19] Under the final plan, an employer would be required to pay 80 percent of the average premium in an alliance, except that the employer's actual cost would be capped as a percentage of payroll. The cap would be 3.5 percent of wages for firms with average annual wages under $12,000 and fewer than 25 workers, rising in stages through a graduated scale to 7.9 percent for larger firms with higher average wages. The federal government would subsidize the purchasing alliances to the extent that the caps on employer contributions limited the funds to pay for coverage. As a little reflection will show, the capped premium had much the same incidence as a payroll tax graduated according to firm size and average wages, but the capped premium had the singular advantage of being called a premium rather than a tax. Unfortunately for the administration, however, when the plan was made public, the caps might as well have been treated as classified information. What employers and the public learned was that the employer share was 80 percent of the premium. Small businesses would have paid far less. In fact, all employers, even large ones, would have paid only about 57 percent of the premium for family coverage (80 percent divided by the number of workers per household in a region, which nationally averaged 1.4).

An additional wrinkle affected the share that consumers would pay. If employer payments covered 80 percent of premium, wouldn't consumers pay 20 percent of their insurance plan? Not exactly. Employers' total contributions would cover 80 percent of the *average* plan. The consumers' premium would depend on the *specific* plan they chose. Suppose, for argument's sake, the average premium in an alliance was $100 a month. A consumer who chose a low-cost plan costing $80 would pay nothing. A consumer who chose a high-cost plan costing $120 would pay $40, or one-third of the premium. This was the basic mechanism for generating price competition. Advocates of managed competition wanted the federal government to limit the tax exclusion of employer contributions to the premium of the low-cost plan ($80 in our example), so that consumers would have to pay the full freight for a more expensive option. Provisions to limit the tax exclusion were in early drafts of the Clinton plan, but the president decided against that approach (though the *New York Times* and other newspapers mistakenly reported the contrary, causing friction between the president and the labor movement).

Another set of questions concerned the scope and power of the purchasing alliances. The alliances could be set up with the limited purpose of enabling people who bought insurance individually or through small firms to acquire insurance coverage on the same terms as large employers. Alternatively, the alliances could have the more ambitious goal of pooling risk on a community-wide basis, breaking the linkage of health insurance to jobs, and serving as a way to budget health expenditures. The latter course would make possible a comprehensive system of cost containment, which had been Clinton's aim from the beginning. For example, Congress could set an allowable rate of increase in the average insurance premium in the alliances, indexing that rate to the growth rate of the economy. Clinton decided in favor of broad alliances capable of setting limits on health costs.

Initially, the advocates of managed competition within a budget had thought of the budget as a back-up mechanism, to go into effect only when and where competition proved inadequate. But the White House was concerned about how the Congressional Budget Office would "score" its proposal—that is, the impact that CBO would forecast on both federal costs and overall health expenditures. And because CBO would not credit managed competition with substantial savings, the White House found itself under pressure to tighten up the regulatory features of its proposal, including the budget cap. As a result, the final plan emphasized top-down regulation far more than its proponents originally expected or wanted. But the goal of long-run deficit reduction was so central to Clinton's vision for reform that he accepted that shift. And, in any event, Magaziner and the Clintons expected that Congress in the end would scale back both the generosity of the program and the regulations.[20]

The initial release of the health plan in early September 1993 was not planned, and it is hard to imagine how it could have been handled more ineptly. In early September, while being briefed by Hillary Clinton, Rep. Pete Stark demanded to see the president's proposal. Since Stark chaired the health subcommittee of Ways and Means, the First Lady agreed. But the White House did not yet have a final bill or a lucid exposition of it. Instead, it sent a technical outline of the plan, listing each of its detailed provisions, but without any overall explanation of the framework or the rationale. Soon fax machines were relaying copies in all directions, and the Clinton health plan was published in what seemed to be numbing complexity. When architects release plans for a building, they ordinarily present an artist's rendering or a physical model to the public. The Clinton White House released its health plan in the form of engineering specifications.[21] The impression that the proposal was impossibly complicated was firmly established at that moment.

Nonetheless, all the many missteps of the administration seemed to recede in importance when President Clinton introduced his health plan to the nation in a speech to a joint session of Congress on September 22,

1993. The president began by highlighting the problems that had driven the reform effort:

> Millions of Americans are just a pink slip away from losing their health insurance and one serious illness away from losing all their savings. Millions more are locked into the jobs they have now just because they or someone in their family has once been sick and they have what is called the preexisting condition. And on any given day, over 37 million Americans, most of them working people and their little children, have no health insurance at all.
>
> And in spite of all this, our medical bills are growing at over twice the rate of inflation, and the United States spends over a third more of its income on health care than any other nation on Earth. And the gap is growing . . .

At the heart of the speech was the president's presentation of six central principles of reform, beginning with security, and its most memorable moment came when he held up a Health Security card:

> Under our plan, every American would receive a health care security card that will guarantee a comprehensive package of benefits over the course of an entire lifetime, roughly comparable to the benefit package offered by most Fortune 500 companies. This health care security card will offer this package of benefits in a way that can never be taken away. So let us agree on this: Whatever else we disagree on, before this Congress finishes its work next year, you will pass and I will sign legislation to guarantee this security to every citizen of this country.
>
> With this card, if you lose your job or you switch jobs, you're covered. If you leave your job to start a small business, you're covered. If you're an early retiree, you're covered. If someone in your family has unfortunately had an illness that qualifies as a preexisting condition, you're still covered. If you get sick or a member of your family gets sick, even if it's a life-threatening illness, you're covered. And if an insurance company tries to drop you for any reason, you will still be covered, because that will be illegal. This card will give comprehensive coverage. It will cover people for hospital care, doctor visits, emergency and lab services, diagnostic services like Pap smears and mammograms and cholesterol tests, substance abuse, and mental health treatment.

If many people did not realize that Clinton was proposing a system that relied on private insurers, they could be forgiven since he alluded to that aspect of the proposal only indirectly. And in the coda to the speech, he compared the effort to pass Health Security to the establishment of Social Security, which he framed as Franklin Roosevelt had, as a step toward freedom—that is, freedom from fear:

> . . . now it is our turn to strike a blow for freedom in this country, the freedom of Americans to live without fear that their own Nation's health care system won't be there for them when they need it. It's hard to believe that there was once a time in this century when that kind of fear gripped old age, when retirement was nearly synonymous with poverty and older Americans died in the street. That's unthinkable today, because over a half a century ago Americans had the courage to change, to create a Social Security System that ensures that no Americans will be forgotten in their later years.
>
> Forty years from now, our grandchildren will also find it unthinkable that there was a time in this country when hardworking families lost their homes, their savings, their businesses, lost everything simply because their children got sick or because they had to change jobs. Our grandchildren will find such things unthinkable tomorrow if we have the courage to change today.

It was a powerful speech, and the initial reception was overwhelmingly positive. The same political analysts who would later say Clinton was a fool to have ever proposed universal coverage were ecstatic when he proposed it. Early polls showed huge margins in support of the president's health plan.

Strangely, however, Clinton's address included little about the plan he was proposing. The speech did have a few lines about how the plan would be paid for, emphasizing that employers would be required to contribute to health coverage. But there was nothing about how consumers would choose a plan or any of the other arrangements. On the morning of the speech, Clinton recognized there was too little specifically about the health plan, and at his instruction, I was brought in that afternoon to work on revisions with the principal speech-writers, Paul Begala and Jeremy Rosner. But even if I had anticipated the problems with the speech (which I did not), it was too late to make big changes; the final text stuck to broad principles and never explained how the proposal would work. Still, watching from the gallery of the House, I was thrilled with the speech, and later that evening at the White House I asked the president to sign one of the Health Security cards that had been made up for the occasion. He did sign it on the back where the cardholder's signature would ordinarily go, but I should have known that evening something was about to go wrong. The president had signed the card upside down.

CHAPTER 4

Getting to No, 1994

NO PRESIDENT BEFORE BILL CLINTON HAD risked so much on health-care reform. Franklin Roosevelt put off proposing national health insurance because he wasn't willing to take the political risk it entailed; Harry Truman endorsed the principle but never submitted legislation, knowing it was certain to be defeated. Richard Nixon and Jimmy Carter backed into proposals defensively. Clinton made health-care reform a central commitment immediately on becoming president, and he put his personal signature on the issue by developing a bill in the White House. His wife's role in the process raised the ante. Even as difficulties emerged, the president doubled-down on his gamble when in his State of the Union Address in January 1994 he told members of Congress he would veto any legislation that fell short of universal coverage.

No wonder, then, that the collapse of health-care reform is usually told as a failure of Bill and Hillary Clinton (and their advisers), which it certainly was. But that is not the whole story. The defeat of reform was also a result of deals that were never closed, of compromises never reached, of backpedaling by Republicans, moderate Democrats, and key interest groups that abandoned proposals they had earlier endorsed. All those alternatives, including a series of consensus-building efforts in Congress, also died. The historical question is as much why the center failed as why Clinton did and why Republicans decided their interest lay in defeating a Democratic president rather than in compromising with him. "We've killed health care reform," Senator Bob Packwood told his Republican colleagues in September 1994. "Now we've got to make sure our fingerprints are not on it."[1] The Republicans enjoyed a double triumph, not just killing reform but watching the jurors find the president guilty. It was the political equivalent of the perfect crime.

At the beginning of Clinton's presidency, many observers thought health-care reform was unstoppable. Rising health-care costs and deteriorating coverage seemed to create overwhelming pressures on the government to act. Proposals for reform came from influential business organizations as well as health-care interest groups that had generally opposed national health insurance. So wide was the support for health reform that many in Congress and the new administration were confident they could find a basis for compromise.

But that reading of the situation turned out to be wrong. No economic imperative compelled action by the government; no political imperative forced the supporters of competing visions of reform to resolve their differences. None of the strategies devised by Clinton or congressional leaders could bridge the fissures among Democratic factions, moderate Republicans, and influential interest groups, especially on such critical issues as financing. While the supporters of reform fought over alternatives, the opponents took advantage of delay and confusion and, seeing the issue as a decisive ideological test, turned business groups, elite opinion, and a large part of the public from embracing change to rejecting it.

The Democrats' Disorder

The conflicts over health reform that split the Democrats before the 1992 election spilled over into the Clinton administration and the new Congress. On the left, progressive Democrats continued to favor a single-payer system or the opening of a new Medicare option to the under-65 population, while on the party's right flank, a group of conservatives adopted the model of managed competition proposed by Enthoven and the Jackson Hole Group. The hybrid approach that Clinton had adopted during the campaign was neither widely shared nor even well understood in his own party. Wary of a comprehensive program of any kind, some influential Democrats in both Congress and Clinton's own cabinet favored only limited insurance-market reforms and a modest expansion of access. Constant in-fighting among these factions resulted in hostile leaks to the press from inside the administration and Congress, disparaging comments about the feasibility of different options or the integrity of cost estimates, and the proliferation of options until not even the policy experts could keep them straight. The in-fighting helped mightily to confuse the public and slow the momentum of reform.

The Clinton health plan had a doubly reinforced method of cost containment: stronger incentives for consumers and health-care providers to make cost-conscious choices, plus a cap on expenditure growth, which took the form of a limit on increases in the average premium in the purchasing alliances. The general idea of "competition within a budget" was to combine market and regulatory approaches to attract support from conservatives and liberals.

But the synthesis was also doubly heretical. Any reliance on private health insurance was heresy to many on the left and to some in the Democratic health-policy establishment. Any regulation of health insurance rates was heresy to advocates of managed competition. The rise of managed care had produced a deep rift among Democrats. Those who favored the Clinton plan or pure managed competition accepted HMOs and other forms of managed care as a positive force or a necessary evil to carry out systemic reforms, control costs, and make universal coverage affordable. But many progressives saw single-payer as a way of avoiding managed care and regarded the Clinton plan as totally unacceptable.

The splintering of views about health care was evident among Democrats in both houses of Congress. The main bastion of progressive strength was in the House, where Rep. Martin Russo had introduced a single-payer bill calling for a federal insurance program to provide comprehensive coverage with no out-of-pocket payments, to be paid for through increased payroll and income taxes. According to CBO estimates, the bill would increase the demand for health care significantly, but total national health expenditures, public and private, would remain about the same because of administrative savings.[2] Another proposal from the left, introduced by Rep. Stark, called for the expansion of Medicaid to cover more low-income people and the establishment of a new, premium-financed Part C in Medicare for the under-65 population.[3] This was a version of play-or-pay: employers could either "play" by providing private insurance for their workers or pay a share of the premiums for the new Medicare program. Both the Russo and Stark bills included federal controls on health expenditures.

The House also included a significant number of conservative Democrats, members of the Conservative Democratic Forum, who lined up behind a managed-competition bill introduced by Rep. Jim Cooper of Tennessee. Although Cooper himself was just fifteenth in seniority on the critical Energy and Commerce Committee, his bill served as a rallying point for center-right critics of the Clinton plan and played an outsized role in both the congressional battle and the national debate over health reform.

The Cooper plan was based on the Jackson Hole framework for managed competition with two crucial omissions: it did not include an employer mandate or an individual mandate and consequently did not provide for universal coverage. While these omissions may have suggested that Cooper's proposal was minimalist, it would have radically reshaped health insurance. Like the Jackson Hole proposal, the Cooper bill called for a National Health Board to supervise the health insurance market and establish a uniform benefit package, uniform deductibles and cost-sharing, and criteria for accountable health plans. States would set up "regional health purchasing cooperatives" to enable individuals and employers with up to 100 workers to buy insurance on better terms, and the tax exclusion of employer contributions for health insurance would be limited to the low-cost accountable health plan in a region. Employers would not have to provide health coverage to their workers, but if they chose to do so and had fewer than 100 employees, they would have to use the purchasing cooperatives. The co-ops would also serve people without a connection to the labor force.

The Cooper bill did not change Medicare, but it replaced Medicaid with federal aid to the poor to purchase a private plan through the regional cooperatives. Individuals with income below the federal poverty level could enroll in an accountable health plan without paying any premium and with only nominal co-payments, while those with incomes up to 200 percent of the poverty level would receive subsidies on a sliding scale. Although the federal government would assume full responsibility for financing medical care for the poor, it would turn over to the states the responsibility for financing long-term care in nursing homes. Cooper proposed to pay for the new federal costs by repealing the limit (at that time $135,000) on wages subject to the Medicare hospital insurance tax. The CBO estimated that the plan would reduce the uninsured population by about 40 percent, down from 39 million to 24 million, while having little impact on the federal deficit (increasing it slightly at first, then cutting it).[4]

From the standpoint of the administration, the range of views among House Democrats presented a difficult challenge. The single-payer and Stark bills both called for universal coverage without managed competition, while the Cooper bill called for managed competition without universal coverage. The Clinton effort to achieve universal coverage with managed competition did not have a strong base of support in the House. Russo had more than 70 co-sponsors for his single-payer plan; Stark's bill was co-sponsored by Majority Leader Richard Gephardt and had the backing of the Ways and Means Committee. But with more than 50 co-sponsors, Cooper had enough votes to deny the Democrats a majority if they were unable to reach a compromise with him. The redoubtable chair of the Energy and Commerce Committee, Rep. John Dingell, whose father had co-sponsored the original national health insurance bill of the 1940s, was unable to report out a bill because of Cooper's opposition.[5]

The Senate posed equally serious difficulties, though for different reasons. Senator Byrd's declaration in early March that health reform could not go into the budget bill meant health reform could be filibustered and therefore might require 60 votes, not 50. Clinton later told journalists David Broder and Haynes Johnson that he should have realized that it would be impossible to pass the full health plan that year once Senator Byrd made his position known. "This is entirely my mistake, no one else's," Clinton said, conceding that he should have scaled back the proposal. "I set the Congress up for failure."[6]

With only 56 Democrats in the Senate—and some of them doubtful supporters of any substantial health reform—the main hope for passage of legislation lay in a compromise with the moderate Republicans who supported the bill introduced by Senator Chafee. Like the Clinton proposal, the Chafee bill established a right to health insurance for every citizen and legal resident of the United States, though it did not put that right into effect until 2005. Although the bill did not require employers to pay for health coverage, it required them to offer their employees the opportunity to enroll in either a catastrophic or a standard insurance plan. It also authorized firms to establish joint purchasing groups. People with low incomes who were not eligible for Medicaid would receive vouchers for health insurance, and in 2005 everyone would be required to carry coverage. The general model for the bill, including the original idea for the individual mandate, came from a proposal by the economist Mark V. Pauly and his colleagues for "responsible national health insurance."[7]

The Chafee bill encouraged Senate Majority Leader George Mitchell and other Democrats to believe that a compromise was in reach. Two committees in the Senate would play the central role. Senator Kennedy's health committee would be certain to act favorably, but the Senate Finance Committee was a different story. The Democrats on Finance were more conservative, and the committee's chairman, Daniel P. Moynihan, was uninterested in health reform. He did not hold hearings before the fall or establish a working relationship with Kennedy, and he made no effort to build consensus within his own committee. "I think that Moynihan never understood the health care bill, never tried terribly hard," one of his aides said later. "There he was, chairman of Finance, facing an incredibly complicated bill. He decided he was too old and set in his ways to spend six months learning health care. It's sort of a joke among Moynihan staff that the one part of the bill he engaged and got into was the protection of medical schools."[8] One of the original neoconservatives, Moynihan also did not share the basic assumptions of other Democrats that the health insurance system needed fundamental reform; he thought America's high health-care costs were unavoidable and that the poor were able to get health care. "We do have universal health care in the country, actually," he said, since the poor could get care in emergency rooms.[9]

If Clinton had left health-care reform to Congress, legislation would likely have been still-born because of the discord among Democrats and the absence of effective consensus-builders in key committees. Congressional leaders told Clinton he would have to jump-start the process because they recognized the internal barriers that health-care reform faced.

In trying to navigate the political terrain and build public support, the Clinton strategy took three political turns—or rather, it took two turns but was never able to complete the third. The first turn, a move to the center right, had taken place in the final stretch of the 1992 campaign when Clinton embraced managed competition within a budget. The second turn—a move left—came in the period between January and October 1993, when the president had sought to consolidate support among the many Democrats and constituency groups unhappy about the adoption of managed competition. It was in this period that Clinton opted for a comprehensive benefit package and a number of expensive elements designed to appeal to older Americans: a prescription-drug benefit to be added to Medicare, a new program of home-based long-term care for the elderly and disabled, and generous health insurance subsidies for early retirees. The bigger the program, however, the tighter the cost controls would also have to be.

Two theories in favor of this bigger, tighter program had considerable influence within the administration. One argument, the enthusiasm theory, held that since there would be fierce opponents of reform, Democrats needed equally passionate supporters. Health-care reform had to give ordinary people something worth fighting for. A minimal program of bare-bones insurance or a program that was directed only toward the poor would fail to appeal to the middle class that had elected Clinton. The president also had to include significant benefits for the elderly to give them a reason to support his plan.

A second argument, the bargaining-chip theory, held that the administration should go to Congress with a big program intentionally including elements that could be bargained away later. Some benefits could be cut, the budget caps relaxed, the alliances scaled back or sacrificed entirely. At one strategy meeting in the White House, Magaziner likened the process to peeling off the outer layers of an onion without harming the core: the president could trade away elements of the health plan without damaging its central features—universal coverage, consumer choice, and a backup system of cost containment. The paradigm was a complex negotiation: "You don't go into a negotiation with your final offer on the table." By proposing a comprehensive plan, Clinton would show he appreciated the legitimate concerns of diverse groups.

The final lap would necessarily require a turn right; the question was only when this turn would come and how far it would go. There was no other way to pass a bill than to get conservative Democrats and moderate Republicans on board. Democratic congressional leaders, however, did not want the administration to make those concessions; they wanted to do the bargaining themselves. To get past the senior gatekeepers in Congress such as Stark, it would also be impolitic to negotiate first with a junior congressman from Tennessee, Jim Cooper. Compromise with conservative Democrats would have to come in the later stages of congressional deliberation.

To say these judgments about strategy were mistaken is an understatement; they proved to be a disaster. Despite the comprehensive benefit package and the extras such as prescription drug coverage for the elderly, the administration did not receive passionate support from the groups it was counting on. The Clinton plan did succeed, however, in mobilizing the opposition. The scale of the program and its regulatory features also caused sympathetic groups in the business community and opinion leaders in the media to think twice about support for reform. Because the administration had failed to edit the plan down to its essentials and find familiar ways to convey it, many people couldn't understand what the president was proposing.

The original political impulse behind the managed-competition strategy was to find common ground with moderates and conservatives. Instead, much of the rhetoric used to defend the president's plan, beginning with his speech to Congress, made it sound almost as if it were a single-payer proposal. Although the administration repeatedly sought to link the Health Security plan to the concerns of the middle class, universal coverage became the one clear theme, suggesting a focus on the poor. The president had invested so much in the proposal that one might have expected a more sustained and consistent effort to explain it. But after Hillary Clinton gave a bravura performance at the initial congressional hearings, the White House focused entirely on the principles of reform and made little effort to defend the specifics of the proposal. In fact, it never released the back-up analyses explaining the rationale for the various elements in the plan. The president's political advisers insisted that it would be counterproductive for him to focus on the mechanics of reform, so instead the White House left the content of its proposal to be defined by its opponents.[10] The administration had gone to the trouble of writing a bill and then left it like a foundling on the doorstep of Congress.

On the political calendar, health care gave way to other priorities. Before he addressed Congress about health care, Clinton had necessarily concentrated on economic and budgetary policy. The budget battle, however, prejudiced the outcome on health-care reform by using up a lot of the president's political capital. The health legislation went to Congress *after* the president had already asked members of his party to cast difficult votes for tax increases and budget cuts as well as gun control and other measures that many of them knew might doom their reelection chances. Once Democrats voted for one set of tax increases, persuading them to vote for an employer mandate or any other method of financing expanded health coverage was going to be difficult, if not impossible.

Even after the president's speech in September and the introduction of the health bill the next month, Clinton decided to give priority to Senate approval of the North American Free Trade Agreement. Some analysts suggested that NAFTA would help health care by earning the president support from business and opinion leaders, and Clinton did enjoy high approval ratings as 1993 came to an end. NAFTA, however, seriously undermined the president's popularity among the unions and other organizations that had the ability to mobilize grass-roots support for health reform.

Delaying health care until the beginning of 1994 also had unforeseen consequences because of unrelated political developments. The new year began with a feeding frenzy in the press over "Whitewater"—a long-failed Arkansas real-estate investment of the Clintons that became the focus of a series of breathless revelations undermining trust in both the president and his wife. As the Clintons had personalized the health-care issue, so the opponents now attached it to them personally as confidence in their integrity fell. If there ever was a season of opportunity for health-care reform, it was ending.

The Big Turnabout

The prospects for health-care reform rested largely on the Democrats' ability to win support from two groups who were not their usual political allies—moderate Republicans and business leaders. During 1993, senior figures in the Republican Party, including the Senate minority leader, Bob Dole, indicated a readiness to compromise, and the White House seemed to make progress in negotiations with business groups. These signals were critical in giving the White House confidence to proceed.

The idea of a bipartisan bill was not outlandish. During the twentieth century, Republicans had twice provided major backing for publicly financed health insurance—in the Progressive era, when state-level reforms enjoyed support from Progressive Republicans in the Theodore Roosevelt mold, and in the early 1970s, when Nixon was president. Since the Nixon era, the party's center of gravity had moved to the right, and by the early 1990s there was no chance of GOP support for reform in the House, where Rep. Newt Gingrich was already effectively in control of the Republican caucus, awaiting the retirement of the Minority Leader Robert Michel and organizing all-out opposition to the administration. But the Senate still included a substantial group of moderate Republicans inclined to work with Democrats on health care. One Republican, Jim Jeffords (Vermont), endorsed the Clinton plan (and subsequently switched parties). The 20 co-sponsors of Chafee's bill included John Danforth (Missouri), Pete Domenici (New Mexico), Dave Durenberger (Minnesota), Mark Hatfield (Oregon), Nancy Kassebaum (Kansas), and Arlen Specter (Pennsylvania), all of whom had a record of supporting bipartisan legislation. Originally, the Chafee bill also had a number of conservative co-sponsors, such as Robert Bennett and Orrin Hatch (Utah), Alan Simpson (Wyoming), and Lauch Faircloth (North Carolina).

The battle over health-care reform, however, would prove to be a critical moment in the ideological sorting out of the Republican Party. The turn away from any Republican partnership in reform began with a December 2, 1993, memo to party leaders from conservative strategist Bill Kristol. The administration's pattern, Kristol warned, was to seek compromises in Congress, but Republicans should resist any "urge to negotiate a 'least bad' compromise with the Democrats, and thereby gain momentary public credit for helping the president 'do something' about health care." Kristol continued: "Passage of the Clinton health care plan, in any form, would guarantee and likely make permanent an unprecedented federal intrusion into and disruption of the American economy—and the establishment of the largest federal entitlement program since Social Security." The Clinton proposal was also "a serious political threat to the Republican Party." It would "help Democratic prospects in 1996. But the long-term political effects of a successful Clinton health care bill will be even worse—much worse. . . . It will revive the reputation of the party that spends and regulates, the Democrats, as the generous protector of middle-class interests." Republicans had to "adopt an aggressive and uncompromising counterstrategy" to "delegitimize" the Clinton proposal and bring about its "unqualified political defeat."[11]

Kristol discerned a pattern in public opinion surveys that could provide a basis for bringing about that defeat. The initially "strong public support" for the Clinton plan was fading. A *Washington Post* poll in late September had respondents approving the plan by 56 percent to 24 percent, but by mid-November the margin of approval was only 46 percent to 43 percent. Moreover, while polls showed overwhelming agreement that the system needed fundamental reform, the great majority were satisfied with their own medical care. Kristol counseled, therefore, that Republicans should say that there was no health care crisis and that the Clinton plan would damage the quality of medical care most people had. Within a short time, many Republicans who had previously taken a conciliatory stance toward Democratic proposals were repeating Kristol's arguments.

The case against making any concessions received another boost the next month with the publication of a pair of articles by Betsy McCaughey, a researcher at a conservative think tank, who claimed that the Clinton bill "will prevent you from going outside the system to buy basic health coverage you think is better. The doctor can be paid only by the plan, not by you." In fact, the legislation stated right at the beginning, "Nothing in this Act shall be construed as prohibiting the following: (1) An individual from purchasing any health care services." McCaughey had twisted the meaning of a provision that barred doctors from double-billing patients for services that an insurer was already required to pay for. But her charges were widely circulated through the media and contributed to the broader erosion of trust in the Clintons brought about by the Whitewater stories that were dominating the news at the time.[12]

It was in that atmosphere that the Clinton reform effort suffered its most serious blow: the loss of support of business groups. Historically, with only a few exceptions, American business leaders had never supported national health insurance. But the steep rise in the cost of employee health benefits had persuaded many executives that federal intervention was necessary. Moreover, both health-care interest groups and employers frustrated with rising costs were receptive to an approach to reform that sought to achieve universal coverage through private health plans.[13]

The days when the AMA served as the lead opponent of government health programs were over. The association had endorsed an employer mandate as the primary means for financing universal coverage, and its leaders had cooperative relations with the Clinton White House. The American College of Physicians, the pediatricians, neurologists, and family practitioners, as well as the American Nursing Association, retail pharmacists, and other provider groups backed the administration's proposal. Both the American Hospital Association and the Catholic Hospital Association had developed proposals for universal coverage that were similar to the Clinton health plan (though they opposed the cuts in future increases in Medicare hospital payments that were part of the Clinton plan's financing). The big insurance companies initially did not reject the administration's general framework.

Some of the nation's biggest employers also had endorsed comprehensive reforms aimed at achieving cost containment and universal coverage. In 1991, a group called the National Leadership Coalition for Health Care Reform, representing major corporations and labor unions, had endorsed a play-or-pay plan for universal coverage, including an employer mandate and price controls on health services. The view of business, however, was far from unanimous; some companies quit the coalition when it adopted its health-care proposal. The corporations remaining in the coalition came from the manufacturing, utilities, media, and banking industries and had long offered generous health benefits that were now soaring in cost. In their

view, they were covering the cost of their employees' entire families, including spouses who often worked for businesses that failed to provide health
coverage, as well as paying for the bad debt left at hospitals by the uninsured, many of whom had jobs too. As these companies saw it, a universal
insurance program with an employer mandate could spread the costs of
health care more fairly and possibly relieve them of the burden of health
benefits for early retirees.

These kinds of considerations motivated early support for health reform
in such big-business groups as the National Association of Manufacturers,
the Washington Business Group on Health, and the Business Roundtable.
The most surprising convert to the cause of reform was the United States
Chamber of Commerce, a group that predominantly represented firms with
fewer than 100 employees and had long been a reliable opponent of government social programs. Since 1991, however, the Chamber had turned toward
more centrist leadership; in early 1993, for example, it had not opposed the
Family and Medical Leave Act. Under the Chamber's Health Committee,
Robert Patricelli, a benefits manager, had created a subgroup representing
employers that paid for health benefits. Patricelli's group recommended that
the Chamber back universal health coverage, including an employer mandate for 50 percent of the premiums, and in March 1993 the Chamber's
board unanimously approved that position. That year the Chamber's leadership met frequently with Magaziner, seeking subsidies for small business as
well as other provisions. The schedule for capping employers' premium obligations, ranging from 3.2 percent of payroll for small, low-wage firms to
7.9 percent of payroll for larger firms with higher wages, resulted from proposals that the Chamber made. The president cited the Chamber's support
for reform in his speech to Congress.

But not all employer groups took a friendly view. The Chamber's chief
rival in representing small-business interests, the National Federation of
Independent Business, immediately started agitating against an employer
mandate. The members of the NFIB were less likely than members of the
Chamber to provide health benefits, and the NFIB's leaders were dead-set
against any compromise with the administration. Early in 1993 the organization began sending out alerts to small-business owners about the danger
of a federal mandate that would force them to provide health insurance to

their workers. The NFIB focused its campaigns on states with senators or representatives on key committees; one such effort, in Montana, targeted Max Baucus, a Democrat who was second in seniority on the Senate Finance Committee.

Another early interest-group opponent of the administration was the Health Insurance Association of America, the industry lobbying group dominated not by the Big Five health insurance companies, but by the smaller ones, which saw the proposed market reforms as a direct threat. Their business model depended on medical underwriting—that is, cherry-picking the healthy and denying coverage to the sick—which the reformed system would make impossible. During 1993 HIAA began an advertising campaign intended to stoke doubts about the Clinton health plan. In the fall, the ads showed a couple at a kitchen table, saying the reforms would take away consumer choices. "They choose, we lose" was the tag line, which would have been an apt description of what the insurers did in choosing whether to cover people with chronic illnesses. These "Harry and Louise" ads became important symbols of opposition, though according to communications scholar Kathleen Hall Jamieson, the evidence indicates they had a "negligible" impact on public opinion.[14]

Yet another source of business opposition to the Clinton health plan was the tobacco industry. Although the industry was mainly concerned about the proposed 75-cent cigarette tax, it poured its resources into conservative organizations opposing health-care reform as a whole. Documents from the Tobacco Institute (uncovered in unrelated litigation) show that the industry also gave money to single-payer groups to attack the Clinton plan from the left and specifically to attack the cigarette tax as falling disproportionately on the poor.[15]

If the Democrats had been able to hold the support of the major business organizations like the Chamber of Commerce, they might have been able to overcome the opposition of the NFIB, small insurers, and tobacco companies. Conservative Republican leaders, however, began a concerted campaign to turn around the position of the major conciliatory business groups. Lobbyists usually lobby politicians, but in this case, the politicians lobbied the lobbyists. Representative John Boehner, head of the 75-member Conservative Opportunity Society in the House, told the Chamber's national leaders that they had a duty to oppose the administration, and he and other House Republicans contacted local Chambers, urging them to disaffiliate from the national organization. Before the Chamber's representatives were scheduled to testify in February, conservative Republicans "read them the riot act."[16] Conservative business groups joined in the campaign, and the National American Wholesale Grocers' Association resigned from the Chamber.

In early February, the Chamber and other business organizations reversed direction. In a three-day period, the Business Roundtable announced that it would support the Cooper plan, the National Association of Manufacturers said it would oppose the Clinton plan, and the Chamber withdrew its support for an employer mandate and then joined the opposition to any reform proposal.

What explains the reversal? Business was divided and ambivalent from the start; support for government intervention in health care conflicted with the general corporate preference for a minimalist state. Some aspects of the Clinton plan fed that ambivalence; employers were generally opposed, for example, to the inclusion in the purchasing alliances of all firms with up to 5,000 employees. Although the White House tried to assure business that Congress would scale back such provisions, the business groups did not trust the Democrats. The Clinton plan and other reform proposals faced inherent difficulties in trying to mobilize both public and employer support. The promises of guaranteed, comprehensive insurance that were aimed at generating popular enthusiasm undercut the ability to bring business on board.

Ideology and trust influence the calculus of interests. Many people have written about the politics of health reform on the basis of which groups would "win" and which would "lose" under different approaches. As expected, the "losers"—for example, insurance brokers, whom the alliances would have displaced—resisted health-care reform, but the "winners" didn't necessarily support it. Many companies or industries that would have had net gains from the legislation focused on lesser provisions that hurt them or on the risk that the balance of effects would turn negative as legislation moved through Congress. During 1993 and early 1994, many winners used their influence to change provisions that adversely affected them and devoted little energy to ensuring that legislation would pass. Some winners opposed the Clinton plan outright. For example, the manufacturing sector would have seen its health insurance costs go down dramatically. But some provisions, like the generosity of the benefit package, would have raised employer costs; the early retiree provisions were unlikely to make it through Congress; and the expansion of government authority posed the risk of new burdens in the future. So although individual companies backed the Clinton plan, the National Association of Manufacturers came out against it.

Finally, and more fundamentally, business never became a strong supporter of health reform because the rising cost of employee benefits ultimately does not come out of profits. If it did, business would long ago have been far more aggressive in controlling health insurance costs. Although employers may find it difficult to offset rapid rises in the cost of health benefits in the short run, they can adjust wages and other benefits over a longer period. The spurt in private health insurance costs in the late 1980s helped generate a wave of business support for reform. But health care inflation eased in 1993 and 1994, and some employers came to believe that managed care provided them with a long-term solution. Prodded by the Republicans, business representatives worried less about the costs of health care and more about the wider ramifications of expanded government authority.

After business backtracked from its earlier support of reform, Senate Republicans reassessed their position. Going into a meeting with their Senate colleagues in Annapolis, Maryland, in early March, Dole and Chafee still expected they would come out with a position in support of reform. But the opponents of compromise dominated the meeting—Senator Phil Gramm called the Chafee bill "socialism with a smile"—and by the end of the month, Dole had abandoned the Chafee bill. He then co-sponsored a bill with Packwood and within weeks abandoned that as well.[17]

Overconfident about the momentum of reform, the White House had wrongly assumed that the leading Republicans and key interest groups that had endorsed significant change would not only maintain their positions but also move closer to the administration in a final bargain. By spring 1994, however, Republicans were already anticipating big midterm

election gains and saw no reason to make a deal. Killing reform in the
103rd Congress, they had decided, was good politics.

The Collapse of Congressional Compromise

When Clinton became president, there seemed to be the makings of
a consensus around the principles of universal coverage and managed
competition. The Clinton, Cooper, and Chafee proposals all called for consumer choice among competing health plans, the establishment of health
insurance purchasing cooperatives, a standard benefit package set or interpreted by a national board, similar reforms of the insurance market, and
premium subsidies for low-income families. The Chafee and Clinton plans
included mandates to make them universal; Cooper saw that as a second
step sometime in the future. By adopting a managed-competition framework, it seemed, the president was laying the basis for eventual compromise with Cooper and Chafee. If the administration started out with a
structurally similar plan, it would be much easier to split the difference on
any number of provisions.

But the sharply partisan climate of 1994 and fear-mongering by the opposition were hardly conducive to splitting differences. The Republicans
who agreed with Kristol's political assessment and the interest groups that
benefited from the status quo did not want to see compromise succeed.
Despite insisting he was flexible, Clinton boxed himself into a corner by
threatening to veto any bill that fell short of universal coverage.

The failure of congressional compromise also stemmed, however, from
the weaknesses of the centrist proposals. While rejecting an employer mandate, the Cooper and Chafee plans included no other source of revenue capable of financing the broadened coverage each called for. Because the
Cooper plan also had no individual mandate (or substitute mechanism),
the individuals who signed up for insurance were sure to have disproportionately high health costs; those costs would drive up premiums in the regional purchasing cooperatives, raise the cost of subsidies for low-income
enrollees, and lead small employers to demand that they be allowed to get
out of the cooperatives. The Chafee plan had nowhere near enough revenue
to pay for the subsidies it envisioned for households with incomes up to 240

percent of the poverty level. These inadequacies were typical of moderate and conservative proposals. The reform plan that President Bush presented in February 1992, for example, included no financing provisions at all. Dole backed out of the Chafee bill and later out of the bill he co-sponsored with Packwood when he saw the fiscal difficulties they posed.

The employer mandate in the Clinton plan resolved this problem, but at the cost of raising others. If there is a simple answer to the question, "Why did universal coverage fail?" it's that Congress would not enact the employer mandate in any form, and when the mandate failed, so did universal coverage, because there was no willingness to raise taxes to pay for expanded coverage. At the inception of the debate, the employer mandate enjoyed more interest-group support than ever before. It was by far the most plausible financing strategy for expanded coverage; after all, Nixon had proposed it, and it was approved by a wide margin in public opinion polls. But while groups like the AMA and the health insurers had accepted a mandate as preferable to a tax-financed system, they would never fight for it, nor would other interest groups. On the other hand, the NFIB fiercely resisted the mandate and targeted its efforts strategically to districts of swing members of key committees. When the employer mandate was defeated in the Senate Finance Committee, Baucus was one of those who voted against it.

Employer contributions were the kind of issue perfectly suited to legislative bargaining. Instead of an 80 percent contribution, the level could have been set at 50 percent. The smallest employers, with fewer than 10 or 20 employees, could have been entirely exempt or paid a minimum rate of 2 or 3 percent of payroll. These were precisely the compromises that Senators Kennedy, Moynihan, Mitchell, and others incorporated into their plans or floated as options. If Clinton had had ten more Democrats in the Senate, as Lyndon Johnson did when Medicare passed in 1965, a deal of this kind might have worked, but the party's margin was too narrow. Even such Democrats as Bob Kerrey, Dianne Feinstein, and Joseph Lieberman—all running for reelection in 1994—would not vote for the mandate in any form.

In his effort to find a majority for a reduced program in August, Senator Mitchell gave up the premium caps, made the alliances voluntary, and deferred the possibility of an employer mandate until 2002. At that point, a mandate for 50 percent of premiums would be triggered only if two conditions were met—coverage hadn't reached 95 percent of the population in a state, and Congress had failed to do anything else to reach that level. These concessions made no difference to the mandate's opponents; nothing would mollify them now. "Sight unseen, Republicans should oppose it" was Kristol's advice regarding Senator Mitchell's attempt to craft a compromise.[18]

In the House, Gephardt had combined the bills that passed the committees on Ways and Means and on Education and Labor into legislation that was far more liberal than Mitchell's. Many Democrats made no secret of their desire to use the Mitchell bill as a stratagem to get the legislation into House-Senate conference and then bring back a much stronger bill to the Senate. It is hard to imagine an approach better designed to increase distrust of Mitchell's proposal among conservative Democrats and moderate Republicans. But Gephardt's bill probably never had any chance of passing the House. Instead of developing a compromise, Gephardt had only slightly revised the Stark bill from Ways and Means. To business interests and conservative Democrats, this was even less palatable than the Clinton plan because they believed its new Medicare Part C for the under-65 population would screw down payment rates, shift costs to private insurance plans, and ultimately bring about a collapse of the private market. By the summer, the only conceivable scenario for passing legislation was that the House would finally defer to a more conservative bill developed in the Senate. The unwillingness of House Democrats to acknowledge this reality was a premonition of coming disaster.

The final act was played out in the Senate and starred the "mainstream group," a bipartisan coalition of roughly 18 senators, led by Chafee and John Breaux of Louisiana. Of all the centrist proposals that included significantly broadened coverage, the mainstream plan was the only one that was fiscally defensible. It financed an extension of coverage up to 91 or 92 percent of the population by imposing a cigarette tax, a tax on high-cost health plans, and cuts in Medicare. Coverage of pregnant women and children would have been nearly universal. The proposal also included insurance-market reforms and voluntary purchasing alliances along the lines of the Jackson Hole Group's version of managed competition. For all its flaws, the bill would have been a historic advance.

There was only one problem: it didn't have much public support. It was too big for conservatives, too little for liberals. Democrats in Congress who genuinely wanted a compromise found that hardly any organized constituencies would swallow the bitter pill the mainstream group was offering. The elderly saw the proposal as cutting Medicare without providing anything in return; unions saw it as taxing high-cost health plans—the kind some union members still enjoyed—without the guarantee of coverage "that can't be taken away." Health-care reform that hurt the protected public never had a chance.

From the beginning, the proposals in the center had failed to generate any public excitement. At the time, economists and some conservative intellectuals liked the individual mandate in the Chafee plan and the cap on tax benefits that both the Chafee and Cooper plans originally included, but no one even tried to build public support for these measures. Most of the initial business backing for the Cooper plan seems to have been expedient. Business interests backed Cooper when they feared worse, but they lost interest when the feared alternatives evaporated.

During the spring and summer of 1993, in what may really have been the crucial shift, the nation's elites abandoned health care reform entirely. They had become impatient with its complexity and nervous about its cost. While there was a general swing in the national mood at the same time, elite views were particularly critical. In 1992 and 1993, the Jackson Hole Group and the *New York Times* editorial page seemed to be prodding the nation's establishment into assuming leadership in a restructuring of the health-care market. The Senate mainstream group was this establishment's congressional incarnation. The effort might have actually succeeded if the debate had come to a head in the summer of 1993 instead of the summer of 1994. That moment was lost.

Why *No* Reform?

The Clinton health plan and other alternative approaches to comprehensive reform attempted to escape from what I have referred to as the American health policy trap: a costly and complicated system that has left a growing minority of Americans without financial protection in sickness but has nonetheless satisfied enough people to make it difficult to change. The key elements of the trap are a system of employer-provided insurance that conceals its true costs from those who benefit from it; targeted government programs that protect groups such as the elderly and veterans, who are well organized and enjoy wide public sympathy and believe that, unlike other claimants, they have earned their benefits; and a financing system that has expanded and enriched the health-care industry, creating powerful interests averse to change.

The Clinton plan sought to enlist the elements of society unhappy about rising costs and deteriorating coverage without antagonizing the protected public or the interest groups in the industry. Surveys in the early 1990s showed that the public consistently ranked health-care reform at or near the top of national priorities. The Clinton administration framed its proposal around the concept of "security," calling for health care "that cannot be taken away," so as to appeal not only to the uninsured but also to the larger population who were underinsured, denied coverage of pre-existing conditions, or at risk of periodically losing protection during spells of unemployment. The reliance on employer-funded private coverage and proposals for prescription-drug coverage and other new benefits for the elderly were aimed at obtaining the support of the protected public. By sticking with private health plans, the administration hoped to win over or at least neutralize the health-care and insurance industries as well as people satisfied with private coverage. And by calling for managed competition within a budget, it sought to rally business and other elite groups concerned about the rising cost of employee health benefits and government health programs.

President Clinton, however, could not obtain any reform legislation from Congress without the votes of Republican moderates in the Senate and conservative Democrats in the House. If he had immediately embraced a position close to theirs in January 1993, Clinton might have had a shot at passing a bill, though at the cost of defaulting on his campaign promises and causing a revolt within his own party. Instead, after moving right by adopting managed competition during his campaign, Clinton moved left during his first year in making choices about such issues as the guaranteed benefit package, hoping to build enough public support to push Republican moderates and conservative Democrats into a negotiation. The strategy was a high-stakes gamble, and it didn't work. Although the Clinton plan had wide backing from the public and from business when it was introduced, both of those sources of support proved vulnerable to erosion, undermining the administration's capacity to drive a final compromise.

Public support eroded, first of all, because of the disarray of the Democrats and delays in action on health reform. "For God's sake, don't let dead cats stand on your porch," Lyndon Johnson told Wilbur Mills in 1965, urging him not to let the debate on Medicare get strung out.[19] Long experience in Congress, if not with dead cats, had taught Johnson that even popular bills can lose support if the process gets mired down amid confusing details and alternatives.

Second, the decision to design a proposal inside the White House and put the Clinton label on it led to the confusion of public feelings about the president and his wife with the issue of health care. Opinion about health reform was not logically related to opinion about gays in the military, the role of women in society, or Whitewater. But the identification of the Clintons with the health plan became so strong that sentiments crossed over. The *Wall Street Journal* reported showing the same description of a health reform plan to focus groups with and without the Clinton label. Without the label, the plan won more than 70 percent support; with the label, approval dropped 30 to 40 points.[20] It seems likely that when polls asked for opinions about the "Clinton health plan," they tapped general feelings about the Clintons rather than specific preferences about health policy. The decline of support for the Clinton plan should be interpreted with this in mind. According to the Roper surveys, while 59 percent of respondents supported "President Clinton's plan to reform health care" and 33 percent opposed it in late September 1993, the supporters had slipped to 44 percent and opponents risen to 49 percent by late June 1994.[21] Support for complex policy changes requires a foundation of trust, and although Whitewater and the other scandals of Clinton's first two years never amounted to anything, they undermined trust in his leadership.

Compounding these difficulties, the Clinton administration made several mistakes in developing and presenting its proposal. Critics never failed to mention that the administration's bill was 1,342 pages long, faulting it for complexity. That in itself was not the problem: Congress deals

with many long and complicated pieces of legislation—try reading a bill reforming the tax code—and complexity was already built into health care law
and finance. In fact, for individual consumers and providers, the Clinton
plan would have simplified things a great deal through such features as a
community-wide open-enrollment period, standardized benefit packages,
standardized claims forms, and continuity of coverage regardless of employment. But the proposal undoubtedly seemed complex because of the way it
was initially introduced, the administration's failure to explain clearly how
it would work in practice, and the novelty of the proposal's central innovation, the "alliances" (now called insurance exchanges). The confusion of
"managed competition" with "managed care" added to the befuddlement
and anxiety about reform.

Still, it is a mistake to assume that the causal arrow runs from public
opinion to policy outcome. In 2003 the Republicans would pass Medicare legislation amid overwhelmingly hostile opinion polls. The trajectory
of public opinion on health care in 2009–2010 would repeat the pattern of
1993–1994. Whether public opinion influences public policy depends on,
among other things, what strata of society a policy's support comes from.
In a study of public opinion and national policy decisions between 1981
and 2002, political scientist Martin Gilens finds that on issues where opinion varied according to income level, policy outcomes were strongly related
to the opinion of upper-income people, but not at all to average opinion.
Health care was one of those issues: the support for universal coverage, an
employer mandate, and other provisions of Democratic proposals came
disproportionately from people with incomes at the median and below, and
in line with Gilens' general findings, their preferences were not reflected
in what the government did.[22] Continued majority support for specific
health-care proposals was no guarantee of congressional action; for example, the public's overwhelming support for an employer mandate did not
lead to its adoption. Indeed, the defeat of the employer mandate in the Senate was the single most important reason for the failure to pass any legislation. In this case as in many others, powerful interest-group opposition was
able to derail a popular proposal.

Although it seemed for a while that employers would push for reform,
they reverted to their historic position in the heat of controversy. Clinton

had staked so much on the support of business that the defection of the leading business lobbies represented an enormous blow, especially damaging in light of the need to attract moderate Republicans and conservative Democrats. The efforts to build popular and business support were inherently in tension with one another. The administration hoped to mobilize popular backing with such provisions as the broad benefit package and the requirement that employers pay 80 percent of the average premium, while keeping business support by signaling privately that the president would settle in congressional negotiations for a smaller benefit package and a 50 percent contribution. But business didn't trust Clinton and the Democrats, and conservative Republicans played on that distrust. Rising health costs also do not arouse employers to steady and concerted support for reform because over the long run, according to economic research, employers take the cost of health benefits out of their total labor bill. The effect is to depress cash wages or other benefits, but most employees do not make the connection. The system works badly for small employers (and their workers), who face significantly higher costs for health insurance. But the law has left small-business owners free not to cover their workers at all, and many of them prefer that flexibility to the unknowns of a system regulated and financed by the government.

If business was an inherently unreliable political ally, should Clinton have never sought to win it over? Some on the left believed that if only Clinton had endorsed single-payer or an expansion of Medicare, he would have had a simpler plan, and by rallying the public against the insurance industry, he could have won. But a single-payer plan never stood a chance. Paul Wellstone, single-payer's leading advocate in the Senate, had only four co-sponsors for his bill; reaching 50 votes, much less 60, was inconceivable. In November 1994, California voters defeated a single-payer ballot initiative by a margin of 73 percent to 27 percent, putting to rest the hope of an uprising against the insurance industry.[23] The supporters of single-payer enjoyed the illusion that their plan was simpler and more popular only because the Clinton plan was the lightning rod for criticism.

Another argument that Clinton should have gone for broke comes from Theda Skocpol, who suggests in her book *Boomerang* that the president's health plan gave Republicans the "perfect foil" for an anti-government campaign and contributed to the Republican victories in the congressional elections in 1994. In Skocpol's view, Clinton was unduly concerned about the deficit; rather than emphasizing cost containment, it would have been "politically wiser" for Clinton to have offered a looser, "less fiscally responsible" program.[24] But even if there had been no deficit, any program for universal health insurance in the 1990s had to include strong cost controls. Federal costs for Medicare and Medicaid were projected to grow at a compound rate of 13 percent a year, while revenue was growing less than half as fast. The policy legacy that Clinton confronted was not only the deficit hangover from the Reagan years, but also the failure of earlier health programs to control spending. Like single-payer, a fiscally "loose" plan would have been merely a political gesture without any real chance of passing Congress.

Many factors entered into the Democratic losses in the congressional elections in 1994, as would be true in 2010. Although an economic recovery had begun in 1994, the majority of voters had not felt the benefits. According to an analysis of survey data by Gary Jacobson, "57 percent thought the economy was still in bad shape, and 62 percent of this group voted for the Republican." The losses in the House were concentrated in the South and rural areas, culminating a long turnover of these districts from conservative Democrats to Republicans. Jacobson argues that Republicans benefited from the illusion of unified government. Voters held the Democrats accountable for a failure to perform on health care and other concerns, even though Republican opposition in the Senate was critical in blocking congressional action:

> The illusion of unified government put the onus of failure on the Democrats; the reality of divided government let Senate Republicans make sure that the administration would fail. Clinton was elected on a promise of change. Senate Republicans could prevent change, and they did. It was not difficult, for while everyone may agree that change is desirable, rarely do we find ready consensus on what to change to. The health care issue is exhibit A.[25]

The only way for Clinton to have avoided defeat on health care would have been to have moved faster with a smaller program than the one he offered, either by adopting something along the lines of the Chafee proposal immediately after he was elected or by proposing a limited expansion of coverage through changes in Medicare or Medicaid that could have been accomplished through the budget process. But it took the defeat of the Clinton plan for many Democrats to learn that they would have to settle for a lot less in health-care reform than they believed was either just or necessary.

CHAPTER 5

Comes the Counterrevolution, 1995–2006

THE CONSERVATIVE REPUBLICANS WHO swept into power in Congress in January 1995 reframed the national agenda in health care. Instead of covering the uninsured, the priority became cutting taxes and spending. Instead of controlling overall health-care costs, the priority became limiting costs to the government by rolling back the big federal health-care programs. According to the new Speaker of the House, Newt Gingrich, the Republican majority aimed at nothing less than changing the course of American history by dismantling the "welfare state" that Democrats had erected since the New Deal. "One of my key decisions in November of 1994," Gingrich said the following year, "was to launch a revolutionary rather than a reformist effort. A revolutionary launches sixty battles. . . . You spread the attention [of the established order's defenders] so they can't focus. They can beat you on any five things. They can't beat you on sixty."[1]

Launching "sixty battles" would not turn out to be as brilliant a strategy as Gingrich imagined. When he talked about destroying the "welfare state," the former history professor was taking advantage of an ambiguity. To most Americans, "welfare" meant aid to the idle poor, particularly the program of cash assistance to single-parent families. That program had little support, and Republicans would largely succeed in their attack on it. But the many who disapproved of "welfare" in the narrow sense did not necessarily think of Medicare or even Medicaid as belonging in the same category. And when Gingrich summoned them into battle against the "welfare state" in the wider meaning of that phrase, they did not follow.

Much of the struggle over national policy that unfolded during the mid-1990s focused on the federal budget, but the issues at stake were deeper than spending levels. The Republicans wanted to change the framework of policy by adopting a constitutional amendment requiring a balanced budget and by enacting legislation to eliminate or restrict the individual entitlement to benefits under the major federal health programs. Medicaid they wanted to devolve upon the states; Medicare they wanted ultimately to turn into a voucher, which the elderly could use to buy private insurance. The aim was to reduce the liabilities and scope of government and the demands on taxpayers on the grounds that individuals would make better decisions about health care if they had to bear more of the cost. Republicans had a parallel agenda for private insurance, hoping to reform it to curb "overinsurance" and make consumers pay a larger share of medical expenses out of pocket.

The Republican effort to redirect national health policy went through three phases. In the first, self-proclaimed revolutionary phase during 1995 and 1996, the efforts by Gingrich and the Republican Congress to change Medicare and Medicaid took on central importance in a historic confrontation with President Clinton about the role of government. Although slow to respond to the challenge at first, Clinton proved more agile and determined than Gingrich expected, and when the president defied Republican demands and allowed the federal government to be shut down in late 1995, he framed his position as a defense of "Medicare, Medicaid, education, and the environment."[2] With public opinion turning sharply against them, Republican leaders discovered they had overreached and were forced to retreat.

A second and quieter phase began to emerge in mid-1996 as Clinton reached agreement with the Republicans on modest reforms of private health insurance. This new phase came into full flower after Clinton's re-election as the economy grew at a torrid pace, health costs moderated, and the fiscal environment brightened, allowing the administration and Republican leaders to reach bipartisan compromises on health policy and the budget. Although the Republicans did win some victories, they did not significantly reduce federal commitments in health care; in fact, they agreed to a new government health insurance program for children.

A bigger opportunity for conservatives to change the course of federal health policy came in the third phase of GOP power after George W. Bush succeeded Clinton in January 2001. For the first months of the Bush administration (until one Republican senator defected) and then again from 2003 through 2006, Republicans controlled both the legislative and executive branches. But instead of dismantling the welfare state, President Bush and the Republican Congress enlarged it by passing a new Medicare prescription-drug benefit, though they established it on their own terms. The same legislation promoted high-deductible private health insurance, combined with a tax-free health savings account. And Bush continued a process begun by Clinton of giving states waivers of federal Medicaid rules, allowing some states to expand Medicaid coverage and others to reduce it.

Yet the great surprise about the dozen years of Republican control of Congress from 1995 through 2006 was how little change conservatives brought to health care. Grand ambitions were frustrated; the welfare state survived. Like the Clinton health plan in 1994, the major conservative efforts to reshape national health policy met defeat. Even though Congress was in Republican hands, it voted for two new federal health programs— first for children in 1997, then for the elderly in 2003—and nonetheless left the central problems of health costs and coverage unaddressed. But a dozen years of drift did not leave things unchanged. As employer-based coverage eroded and costs rose in the early 2000s, health care became a more daunting economic challenge than ever.

Gingrich and the End of Entitlements

National policy made a U-turn in 1995. After President Clinton had tried to establish a right to health care for all citizens, congressional Republicans in 1995 sought to roll back existing rights under Medicare and Medicaid. Constitutional law in the United States, unlike many other democracies, provides no general right to health care or health insurance. Americans' rights to health care, insofar as they have any, depend on statute, and as of

1995, the two health-care entitlement programs, Medicare and Medicaid, were the primary sources of those rights.[3]

All rights impose obligations on another party. The rights enjoyed by beneficiaries of Medicare and Medicaid impose obligations on government and the taxpayers, and it was those obligations that Republicans wanted to reduce. From a fiscal standpoint, entitlement programs differ from discretionary spending because they do not have fixed, annual budgets. The cost of an entitlement depends on the number of people who qualify for it as well as the volume and price of its benefits. Medicare and Medicaid are not the only federal health-care obligations with no annual limit on costs. Tax expenditures for health insurance—that is, taxes foregone because of medical deductions and the exclusion of employer contributions from taxable income—also have no budgeted limit. The tax expenditures, however, chiefly benefit the privately insured, and the new congressional majority in 1995 did not attempt to limit the cost of those benefits.

The "Contract with America" that the House Republicans adopted during the 1994 campaign made no mention of cuts in Medicare or Medicaid. But the Contract did promise a balanced-budget amendment to the Constitution, and after that amendment failed to pass the Senate, Republican leaders sought to fulfill their commitment to fiscal responsibility by passing a budget that would reach balance in seven years.

By 1995 the federal deficit was already on its way down from the imbalance created by the tax cuts and defense-spending increases adopted during the Reagan administration. In 1990 President George H. W. Bush had agreed to a budget deal with the Democrats that included a tax increase, an unforgiveable apostasy for a Republican in the eyes of conservatives. And in 1993, without a single Republican vote, a Democratic Congress had passed Clinton's first budget, which included an increase in taxes on the highest-income brackets as well as major spending cuts. In the 1994 election Democrats paid heavily for voting for that budget, though it cut the projected deficit from 5 percent to 2.5 percent of GDP, a manageable level that was continuing to fall in 1995 as the economy rebounded.[4] To the Republican congressional leaders, however, nothing less than a balanced budget would do—balanced, that is, in the seventh year (the budget they sent to Clinton actually went back into the red in year eight and thereafter because of tax cuts). And in the name of that goal, they sought fundamental changes in Medicare and Medicaid that would guarantee sharp reductions in the growth of spending for both programs.

If Clinton had not vetoed it, the Republican budget would have effectively converted Medicare from a "defined benefit" to a "defined contribution" program, to use a distinction commonly made among types of pensions. Instead of an open-ended commitment to beneficiaries to pay for specific health services, the federal government would have furnished a fixed amount of money. The budget bill called for hard caps on future Medicare spending and a shift of beneficiaries from the traditional fee-for-service program to private managed-care plans. Health-care costs exceeding the caps would not have been the government's problem; the beneficiaries and providers would have had to absorb the difference. And because the legislation that Republicans sent to Clinton called for cutting future Medicare spending by $270 billion—a 30 percent reduction—the new framework could have shifted much of the burden of rising health costs to the elderly.[5]

The Republican effort broke with long-established patterns in Medicare politics. From 1966 to 1994, as Jonathan Oberlander has argued, the program was run on the basis of a politics of consensus. When changes were introduced, they were typically made with bipartisan support. Under Gingrich's leadership, however, Republicans were willing to challenge the fundamental tenets of the program as part of the general effort to replace the welfare state with their vision of a "conservative opportunity society." As it happened, the budget reconciliation bill adopted by the Republicans called for $245 billion in tax cuts along with the $270 billion in Medicare cuts, and the Democrats used those figures to argue that Republicans were trying to change Medicare so as to cut taxes on the rich. Republicans insisted, on the contrary, that their program was the only way to preserve Medicare from "bankruptcy" and to "modernize" the program.[6]

Since Medicare is part of the federal government, it cannot go bankrupt any more than the Department of Agriculture can. But Medicare Part A (hospital insurance) is financed through a separate trust fund by an earmarked payroll tax, and projections that the trust fund's revenue stream will be inadequate at some future time have periodically triggered an alarm about the program's finances. (The funds for Medicare Part B come from general federal revenues, so it is never subject to crises of this kind.) During the era of consensus politics, Congress resolved problems in Part A financing without much public attention. But in 1995, Haley Barbour, the chair of the Republican National Committee, came across a projection that the hospital trust fund would start running a deficit in 2002, and Republicans seized on that forecast as a reason why transforming the program on the lines they advocated was the only way to save it.[7]

The Republican vision for Medicare was to bring the program into conformity with the shift to managed care in the private market. When Medicare was established in 1965, its provisions for paying health-care providers were the same as the prevailing arrangements in private insurance. But by the early 1990s, Medicare had become a lingering bastion of traditional fee-for-service. Referring to the program as a "dinosaur," leading Republicans called for the introduction of private plans to reduce Medicare spending, though the available evidence did not indicate that private plans would actually save Medicare money. Thanks to its prospective payment system, fee-for-service Medicare was already obtaining heavy discounts from health-care providers. In addition, the enrollees that private managed-care plans attracted among the elderly tended to be relatively healthy. As a result, under the formula it was using, the federal government was paying private plans more for enrollees than it would have cost if those Medicare beneficiaries stayed in the traditional fee-for-service program.[8]

On the advice of pollsters, the congressional Republicans were supposed to avoid any hint of hostility to Medicare and to say their aim was to give the elderly "more options" and to "save" Medicare from bankruptcy. But the Republican leaders undermined their own cause. On October 24, 1995, in the midst of the fight over Medicare, Senator Dole said in a speech to the American Conservative Union: "I was there [in 1965], fighting the fight, voting against Medicare . . . because we knew it wouldn't work." On the same day, Gingrich told a Blue Cross meeting that Medicare should be left to "wither on the vine": "We don't get rid of it in round one because we don't think that's politically smart." Gingrich later insisted that he was referring to the Health Care Financing Administration, which administered the traditional Medicare program, but either way the implication was that the Republican plan would eliminate the Medicare program in its traditional form, even if it wasn't "politically smart" to do that right away.[9]

Just three weeks later the political confrontation between Clinton and the Republicans came to a head. Without an agreement on a budget, the federal government was operating on the basis of short-term "continuing resolutions." By this point, Clinton had accepted the goal of a balanced budget, though not the Republicans' tax and spending cuts. When Republicans wrote their priorities into a continuing resolution that also included an increase in Medicare Part B premiums, Clinton refused to sign it, and at midnight on November 13 the government began the first of two shutdowns. The prominence of Medicare in Clinton's last-minute negotiations with the Republican leadership and in his public response didn't just reflect concerns about health care for the elderly; "Medicare was a metaphor," journalist John F. Harris notes, "for a large set of other worthwhile programs."[10]

What was more surprising than Clinton's frequent invocation and successful defense of Medicare was the outcome of the battle over Medicaid, long thought to be the politically weaker of the two entitlements. The standard view among Democrats was that like other programs serving the poor, Medicaid would always be a poor program for want of middle-class support. But between 1984 and 1990, Democrats in Congress had won legislation decoupling Medicaid from welfare and phasing in Medicaid coverage of all children below the federal poverty level and all children under age six up to 33 percent above the poverty level. The battle of the budget in 1995 showed that Medicaid now had a stronger base of political support than many had believed.

The budget bill adopted by the Republicans in the fall of 1995 called for eliminating the individual, federal entitlement to Medicaid benefits, as Reagan initially had wanted to do in 1981. Instead of guaranteeing a list of minimum services to those who qualified for Medicaid, the federal government would convert the program into a "block grant" to the states, which would then have more flexibility in deciding whom and what to cover. Substituting a block grant for an entitlement was also what the Republicans wanted to do with welfare. The Republican governors were willing to accept less generous federal funding for Medicaid in exchange for more control over it. But strong opposition from the hospitals and other health-care groups resulted in smaller cuts in Medicaid than conservatives originally wanted, and as a result of concessions to moderate Republican senators, the final budget legislation also preserved a residual entitlement for some vulnerable groups. States would have to maintain Medicaid coverage of low-income children under age 13 and pregnant women as well as the disabled, though the states could determine what benefits to provide. None of these changes went into effect, however, because Clinton vetoed the budget bill in 1995.[11]

The next year, Republicans linked their reforms of Medicaid and welfare by combining them in one bill, which they framed as a budget-reconciliation measure so they wouldn't need 60 votes in the Senate to pass it. Their hope was that Clinton would be forced to agree to the limits on Medicaid because of his interest in passing welfare reform before the 1996 election. But the president vetoed this bill too, demanding that the Republicans send him freestanding welfare legislation. In July 1996, the congressional leadership acceded to that demand, and Clinton signed the welfare reform bill over the objection of many of his liberal advisers, ending a federal entitlement to welfare in the narrow sense—that is, to cash assistance.

After vetoing two earlier versions of welfare reform, Clinton was willing to sign the third bill because it maintained the federal entitlement for Medicaid as well as food stamps, and it preserved Medicaid eligibility for individuals who previously qualified for welfare. In the short term, however, loss of contact with welfare agencies disrupted enrollment in Medicaid for many of the poor. No systematic government surveys tracked families leaving welfare, but an analysis of the 1997 Survey of American Families indicates that 49 percent of the women who left welfare and 30 percent of the children were uninsured one year later.[12]

Nonetheless, Clinton's defense of the entitlement for Medicaid but not for welfare was a critical turning point in the relationship of the two programs. Medicaid had begun largely as an offshoot of welfare; eligibility for welfare had meant eligibility for Medicaid. Now the connection was completely severed, and Medicaid could include more low-income two-parent families and single individuals. As one federal analysis argued, the welfare-reform legislation was "an opportunity for states to recast and market Med-

icaid as a freestanding health insurance program for low-income families"
without the stigma of welfare.[13]

Why did welfare and Medicaid meet different fates? Clinton believed the
traditional welfare program was inconsistent with American values because it failed to reward work, and he had championed an increased Earned
Income Tax Credit in 1993 as a more defensible alternative form of assistance to the poor. The EITC also had the advantage of being a purely federal benefit independent of the states, whereas the states determined both
eligibility for welfare and the level of cash assistance. Some states kept that
assistance at so low a level that Clinton did not view the federal entitlement
to welfare as much of an entitlement at all.

In contrast, Medicaid had become the primary means of financing
health care for the poor and could now serve a wider population of low-
wage workers as well as the poor who were unemployed or outside the labor force. Medicaid was also easier to defend because of the groups other
than the poor who supported it. Like food stamps (sustained by the agricultural lobby), Medicaid had powerful defenders (health-care providers),
while welfare had no supporting constituency of similar influence. It
was also not true that Medicaid lacked middle-class backing; much of the
money that went to nursing-home care benefited the middle-class elderly
who had spent down their assets. (The Republican bills included measures
to recover from children the cost of nursing-home care of their elderly
parents.) The mixed interests in Medicaid, however, made a block grant
potentially threatening to the interests of the poor. If Medicaid became a
block grant, Clinton told one of his aides, "the nursing home lobby in every
state legislature will make sure all the Medicaid money goes to old folks in
nursing homes, and poor kids will end up getting screwed."[14]

When the battle of the budget began in 1995, Republicans seemed likely
to terminate the federal guarantee of health coverage that Medicaid provided. Instead, Medicaid emerged in some respects stronger than it had
been before. Many who previously denigrated the program came to appreciate its value. The benefits were broad, including a wider range of preventive services for children than private health insurance typically covered.
No longer tied to welfare, Medicaid had the potential to serve as a general
basis of health insurance for low-income Americans. Instead of expecting

to abolish Medicaid, liberal reformers would now think about how to incorporate it into a system of universal coverage.

From Bold Leaps to Baby Steps

Between 1993 and 1996, a cycle of initiative, miscalculation, and defeat had played out twice as Clinton and the Republicans had each tried—and failed—to recast national health policy according to a grand design. Now both sides became willing to settle for relatively innocuous, small-scale changes. This new incrementalist phase began in the summer of 1996 with the passage of legislation regulating private health insurance, and it continued in the year after Clinton was reelected, when Congress and the president compromised on a comprehensive budget agreement, including a limited program for children's health coverage. In this period, Republicans also won a trial of one of their preferred reforms, medical savings accounts, as well as more private insurance options for Medicare beneficiaries. In the remainder of Clinton's term, however, the two parties were unable to find common ground on measures such as legislation protecting patients' rights or a Clinton proposal to allow people age 55 to 64 to buy into Medicare. The period showed what bipartisan incrementalism in health policy could accomplish—and also what it could not.

Heralded at the time as a major achievement, the 1996 Health Insurance Portability and Accountability Act (HIPAA) epitomized bipartisanship. In the Senate, where it passed 98 to 0, the bill was the joint initiative of the senior Democrat on health-care issues, Ted Kennedy, and Kansas Republican Nancy L. Kassebaum. HIPAA purportedly enabled people to keep their health coverage when leaving a job and banned pre-existing-condition exclusions—except that it did so only for some people under limited conditions. The law did not make insurance "portable" in the common meaning of that term; it provided no right to carry a policy from one job to another. Rather, it prohibited a new insurer from denying coverage in certain circumstances. If a job changer moved from one firm with group health insurance to another firm that also offered group coverage, and if that employee had been insured for 18 continuous months (with no more than 63 days of lapsed coverage between jobs), the new health plan could not deny coverage of a pre-existing condition. Otherwise, the new insurer could deny that coverage for no more than 12 months (a limit that was reduced one month for every month of continuous prior group coverage).[15]

In an early draft, the legislation would also have provided the same protection for people moving from a group plan to an individually purchased policy, but the insurance industry opposed that measure on the grounds that the people who would buy coverage on their own would be relatively unhealthy, raising costs for all individual policies.[16] In the interests of bipartisan consensus, the final legislation included rules for the individual market that were so riddled with loopholes as to nullify any benefit for most consumers. For example, insurers could limit policies meeting the law's requirements to two of their products, which they were free to price at prohibitively expensive levels. States could also establish high-risk pools, also with premiums at unaffordable levels. Two years later, an investigation by the General Accounting Office found that individuals who sought policies under the law were being quoted prices "from 140 percent to 600 percent of the standard rate." Some insurance companies were also penalizing insurance agents for referring the customers with pre-existing conditions whom the law was supposed to protect.[17]

The legislation enjoyed broad backing in Congress partly because it did not regulate the prices insurers could charge or make any effort to control health-care costs. The law's most significant protection was to prohibit group plans from excluding members in poor health or charging them higher premiums. Insofar as it provided any benefits, it provided those benefits to people who already had insurance; it did nothing for the low-wage workers who didn't have jobs with group health benefits or for people who lost a job with health benefits and then couldn't afford coverage while they were unemployed.

"While the Senate bill guarantees the right to purchase health insurance, it doesn't go far enough and address the price of that policy," Rep. Dennis Hastert, the Republican deputy whip, said during the debate on the bill in the House. "Common sense tells every American that the right to purchase a health insurance policy is meaningless if you cannot afford the premium."[18] Hastert was arguing for the Republican proposal for medical savings accounts, which would allow individuals to save money for health care in a tax-free account if they purchased a health insurance policy with a high deductible ($1,500 for an individual; $3,000 for a family)—an idea logically attractive to healthy people in high tax brackets, who could expect to roll over much of their tax savings from one year to the next. The compromise in the final bill provided for a trial of 750,000 medical savings accounts for people in small firms or the individual market. But the legislation failed to deal with the problem of affordability that Hastert had highlighted.

HIPAA did fill a gap in insurance regulation that Congress had created in 1974, when it preempted state regulation of self-insured employer health plans but then failed to set any standards for those plans. Many states had adopted standards for health insurers—22 of them, for example, already limited the duration of pre-existing-condition exclusions, typically to 12 months. But the federal pre-emption had barred the states from applying those standards to self-insured employer plans, which by 1996 covered about half the privately insured.[19] HIPAA also included provisions for facilitating electronic health transactions and improving their security, and it dealt with the privacy of personal health data in an unusual way. Unable to agree on specific rules, Congress set itself a deadline, August 21, 1999, for enacting federal privacy standards, in lieu of which those standards were to be set by the secretary of Health and Human Services. As it turned out, Congress did not meet its own deadline, and the Clinton administration issued the privacy regulations. In the long run, the privacy and security standards turned out to be HIPAA's main legacy even though they received little public attention at the time.

After the Democrats' reverses in 1994, few people had expected Clinton to be reelected in 1996, but by that fall the economy was booming and Clinton easily defeated the Republican nominee Bob Dole, though the GOP held on to control of Congress. Taking full advantage of the Republicans' forays on Medicare, Clinton won elderly voters by a margin of 51 percent to 42 percent—a striking edge because below age 65, the older a voter, the more likely he or she was to vote Republican.[20] On health care, the campaign left Republicans with a bitter aftertaste. Just as Democrats believed that Republicans had "demagogued" the Clinton health plan two years earlier, so Republicans felt that Democrats did the same on Medicare in 1996. The experience seemed to show that for both parties health care held more negative political possibilities than positive ones, a lesson that discouraged large-scale initiatives by either side.

Yet rising federal revenues from economic growth facilitated political bargaining, and as part of a larger budget agreement in 1997, Clinton and Republican congressional leaders reached a deal on a series of health-care issues. The most significant result was a new government insurance program for children in families that were neither poor enough to qualify for Medicaid nor affluent enough to pay for private insurance. The State Children's Health Insurance Plan (originally SCHIP, later CHIP when the name was shortened) did not create a new individual entitlement; instead, it provided grants to the states, which they could use in different ways to extend coverage of children. Carefully calibrated to appeal to both Republicans and Democrats, the program both built on Medicaid and represented an alternative to it.

Since the 1980s, Democrats and moderate Republicans had worked together on incremental expansions of health coverage for low-income children, slowly phasing in Medicaid eligibility for all children in families with incomes below the poverty line and young children in families earning up to 33 percent over the poverty line. Some states had also used waivers of federal Medicaid rules to cover additional children. Once the Clinton plan was defeated in 1994, the interest in children's coverage revived. Just as reformers had developed a program for the elderly after national health insurance was defeated under Truman, so reformers now focused on a sympathetic age group after another loss on universal coverage.[21]

Clinton's original 1997 budget proposal included a child health initiative of only $8.6 billion over five years, an amount that grew to $24 billion in the final budget resolution. Although White House support was critical in passing the final measure, the push for a substantial program with a new design came from Congress, particularly from the Senate, where Kennedy again found a Republican co-sponsor, Orrin Hatch of Utah. Calling for a block grant rather than an entitlement, the Kennedy-Hatch bill appealed to Republicans in Congress as well as governors from both parties, who wanted to create an alternative framework to Medicaid that gave the states more flexibility and did not involve an open-ended budgetary commitment. Some liberals were wary of the proposal precisely because it allowed states flexibility to establish more limited benefits than Medicaid provided and to turn children away once the capped federal funds ran out. Worried about undermining Medicaid, Senators Jay Rockefeller of West Virginia and John Chafee of Rhode Island proposed instead to use the additional funds to expand Medicaid's coverage of children. The final legislation was something of a hybrid. It gave states a choice among three options for use of the new block grants: creating a stand-alone program for children, expanding Medicaid, or doing some mixture of the two. (By 2006, 18 states had stand-alone programs, 11 states and the District of Columbia expanded Medicaid, and 21 states combined the two.)[22] States could use the funds to cover children in families with incomes up to twice the poverty level, and the federal government would pick up a larger share of the cost—on average, about 70 percent—than under Medicaid. An increase in federal cigarette taxes helped to finance the program.

The same budget legislation that established SCHIP also gave states more flexibility in running Medicaid. Previously, states had to get a waiver from the federal government to enroll Medicaid beneficiaries in managed-care plans; under the 1997 budget act, states could require the use of managed care as long as beneficiaries had a choice between two plans. The managed-care plans would also no longer be required to enroll at least 25 percent of their members from non-Medicaid sources. Instead, the plans would have to meet a series of standards for quality assurance, access to care, and patients' rights.[23]

As Congress and the Clinton administration agreed to allow the states to shift Medicaid further toward managed care, so they also agreed on changes in Medicare in the 1997 budget act that at least superficially seemed to achieve what Gingrich had wanted two years earlier by opening up the program to more private insurance options. But the new arrangements for private plans boomeranged. Although more Medicare beneficiaries had been enrolling in managed-care plans during the previous five years, enrollment growth stalled and then reversed under the new "Medicare + Choice" program. As a result of changes that Congress made in the formula for paying private insurers, Medicare was no longer the bonanza for the managed-care industry that it had been, and many insurers cut back the benefits they offered or abandoned the Medicare market entirely.[24]

The 1997 budget agreement made other significant changes in Medicare payment. In the 1980s Congress had replaced cost-based reimbursement with prospective payment for in-patient hospital services and doctors; now it instituted prospective payment for outpatient services, skilled nursing facilities, and home health care. With those changes, the 1997 legislation completed the transition to a system of administered prices, not exactly an ideological triumph for conservatives, but a prudent fiscal measure that contributed to a general slowing of Medicare costs. One cost-containment provision of the 1997 agreement that did not work out called for automatically reducing physician fees if the rise in total expenditures on physicians' services exceeded a "sustainable growth rate." To avoid having those cuts going into effect, which might jeopardize Medicare beneficiaries' access to services, Congress in later years periodically appropriated more money to pay physicians. But with that exception, the government did carry out the measures to control Medicare costs, and those measures helped protect and sustain the program through the next decade.

It wasn't only in Medicare that managed care plans ran into problems during the mid- to late 1990s. A widespread public backlash emerged against managed care that threw into doubt the assumptions of the previous decade about the future of health care and health policy.

The managed-care "revolution" had swept through health care with astonishing speed. Among workers with job-based health coverage, the proportion in managed care had jumped from 27 percent in 1987 to 51 percent in 1993, then to 73 percent in 1995 and to 86 percent in 1998.[25] Conversely, the proportion with traditional, fee-for-service indemnity insurance had fallen to just 14 percent. Where employers offered workers a choice of options, "unmanaged care" tended to become more costly not only because it didn't control the use of services, but also because of adverse selection. The employees who stuck with the traditional option tended to be older or to suffer from chronic conditions (and thus to have relationships with doctors they didn't want to disrupt). For a while, managed care reigned triumphant. Instead of rising at a double-digit rate, health insurance premiums stayed

nearly flat for several years, leading some analysts to conclude that managed care had finally tamed medical inflation. Some of the slowdown, however, was due to a one-time savings in hospital costs, as managed-care plans
reduced admissions and lengths of stay, and to a temporary phase in the
insurance industry when companies held down rates to gain market share.
Under pressure from the insurers, doctors and other providers also made
concessions on prices and accepted new requirements for authorizing tests,
hospital stays, and referrals.

All these measures took a toll on attitudes toward managed care. Patients
and providers alike complained about bureaucratic hassles and paperwork,
and the media were rife with accusations that the plans were denying necessary care. Changes in both the enrolled populations and the managed-
care plans raised the level of tension. In their early development, HMOs
had enrolled members on a voluntary basis. To avoid having unhappy, cap-
tive patients, Kaiser-Permanente, the largest HMO, even insisted that employers offer their workers at least one other insurance option. Now many
employers switched entirely to managed care, and some of the new enrollees (and their doctors) were predictably resentful. In addition, while the
early HMOs had been nonprofit, commercial managed-care plans now
dominated the field, and their interest in making a profit raised suspicions
that they were withholding approval for care out of sheer greed.

Through the late 1990s the managed-care backlash led to changes in
both politics and the marketplace. State governments enacted patients' rights
legislation setting a variety of standards for insurers such as requirements to
offer direct access to gynecologists and obstetricians, to pay for a minimum
hospital stay for childbirth, and to cover emergency care when a prudent lay-
person would reasonably expect harm from lack of immediate medical attention. The state laws typically also required appeals procedures when plans
denied coverage. At the federal level, though, no legislation to protect the privately insured made it through Congress at a time when Republicans were
in the majority and took the side of the insurance industry on key issues.

Employers and insurers also responded to the discontent, loosening
some of the controls that they had imposed earlier. Preferred-provider organizations surged ahead of HMOs to become the dominant form of man-

aged care. Insurers also broadened their networks, often including all the major hospitals in a region, and many plans reduced or dropped requirements for pre-authorization of hospital admissions, diagnostic tests, and specialist referrals. These trends gained momentum in the late 1990s, culminating in a major relaxation of controls in 1999 by United HealthCare.[26]

During the same period, federal policy was stalemated not only on patients' rights but on other health-care issues as well. Conservatives continued to want to privatize Medicare and cut it back. In 1997 Congress created a bipartisan commission on Medicare, co-chaired by a conservative Democrat (Senator John Breaux of Louisiana) and a conservative Republican (Rep. Bill Thomas of Virginia), which two years later called for turning Medicare into a voucher system and for raising the age of eligibility for Medicare from 65 to 67. The commission could hardly have chosen a moment when the public would be less receptive to such ideas. Not only was managed care unpopular, but the growth in Medicare's costs—like those in the private sector—had slowed. In 1998 Medicare costs rose by just 1.5 percent, the smallest increase in the history of the program.

Moreover, the federal budget was moving from deficit to surplus, reducing the drive to cut back government programs. When Clinton began his second term, the Congressional Budget Office was projecting a deficit of $188 billion in 2002; by 1998, the government was running a surplus, and by 2000 the CBO was projecting a surplus of $3.1 trillion for the coming decade. According to an analysis by Alan S. Blinder and Janet L. Yellen, all of the swing in fiscal projections between 1997 and 2000 was due to economic growth and other changes in the economy; the net effect of legislated changes was actually to reduce the surplus.[27]

Amid this rising tide, Clinton proposed that instead of cutting Medicare and raising the age of eligibility, the government add a prescription-drug benefit to the program and open Medicare to people age 55 to 64. Under the latter proposal, 55- to 64-year-olds could obtain coverage for $300 to $400 a month; among that group, those who were 62 to 64 would also pay a surcharge on their Medicare premiums after they reached 65. Critics objected that voluntary Medicare enrollment would attract a high-cost population, but even if the policy required some subsidy, it still had its attraction. With its low administrative costs, Medicare was a relatively inexpensive way to insure people in that age group who were unable to obtain or afford private coverage. But opposition from the health-care industry and conservatives blocked any action.

If political circumstances had been more favorable, the late 1990s might have seen significant progress on a variety of problems, including the un-insured. But while the economic environment was benign, the political environment was poisonous. Amid the congressional impeachment of Clin-ton over the Monica Lewinsky affair, nothing much could get done. Mean-while, the federal Treasury was piling up a huge surplus. Whoever won the 2000 election would have an exceptional opportunity to set a new direction in domestic policy.

A Republican Window

In 2000 the Republicans gained control of both Congress and the White House for the first time since 1954, though it was hardly a decisive victory. George W. Bush was the first candidate in more than a century to become president after losing the national popular vote, and in the Senate the Re-publicans lost four seats, creating a 50–50 tie, broken only by the vice president. While the election did not confer much of a popular mandate, Bush and the Republicans nonetheless seized the opportunity and deci-sively changed the nation's direction at home and abroad.

Once in office Bush's priority was cutting taxes, which Congress pro-ceeded to do early in his first term through legislation that dramatically altered the fiscal outlook. Within a year, the federal budget went from sur-plus to deficit, with the benefits of the tax cuts flowing overwhelmingly to the highest earners. When fully phased in, the new rates under Bush provided an average annual cut of $19 (in 2004 dollars) for people in the bottom 20 percent, $652 for those in the middle 20 percent, and $136,398 for those with incomes over $1 million.[28]

For health care as for other issues, the election held important con-sequences. During the campaign, the Democratic nominee Al Gore had called for extending the initiatives of Clinton's second term: covering all children through an expansion of SCHIP, opening up Medicare to people aged 55 to 64, and establishing a prescription-drug benefit for seniors. Under Gore's drug plan, coverage would be free to the elderly with incomes up to 35 percent above the poverty line. Other seniors were to pay monthly premiums between $25 and $44 for coverage by Medicare of half the cost of prescriptions up to $5,000 and all of the cost above that level. Gore proposed to finance the additional cost to the government with $253 billion of the budget surplus over the next 10 years.[29]

Omitted from Medicare at its inception, prescription-drug coverage had appeared on the national agenda several times, its fate always tied to other reforms. Private insurance complicated the politics. Some seniors had coverage for drugs through corporate retiree benefits, Medigap policies, or managed-care plans, but millions remained without any protection while the cost of drugs escalated. Had it not been repealed, the Medicare Catastrophic Coverage Act would have given seniors a prescription-drug benefit. Seniors would also have gotten drug coverage under the health-care legislation proposed by Clinton in 1993. Worried about government regulation of drug prices, the pharmaceutical lobby fought both of those proposals, but in January 2000, the industry withdrew its opposition to a Medicare drug benefit, dramatically improving the prospects for enactment.[30]

During the presidential campaign in the spring of 2000, Bush endorsed the prescription-drug benefit without offering a specific proposal. After Gore seemed to be gaining traction on the issue in September and demanded that Bush "put up or shut up," Bush proposed a plan of his own—to convert Medicare into a system of competing private insurance plans that would include prescription drugs in their benefits. At one of the presidential debates that fall, the first question was about prescription coverage, and Bush accused the Democrats of failing to pass a drug benefit during the previous eight years and pledged that if elected, he would deliver. Not all campaign promises influence policy after an election. But in light of Florida's importance to his presidency, Bush had good reason to carry through on a commitment that mattered to elderly voters.

Although Congress gave Bush his tax cut, Republicans lost control of the Senate in late May when Vermont Senator Jim Jeffords defected. But they took it back in the 2002 election by a margin of 51 to 49, enough to put Bush in a position to win passage of a prescription-drug benefit and make it the first federal health-care entitlement program with a Republican stamp.

Despite his announced intention not to raise the deficit further, Bush committed himself to spend $400 billion over 10 years on the program. Under the outline he gave Congress, the elderly would get full drug coverage only if they left traditional Medicare and enrolled in a private insurance plan. Not even the Republican majority in Congress, however, would go along with that approach. In the Senate, a bipartisan bill emerged from the Finance Committee, where the chairman, Republican Charles Grassley of Iowa, worked closely with two Democrats, Breaux of Louisiana and Max Baucus of Montana. Under the committee's bill, the elderly who sought subsidized prescription coverage through Medicare would have a choice. They could stay in traditional Medicare and sign up for a stand-alone drug plan offered by a private insurer, or they could opt for a private managed-care plan for all their health coverage, including a drug benefit. The Senate bill provided for a "fallback" government drug-benefit plan in the event that multiple private stand-alone drug plans were not available in an area. The rationale for this fallback plan was that private insurers did not sell drug-only insurance at the time, and the insurance industry itself was skeptical about the feasibility of such policies. Consequently, the government would offer drug coverage directly in case a private market did not materialize. The Finance Committee's bill passed the Senate 76 to 21.

Passage of the legislation was more difficult in the House, where the Republican leadership ultimately prevailed, 216 to 215, with a bill that included a concession to solidify support among conservatives: a subsidy estimated to cost $174 billion for tax-exempt health savings accounts (an expanded version of the earlier medical savings accounts). But compromise between the House and Senate proved difficult, ultimately requiring the intercession of the House and Senate Republican leaders. And when the legislation went back for final votes, it faced sharp opposition. In the Senate, most Democrats opposed the revised measure (which, among other things, lacked a public fall-back plan), but they did not resort to a filibuster, and the bill passed 54 to 44. (This was in keeping with the apparently unwritten rule for health legislation that the requisite majority was only 51 for a Republican bill but 60 for a Democratic one.) In the House, the vote came at 3 a.m. on November 22. After the 15 minutes normally allowed for voting, the bill seemed headed for defeat, but Republican leaders kept the vote open until 5:55 a.m. while they arm-twisted uncooperative members of their own party—doing "the kind of horse-trading that has always been part of politics," presidential adviser Karl Rove later delicately called it—eventually turning around enough votes to win passage 220 to 215.[31]

The legislation might not have passed if the administration had divulged its own internal estimates of the cost. What Congress knew at the time it voted was that CBO had projected a cost of $395 billion over 10 years; Congress didn't know that the chief actuary of Medicare had made a higher estimate and been ordered not to release it. Soon after the bill was enacted, the Office of Management and Budget raised the projected cost by 35 percent to $534 billion. In passing the drug program, moreover, Congress had suspended its normal budget rules. The legislation provided no financing whatsoever for the additional cost, even though the surplus inherited by Bush had already vanished. Neither the Clinton administration in 1993 nor the Obama administration in 2009 had the nerve to propose an expanded health-care entitlement without paying for it. But the Republicans in 2003 did exactly that in the single most important health-care legislation passed by Congress in a period that had begun in 1995 with Gingrich and other Republicans promising to overturn the welfare state and require a balanced budget.

The Medicare Prescription Drug, Improvement, and Modernization Act—known generally as the Medicare Modernization Act (MMA)—may be thought of as having three distinct parts: prescription-drug coverage, new provisions for private insurance options in Medicare, and tax incentives for health savings accounts (HSAs). Each part reflected distinctive political and ideological concerns.

The new prescription-drug coverage, unlike the rest of Medicare, was to come entirely through private insurance. Though individual insurers could bargain with pharmaceutical companies, the law barred the government from negotiating directly with the drug industry over prices. As a result, the elderly (and the Medicare program) would pay higher prices for drugs than did the Veterans Administration or people in countries such as Canada whose governments negotiate on their behalf. On all its major concerns, the pharmaceutical industry got everything it wanted from the legislation.

As a result, however, the billions of dollars spent on the program could not go as far in providing coverage as they might have. If Medicare beneficiaries signed up for Part D (as the new prescription program was called) when it went into effect in 2006, they would pay $35 in monthly premiums, an annual deductible of $250, one-fourth of the cost of drugs between $250 and $2,250, *all* of the cost from $2,250 to $5,100 (the so-called "donut hole"), and 5 percent of the cost above that level. In other words, out of the first $5,100 in yearly drug costs, they would have to pay $4,020 (79 percent) out of pocket. The legislation also barred them from purchasing supplemental "wraparound" coverage to reduce any of this amount.[32]

But, instead of buying the stand-alone drug policy to go with traditional Medicare, the elderly could enroll instead in a private insurance plan that would cover drugs along with other health costs. To make that switch more attractive, the legislation introduced provisions for deliberately paying private insurers more than it cost Medicare to cover the same beneficiaries. By 2008, according to an analysis by the commission created by Congress to review Medicare payments, the plans were being paid an extra $1,100 per beneficiary per year.[33] The plans—renamed Medicare Advantage plans—used some of this money to provide extra benefits to their enrollees, including better prescription-drug coverage. In effect, the legislation ultimately achieved what Bush intended at the beginning: to shift more of the elderly into private insurance. (About one-fourth enrolled in Medicare Advantage plans by 2008.) In 1995 Gingrich had claimed that private insurance plans would reduce Medicare's costs, indeed, stave off bankruptcy. Actually, the private plans had turned out to raise costs because they skimmed off the healthier elderly. Now Congress and the Bush administration could hardly even pretend to be saving money for Medicare; the new payment provisions were a straight-forward give-away.

Ideologically, the establishment of a new entitlement to prescription drugs under Medicare offended many conservatives, but the political logic was clear. Republicans had long been trying to take Medicare as an issue away from the Democrats. Gingrich thought he could win over the elderly by promising to save Medicare at a time when he was trying to cut it. Bush tried the more promising path of expanding the program. But providing windfall gains to the pharmaceutical and insurance industries had the unfortunate result of leaving the program with an unappealing benefit package. At the time Bush signed the bill, polls showed only 26 percent of seniors approved of the program, with 47 percent against and the rest undecided. Among the public as a whole, opinion ran against the legislation 56 percent to 39 percent.[34] Once again, the negative political possibilities of health care seemed to be greater than the positive ones.

The final element of the Medicare Modernization Act, unrelated to Medicare, was an expansion of tax-advantaged savings accounts linked to a high-deductible private insurance policy. In their first incarnation as "medical savings accounts," this new form of health insurance did not attract much interest. The number of accounts established never came close to the 750,000 allowed by Congress in 1996 when it authorized a demonstration, which was limited to the self-employed and employees of small businesses. Although Congress had called for an official evaluation of the trial, the accounts had so few takers that no evaluation was ever carried out. One analysis of tax data for 2001, however, found that the people who established the accounts were disproportionately high-income, and half of the accounts ended the same year they began.[35]

Despite this tepid debut, Congress expanded the program in 2003. Under the law, people could have a tax-advantaged health savings account (HSA) as of 2004 if they bought health insurance with a deductible of at least $1,000 for an individual or $2,000 for a family. Previously, either the employer or the employee could make deposits into the account; under the new rules, both could do so, up to the amount of the deductible (a limit that was later relaxed). A ruling by the IRS also opened another tax-advantaged savings option, a "health reimbursement arrangement" (HRA).

The advocates of tax-sheltered savings options with high-deductible insurance presented them as the conservative answer to rising health costs. In this view, because of the high deductible, consumers would have more money of their own at stake in paying for health care and an incentive to shop around for the best bargains. The high-deductible would deter "moral hazard" (the problem that insurance encourages the use of services and therefore raises total costs). The name that advocates gave to this approach, "consumer-driven health care," highlighted a seeming contrast with managed care. Instead of top-down controls, the consumer-driven alternative would put individual patients in the driver's seat—market-oriented conservative populism at work.

In practice, however, things did not work out as imagined. The number of high-deductible health plans with a savings option did increase— to 6.1 million by January 2008, still a small proportion of those with insurance—but the high-deductible plans were merged into managed care rather than becoming an alternative to it. As James C. Robinson and Paul B. Ginsburg observe, insurers offering high-deductible plans have typically employed standard managed-care controls ("disease management for enrollees with chronic conditions; case management for enrollees with complex . . . conditions; and utilization management for patients using particularly costly drugs, devices, or procedures"). Rather than leaving consumers to bargain with providers, the insurers have used preferred-provider networks, with prices negotiated not by individual consumers but by the insurer (often based on Medicare's administered prices).[36] The HSAs were supposed to unleash consumers to drive health care; instead, they have resulted in the combination of two forms of restraint on consumers' use of services: the high deductible at the front end, managed care thereafter.

None of this ought to be surprising. Health-care spending is highly concentrated in a small proportion of high-cost cases. In any given year, the most costly 5 percent of people account for more than 50 percent of health-care costs, and the top 10 percent of people account for 70 percent of costs—and most of the spending on their care takes place above the deductibles even in high-deductible plans.[37] To control the cost of these policies, insurers could not rely on the deductibles alone. Furthermore, once patients are in the health-care system, doctors and other health-care providers make most of the decisions critically affecting costs. The theory of consumer-driven care rests on a conception of the patient as economic man that does not fit the realities of illness, especially the conditions under which the greatest health-care costs are generated.[38]

It is also not even clear that the combination of HSAs and high-deductible plans significantly increases cost-sharing compared with what consumers otherwise face. The main evidence that cost-sharing restrains health spending comes from an experiment in the 1970s that compared an insurance plan with high cost-sharing to a plan that had none.[39] But by the early 2000s, deductibles and co-insurance had risen sharply throughout the insurance market. In the PPOs that dominate the market, consumers have to pay out-of-pocket costs with after-tax dollars; HSAs and HRAs reduce sensitivity to costs by allowing the use of pre-tax dollars to cover those expenses. In the United States, it does not take all that much medical care to reach the point where the up-front cost-sharing becomes irrelevant. Many high-deductible plans even include a maximum limit on out-of-pocket costs (as of 2005, these averaged $2,551). If consumers know they are going to hit their out-of-pocket maximum, they will also have no incentive to economize even on the amount below the limit because they will incur that cost regardless.[40]

But high-deductible plans with a savings option may spread because they are more attractive to the healthy. Without government regulation, the cost of any insurance plan depends on who signs up for it. Not only do the most costly 10 percent of people account for 70 percent of total health costs in a population, but the least expensive 50 percent of people account for only 3 percent of costs. An insurance plan that draws chiefly from this low-cost population will have an advantage in the free market. If employers offer a choice between low-and high-deductible plans, the high-deductible option will tend to attract employees expecting low costs, who can then roll over their savings to the next year. Consumers who expect major expenses (for example, when they are planning an elective procedure, expecting a baby, or have just been diagnosed with a costly medical condition) will tend to opt for a low-deductible plan. But because of adverse selection of this kind, low-deductible options will become increasingly expensive, driving away more healthy people. When managed care plans grew during the 1980s and 1990s, they attracted younger, healthier employees who didn't have ongoing relationships with doctors. Adverse selection then helped to kill off fee-for-service. Adverse selection may now do the same to low-deductible health insurance.

HSAs also seem likely to spread for other reasons at both the low and high ends of the labor market. At the low end, employers can use high-deductible plans to cut the cost of premiums, leaving their employees to make contributions to the HSAs. A survey of small business found that some firms were using high-deductible plans with HSAs as a "last ditch" effort to provide their workers some kind of insurance. The same survey also found that small employers with highly paid professionals "view HSAs as attractive options because of their value as tax-favored savings vehicles."[41]

In fact, HSAs should appeal to high earners even if they have no intention of using the money for health care. Deposits in HSAs reduce taxable income dollar-for-dollar and accumulate tax-free, and after age 65 they can be withdrawn for any purpose without penalty. The HSAs may not do much to control health care costs, but they are an excellent means of sheltering income from taxes. In 2006, thanks to legislation sponsored by Republicans Eric Cantor and Paul Ryan, Congress relaxed the earlier limit on HSA contributions, enabling people to contribute up to $2,700 per individual and $5,450 per family, even if the deductibles in their health insurance are lower. High earners who don't take advantage of opportunities to use HSAs to reduce their taxes do not have good financial consultants.

Aside from the distribution of drug discount cards to the low-income elderly in mid-2004 (in time for Bush's reelection campaign), the introduction of the new Medicare prescription drug benefit came on January 1, 2006. Unfortunately, the administration had not anticipated the difficulties that 25 million seniors and 60,000 retail pharmacies would have in dealing not with one schedule of benefits, but with 1,429 new private drug plans offered through Medicare. What ensued was a fiasco. Because plans had different formularies, seniors had sometimes signed up with insurers that did not offer the drugs they had been prescribed. Many of the elderly had not yet received their insurance cards and were confused by how the program worked. In a poll that January, 77 percent of seniors said the prescription drug program was "too complicated."[42] As Atul Gawande writes, "Tens of thousands were unable to get their prescriptions filled, many for essential drugs like insulin, inhalers, and blood-pressure medications. The result was a public-health crisis in thirty-seven states, which had to provide emergency pharmacy payments for the frail. We will never know how many were harmed, but it is likely that the program killed people."[43]

Whether the disastrous implementation of the prescription drug program was a factor in the Republicans' loss of Congress in November 2006 is difficult to say. Health care was only the fourth or fifth top-ranked issue in polls. At the beginning of 2006, seniors disapproved of the prescription-drug program by a two-to-one margin, but support increased through the year and, according to one poll, tipped in favor of the program by November. But in other surveys that fall, voters said they trusted the Democrats more than Republicans on all health-care issues, including Medicare prescription drugs.[44]

The difficulties surrounding the introduction of the prescription-drug benefit in 2006 would later affect the view of Democrats in 2010 about the implementation of the new health exchanges under the Affordable Care Act. Worried that similar problems might complicate their reelection efforts in 2012, Democrats in Congress decided it would be better to defer implementation until 2014, even though that long delay put the legislation at risk of being overturned in the event a new president took office in January 2013.

Return to Crisis

Rising health-care costs came back with a vengeance in the early 2000s, pitching the United States back into the thick of the problems that some thought the marketplace was resolving during the previous decade. Two developments—stagnant incomes for the majority of people and a shift of health outlays from employers to workers—heightened the pressures. While the economy grew from 2000 to 2006, the gains from economic growth, like the Bush tax breaks, went to people at the top. Real median household income fell 3 percent in a period when the average annual premiums for employer-sponsored family coverage rose 87 percent, from $6,348 to $11,480.[45] At the same time, employers were also reducing the level of coverage in an average plan through higher deductibles and other changes. So the rise in health-care costs hit many of those even in the protected public.

These developments had predictable effects. As health costs soared, fewer firms offered health insurance, more people became uninsured, and the financial stress of health care increased. From 2000 and 2006, the proportion of firms offering health insurance fell from 69 percent to 61 percent, and the number of workers with health insurance benefits dropped by about 6 million.[46] Despite growth in Medicaid, the number uninsured at any one time rose from 40 to 45 million, to about 15.3 percent of the population. From 2001 to 2006, the share of Americans experiencing a high financial burden from health costs—defined as spending more than 10 percent of pre-tax income on insurance premiums and out-of-pocket expenses—rose by one percentage point per year, reaching 19 percent in 2006.[47] Part of this increase in financial burden reflected the more limited coverage that the insured were receiving. According to one measure, underinsurance—that is, being exposed to high costs despite having health coverage—increased by 60 percent between 2003 and 2007.[48]

The one bright spot in this otherwise grim picture was an improvement in access to health insurance and health care for children. The new SCHIP program covered 6.1 million children by 1994. Roughly 20 million children had also been added to Medicaid since the mid-1980s as a result of the federally mandated expansion of Medicaid coverage to poor children. Some liberals had feared that SCHIP would undermine Medicaid, but because states had to screen children for Medicaid eligibility before determining whether they qualified for the new program, SCHIP indirectly spurred the enrollment of more children in Medicaid too. These increases in public coverage reduced the proportion of uninsured children from 22.3 percent to 14.9 percent between 1997 and 2005. Republicans objected that SCHIP was "crowding out" private coverage of children, but the evidence indicates that only a minority of children in SCHIP would have otherwise had private insurance, and even those children would have had far more limited coverage than they had through SCHIP.[49]

In contrast, the programs adopted during the 12 years of Republican control of Congress did little for working-age adults. Though HIPAA was supposed to end pre-existing-condition exclusions, the law ended the exclusions effectively only for people who moved directly from one employer to another with group health benefits. Most of those who were previously deemed uninsurable on account of pre-existing conditions were still deemed uninsurable. HSAs worked for the affluent and healthy, not exactly the population in need of assistance.

These developments affected Americans in a highly personal way. In surveys sponsored by the Kaiser Family Foundation beginning in 2004, health costs ranked among Americans' main worries about the future. While one-fifth of people said they worried about being the victim of violent crime or a terrorist attack or about losing their job, two-fifths reported being worried about "not being able to afford" health care. In a 2005 survey, 21 percent reported having medical bills that were overdue.[50]

For conservatives, however, the major cause of Americans' problems in health care was "overinsurance." If only Americans had to pay more money out of pocket, consumers would drive health care in the rational way that other markets worked. As it happened, Americans already paid a higher proportion of health-care costs out of pocket than did the people of other rich democracies. Internationally, there was also no relationship between out-of-pocket costs and total health expenditures.[51] Nonetheless, for conservatives the solution lay in privatizing health care in two senses—shifting functions from government to private business and shifting costs to the individual.

Yet even on its own terms, the conservative counterrevolution that Gingrich initiated—the second attempted counterrevolution, if we count the Reagan years—could hardly be judged a success. As in other advanced societies, welfare-state retrenchment generally slowed growth in government spending without reversing it. Health-care programs have been especially difficult for right-wing governments to reverse. Under Margaret Thatcher, Britain's Conservative Party privatized a variety of state enterprises, but not the National Health Service. After Gingrich failed at privatizing Medicare, Bush had more success when he sugar-coated privatization by adding a Medicare prescription drug benefit. But the 2003 Medicare Modernization Act was not exactly a triumph of conservative principle. The drug benefit added a new government entitlement, and the private Medicare Advantage programs cost more than $1,000 extra per beneficiary. The Republican policies might be counted a success if they had at least stabilized the health-care system. But when a dozen years of Republican control of Congress came to an end in November 2006, the problems of cost and coverage were worse than before. The stage was set for new battles in the long-running ideological war over health care.

PART III

ROLLERCOASTER

CHAPTER 6

The Rise of a Reform Consensus,
2006–2008

BY LATE 2006, ECONOMIC AND political developments put comprehensive health-care reform back in play again. During the previous six years, just as in the period before Clinton's election, health-care costs and insurance premiums had risen far more rapidly than incomes, renewing the sense of urgency about reforms that would deal with both costs and coverage. The 2006 election then renewed the sense of political possibility by returning both the House and Senate to the Democrats. As the presidential election cycle got under way, public opinion surveys indicated the Democrats would hold the advantage: George W. Bush's approval ratings sank to levels not seen for a president since shortly before Richard Nixon resigned, and voters preferred the Democrats to the Republicans on a wide range of issues, even taxes, usually a Republican advantage. On health care, the Democrats' edge jumped from 21 to 30 points between 2004 and 2007.[1]

Yet nothing guaranteed that if the Democrats won the White House and increased their control of Congress in 2008, they would be able to pass substantial health-care legislation. Earlier failures haunted activists and politicians alike. The supporters of reform might again split over rival plans and dissipate their energies in internal battles. The interest groups that opposed legislation in the past might once more put their money and influence behind the opposition. Public support for reform could wither if the opponents could again convince people with good insurance that change would come at their expense.

Anticipating these difficulties, a variety of groups began to prepare for the chance that the 2008 election might open another window for reform. Some of these preparations aimed to develop proposals that could win wide support and build consensus between reformers and key interest groups and across party lines. Other efforts strengthened the technical basis for reform; for example, the Congressional Budget Office hired additional staff in health-care finance and undertook a major assessment of policy options to control costs and expand coverage. Still other efforts laid the foundations for a grass-roots network in support of health-care reform. As the campaign for the Democratic presidential nomination got under way, unions and activists also sought to ensure that that all the major candidates would have to deal with health care and commit themselves to a comprehensive reform program.

Even though the two major parties disagreed fundamentally about government's role in health care, the conventional wisdom was that health-care reform would have to be bipartisan. American politics was generally caught between a reality and a hope—the reality of ideological polarization and the yearning for a different kind of politics that transcended partisanship. The two candidates who eventually captured their party's nominations, Barack Obama and John McCain, would both appeal to that yearning for a different politics without being able to create it. The trend toward party polarization was long and deep in the making. Traditionally, political parties in the United States had been broad coalitions that overlapped each other ideologically. The Republicans had included liberals, especially from the Northeast and the Pacific Northwest, and the Democrats had included conservatives, especially from the South. These moderating influences blurred party differences and facilitated bipartisan alliances on specific policies. But by 2009, the ideological alignment of the parties was nearly complete. The shift of the South to the Republicans and the conservative revolution inside the GOP had tilted the party sharply to the right. Liberal Republicans were virtually extinct, and moderate Republicans were on the endangered-species list. A similar process had taken place among the Democrats but not gone as far; the Democratic caucus in Congress still included moderates and even conservatives, though they were less numerous and influential than they had once been. But just as the activist base of the GOP was conservative, the activist base of the Democratic Party was liberal, and as the two parties moved away from each other, fewer centrists remained in Congress capable of building broad coalitions.

The trend toward polarization had complex effects. The growing ideological divergence between the two parties made cooperation between them more difficult. By the same token, each party was more homogenous and therefore more capable of enacting legislation on its own if it had a majority in the House and 60 votes in the Senate. In 2010, that is how comprehensive health-care legislation would pass Congress. But that is not how the model for the legislation began. The model originated in a bipartisan reform that emerged from one of the states, and it was a Republican governor—Mitt Romney of Massachusetts—whose leadership made it possible.

Romney and the Massachusetts Model

In 2006, building on a series of measures it had previously taken, Massachusetts became the first state to achieve near-universal health coverage. Bipartisanship was not an incidental feature of the Massachusetts breakthrough. The state could not have succeeded without assistance from both Democratic and Republican administrations in Washington and without the concurrence of state leaders from both parties. Massachusetts Democrats had long been pursuing universal coverage unsuccessfully through a policy that emphasized a strong employer mandate. That approach drew resistance from business and stood no chance of passage under a Republican governor. The stalemate was broken only when the state's Democrats agreed to compromise on a plan favored by Governor Romney that relied on an individual mandate.

States have long varied sharply in the share of their population without health insurance. The disparities reflect the states' economic and demographic characteristics as well as their institutions and politics. For example, states with more employment in large firms and more unionized workers tend to have higher rates of private coverage because job-based insurance varies directly with firm size and unionization. Race and ethnicity also have an independent effect not reducible to income, industrial mix, or other state characteristics. Relatively larger numbers of African Americans and

Hispanics in a state are associated with lower rates of private coverage, and the same states also tend to have less generous public policies.[2] A primary factor in determining the extent of public coverage through Medicaid is the prevailing ideology in a state—how conservative or liberal its politics and policies generally tend to be.[3] Averaging Census data from 2007 to 2009, the South and Southwest accounted for nearly all the states with uninsured rates higher than the national average; Texas topped the list with 25.5 percent of its population uninsured. In contrast, the six states with the fewest uninsured (under 10 percent) were primarily in New England and the upper Midwest.[4] The one state outside the North with fewer than 10 percent uninsured was Hawaii, which in 1974 had required employers to pay 50 percent of health insurance premiums and then obtained an exemption from ERISA, the federal law passed later the same year blocking state regulation of employee benefit plans.

Medicare, Medicaid, ERISA, federal tax provisions, and other federal laws limit state health policy in some ways and support it in others. To conservative state leaders, Medicaid long represented the most bothersome intrusion, primarily because it gave certain groups among the poor, particularly the disabled, pregnant mothers, and children, an entitlement to medical services that the states had to meet, albeit it with federal assistance. The "unfunded mandates" adopted by Congress beginning in the 1980s that extended mandatory eligibility for low-income children and pregnant women drew particularly sharp conservative objections. In that same decade, however, conservatives at both the national and state levels succeeded in rolling back earlier programs for planning and regulation of hospitals and other facilities. Conservatives also generally favored deregulating the insurance market, which meant, among other things, eliminating state laws requiring health insurers to provide particular kinds of benefits. (Another way of achieving the same result would be to pass a federal law allowing insurers to sell policies across state lines.) Many conservatives in the states saw high-deductible, stripped-down insurance as the solution to the problem of the uninsured. Another policy favored by many conservatives was the establishment of high-risk pools, to be operated for people who were otherwise unable to buy coverage. By the early 1990s, more than 20 states had already established such pools. But because health-care costs are so heavily concentrated in a small percentage of the population—and the pools basically enable people with high costs to share risk with one another—the insurance offered through the pools was unaffordable to the great majority of people turned away by private insurers. As a result, the high-risk pools covered only about 2 percent of the eligible population; by 2003, some 30 state high-risk pools enrolled a total of 173,000 people.[5]

For liberals in the states who wanted to achieve universal coverage, federal policy created major difficulties. The same health policy trap that existed at the national level ensnared the states: Medicare, Medicaid, tax-advantaged employer-based insurance, and other federal programs protected enough of the public, and so benefited the health-care industry, that it was difficult to mobilize support for substantial change, especially any change that involved new taxes. Beginning in the late 1980s, progressive groups organized campaigns for single-payer insurance in the more liberal states but failed in every one, even in Vermont. Federal law also complicated any effort to pass state legislation regarding employer obligations. Under ERISA, any firm that self-insured could free itself of state regulations. As the courts generally interpreted the law, ERISA barred states from requiring self-insured employers to share in the full, community-wide pooling of risk for health costs.[6]

But federal policy also gave the more liberally inclined states at least partial support to expand coverage. Under Medicaid, states had the option to cover more low-income people who fell into the categories eligible for the program. For example, while states had to cover children with disabilities whose families were poor enough to qualify for federal Supplemental Security Income, they had the option of covering additional disabled children in families with incomes up to three times the poverty level. After its enactment in 1997, SCHIP expanded the options for coverage of low-income children and increased the share of costs assumed by the federal government. In addition, states could get "research and demonstration" waivers from federal Medicaid and SCHIP requirements, allowing them to cover low-income groups ordinarily ineligible for both programs—such as childless adults—if they could show savings on their existing beneficiaries so that the federal government would face no higher costs. Under President Clinton, many states received waivers to use managed care to reduce Medicaid costs and expand eligibility. In addition, the federal government also provided payments to states for hospitals bearing a "disproportionate share" of the poor and uninsured, and many states devised accounting gimmicks to increase that money. Through these different routes, states could maximize the flow of federal revenue, potentially covering many of the uninsured. Massachusetts would become the first state to figure out how to build on federal financing to insure nearly all its people.

Massachusetts held peculiar importance in health policy not only because of what it achieved in 2006, but also because of the connections between the state and national politics. Its senior senator, Edward M. Kennedy, had long been the leading Democratic spokesman on health care, and two other Massachusetts Democrats, Governor Michael Dukakis and Senator John Kerry, became candidates for president. Governor Romney ran for the Republican nomination in 2008 and became the Republican candidate in 2012. Hawaii's success with an employer mandate might escape notice or be dismissed as an anomaly far off in the Pacific, but the Bay State—home of the American Revolution—had too high a national profile to be ignored.

Massachusetts didn't make it to universal coverage on the first try. In April 1988, while he was campaigning for the Democratic presidential nomination, Governor Dukakis signed legislation widely understood at the time to be the first in any state to guarantee health insurance for all. The law relied on a mandate, scheduled to take effect in 1992, requiring employers to provide insurance to their workers or pay a tax of up to $1,680 per employee (12 percent on the first $14,000 in wages). Other provisions provided coverage for the unemployed, college students, and the disabled and raised payments to hospitals (which had helped derail Dukakis' original bill).[7] By 1991, however, the state had a Republican governor, William Weld, who opposed the employer requirement, and amid a recession and fiscal crisis, support for the mandate collapsed. But rather than repeal the law, the Democratic legislature postponed the mandate while maintaining other provisions that expanded coverage.

The legislature's decision to keep the employer mandate on the books became important in a second phase of reform. In 1993 Weld sought a federal waiver to allow the state to move Medicaid beneficiaries into managed care and use the savings to expand coverage. Concerned that the managed-care plans might drain revenues from safety-net hospitals, the Clinton administration suggested that the state ask for a supplemental sum to protect those institutions. The waiver, approved in 1995, included an initial $100 million for that purpose. The state legislature then sought to enlarge the program further, voting for a 25-cents-a-pack tax on cigarettes to expand Medicaid coverage for children in families initially with incomes up to 133 percent, then to 200 percent, of the federal poverty level. Governor Weld vetoed that bill, but according to John McDonough, who chaired one of the key legislative committees at the time, Democrats then proposed a deal to business, offering to repeal the old employer mandate in exchange for business support of the cigarette tax. Business groups accepted the bargain, and in 1996 the legislature overrode Weld's veto.[8] The idea of financing expanded children's health coverage with a tobacco tax became the basis for Senator Edward M. Kennedy's proposal for a national children's health insurance program, which Congress enacted the next year.

As a result of these measures, the uninsured population in Massachusetts fell significantly—state surveys showed a drop of almost one-half between 1995 and 2000—but whether the state could continue on that course was unclear. Although the Bush administration renewed the Medicaid waiver in 2002, the renewal was only for three years. By 2003, a new effort to achieve universal coverage was under way, initiated by Andrew Dreyfus, president of the Massachusetts Blue Cross Blue Shield Foundation, who commissioned studies on the state's uninsured from a Washington research organization, the Urban Institute. Dreyfus also began bringing together the state's medical, business, and political leaders at periodic meetings to spur another effort at reform.[9]

That same year, Romney became the fourth Republican in a row to serve as governor in a predominantly Democratic state. Like George W. Bush, Romney was the conservative son of a more centrist Republican father, but as a governor he had to get his programs and budget approved in a political climate more liberal than Bush's Texas. A career in management consulting had also given Romney long experience as a practical problem-solver. Although he had not campaigned on health care, Romney began to focus on the problem during 2003 at the suggestion of one of his friends, Tom Stemberg, the founder of Staples. The first effort in Romney's administration to come up with an initiative for the governor proposed an expansion of Medicaid, but Romney was not about to go in that direction. After having publicly committed himself to offer a new policy, however, the governor needed to develop a plan.

As a result, in the spring of 2004, Romney turned to a new team led by Tim Murphy, a former investment banker who had joined the governor's budget office and then became his director of policy. For the next nine months, Murphy worked closely with Romney, trying to bring a fresh perspective to health care, "unencumbered" by the past or by any interest-group connections.[10] In the governor's view, according to Murphy, there already was a lot of money for the uninsured in the system, but it was poorly allocated, and the insurance market did not work well for small business. As Murphy saw it, he had to "follow the money" and penetrate the "opaque financial arrangements" in health care. The state had a large uncompensated care pool, which paid hospitals for charity care. What if instead of going to institutions that money went to individuals to help them afford insurance? In some cases, hospitals were drawing on the uncompensated care pool for uninsured patients even though the patients were eligible for Medicaid, which would have been a better choice for the state because of federal matching funds. An online gateway to state programs could solve that problem by automatically enrolling such patients in Medicaid. Of the 500,000 uninsured, roughly 20 percent were eligible for Medicaid and should be enrolled, another 40 percent had incomes under three times the poverty level and could pay part of the cost of insurance, and the remaining 40 percent had incomes over that level and could afford coverage if the market were organized more efficiently and gave them the chance to buy insurance that made sense for them. A successful policy needed to address the challenges for each of these groups.

In the midst of this process—Murphy and his team were testing out their ideas in collaborative discussions with stakeholders in the system—the state's leaders had a new and urgent reason to take action on health-care finance. In the fall of 2004, Bush administration officials indicated that while they would renew Massachusetts' basic Medicaid waiver, they objected to the supplemental sum for safety-net providers, which thanks to creative accounting by the state had grown to $396 million.[11] Rather than surrender those funds and bring on a state budget crisis, Romney decided to try to keep the federal aid on the basis of a market-oriented plan that would cover virtually all the remaining uninsured.

To address the problems in the insurance market for individuals and small groups, Murphy turned to the leading conservative think tank, the Heritage Foundation, which had been working on an idea for an insurance exchange to create a more efficient market with lower transaction costs. "Mitt got it," Murphy says. Romney also wanted to reduce regulatory requirements in state insurance law that raised private premiums. So his plan—developed with advice from Heritage and cost estimates by MIT economist Jonathan Gruber—proposed to eliminate state mandates and make insurance with high deductibles and other limits available through an exchange to individuals as well as firms with fewer than 50 workers. The funds in the state's uncompensated care pool—$538 million in 2005—could then help pay for premium subsidies for people with incomes under three times the poverty level. The final question was whether there should be an individual mandate—a requirement for all adults to purchase at least a minimum, low-cost, high-deductible policy. At a meeting with both political and policy advisers, according to Murphy, the question arose as to whether the mandate was "consistent with our principles," and the answer was that it was appropriate to insist on "personal responsibility." According to Gruber, some of the governor's advisers were wary, telling Romney, in effect, "You can't do this as a Republican," but Gruber saw the governor as being in "management-consultant mode."[12] Here was a way to avert a state budget crisis and solve the problem of the uninsured on the basis of what Romney believed to be conservative principles. Some observers speculated that he hoped to rise to the presidency on the basis of the program.

Working with Senator Kennedy, Romney persuaded the Bush administration in January 2005 to approve the full Medicaid waiver. The one proviso was that the state had to pass legislation to comply with federal requirements by July 2006.[13] That deadline effectively put the state under an ultimatum: come up with a plan for expanded health coverage or lose hundreds of millions in federal aid. To help force the issue, a coalition of advocacy organizations began circulating petitions for a ballot initiative on universal health care.

When Romney released his detailed proposal in June 2005, he was emphatic in his defense of the individual mandate. "It's the ultimate conservative idea, which is that people have responsibility for their own care, and they don't look to government . . . if they can afford to take care of themselves," he told reporters after a speech introducing the proposal. Calling for tax penalties, including garnishment of wages, if someone refused to comply, Romney said, "No more 'free riding,' if you will, where an individual says: 'I'm not going to pay, even though I can afford it.' "[14] Romney's proposal did include an alternative to buying health insurance: individuals could post a $10,000 bond with the state to show they had the wherewithal to pay for their own health care. And the minimum policy satisfying the mandate would need to cover only catastrophic health costs. "We embraced the mandate under that structure," Murphy says, although the legislation Romney ultimately signed did not include either the bond alternative or a provision for catastrophic-only coverage.

The individual-mandate approach received support from another quarter, the Urban Institute group commissioned by Dreyfus of the Blue Cross Foundation. According to John Holahan, one of the institute's economists, although their evaluation of policy options included an employer mandate, they saw it as a dead end and urged Dreyfus to push for an individual mandate instead.[15] Like Romney, the Urban Institute team said that a high-deductible policy should count as the minimum required coverage. Their proposal recommended that besides enacting either an individual or an employer mandate (or both), the state expand MassHealth, its combined Medicaid/SCHIP program, to take advantage of federal matching funds. For low-income people not eligible for those programs, the state would need to provide income-related tax credits to make insurance more affordable. The plan also proposed a new purchasing pool to cut costs and improve choices for individuals and small groups; government-funded reinsurance would spread the risk of very high-cost cases.[16]

Each chamber of the state legislature took its own approach. In November 2005 the Massachusetts House approved a bill imposing both an individual and an employer mandate; the latter required firms with more than 10 workers to provide insurance or to pay a tax of 5 to 7 percent of wages, depending on firm size. The House bill also expanded Medicaid eligibility, established an insurance exchange, and provided income-related subsidies up to 300 percent of poverty for adults ineligible for Medicaid.[17] A few days later, the Massachusetts Senate rejected any kind of mandate, voting instead for a modest expansion of Medicaid and the creation of an insurance exchange without any subsidies.[18] Then everything came to a halt: from November to late February, the governor and the two houses of the legislature seemed at an impasse.[19] As it had since 1988, the issue that dominated the Massachusetts political debate about health coverage was the employer mandate. But, according to the *Boston Globe*, a private meeting on March 1 broke the stalemate:

> In a scene right out of the days of the Vault, the secretive group of Boston business executives that for decades influenced public policy, Jack Connors, chairman of Partners HealthCare, convened a March 1 meeting of local powerbrokers to deal with a crisis in the healthcare industry.
>
> Sweeping legislation to expand health coverage and set aside hundreds of millions of dollars in new payments for Massachusetts hospitals appeared near death, a casualty of conflicting agendas and egos on Beacon Hill. It was up to these business leaders to forge a compromise.
>
> "There were a number of us in the business community and in the healthcare field who wanted to be sure that we didn't miss this opportunity," said Peter Meade, executive vice president of Blue Cross and Blue Shield of Massachusetts, and one of the select few invited to the meeting at Connors's advertising agency, Hill Holliday.
>
> The quiet gathering in a John Hancock Tower conference room underscored a changing of the guard: Hospital and healthcare executives have replaced the barons of banking at the pinnacle of power in Boston.[20]

The *Globe*'s description lends itself to a conspiratorial interpretation of the Massachusetts reforms. But the reforms the legislature then adopted also enjoyed overwhelming support in public opinion polls.[21] Under the compromise worked out at the March 1 meeting, firms with more than 10 workers that did not provide health insurance would have to pay an assessment of $295 per employee. Within two days, the House and Senate leaders were saying the legislation was back on track, and the next month it passed the Senate unanimously and the House with only two dissenting votes. Romney signed the law and took full credit for it.[22] As a symbolic gesture, he vetoed the $295 assessment on employers who didn't provide coverage, knowing that the legislature would override him on that score. He was about to enter the race for the Republican presidential nomination and didn't want to be vulnerable to the charge that he had raised taxes.

Besides the individual mandate and employer assessment, the final compromise legislation consisted of several basic elements. It expanded MassHealth for children, though not for adults, in families earning up to three times the poverty level. It established a new public authority to be called the Commonwealth Health Insurance Connector, which would operate an insurance exchange as well as a subsidized program for adults otherwise without coverage if their incomes were below three times the poverty level (at that time roughly $30,000 for an individual). It required employers to set up a so-called "Section 125 plan," which would allow workers to make pre-tax payments for health insurance even if the firm did not offer coverage.

The legislation left critical decisions about the design of the program to the board of the Connector, and it set a demanding timetable for implementation. The individual mandate did not go into effect for a year. But starting from scratch, with no employees in the late spring of 2006, the executive director of the insurance exchange, Jon Kingsdale, had only four months until the beginning of October, when the new subsidized insurance program, Commonwealth Care, was slated to open for enrollment by the uninsured poor who weren't eligible for Medicaid. The rush to implement the law could have led to a shipwreck. But, according to Kingsdale, several features of the Massachusetts political and health-care environment contributed to a successful startup. The program enjoyed total support from both of the major political parties as well as business leaders and health-care institutions. The dominant health insurers in the state, including the managed-care plans serving low-income groups, cooperated fully. And the state government had already built the technical foundations for easy on-line consumer access, the Virtual Gateway for enrollment in state programs, which the Connector was able to use so that people could determine eligibility for its new subsidized insurance coverage in less than half an hour.[23]

Besides the subsidized program, the Connector would operate a second exchange, Commonwealth Choice, where anyone else without insurance could buy a policy to meet the July 1, 2007, deadline, when the mandate went into effect. While calling for the mandate, Romney had also promised to reduce the premiums for insurance, and it was up to the Connector to make good on that promise. A key question was what constituted the minimum "creditable" coverage an individual needed to have to satisfy the mandate; Romney had given $200 as an estimate of what he thought the minimum policy should cost, and the Connector was able to bring in bids in that range for insurance with deductibles of $2,000 for an individual and $4,000 for a family. The policies still covered the full array of medical services, including prescription drugs.[24] Before the Connector, according to Kingsdale, a 37-year-old in the Boston area would have had to pay $335 a month for the least expensive policy, which had a $5,000 deductible; now policies were available for as little as $175 and a deductible less than half as large.[25] These were the lowest-cost "bronze" level policies; the exchange also offered "silver" and "gold" policies with more complete coverage at higher premiums, as well as an especially low-cost, high-deductible policy for young adults.

Within a year, according to surveys conducted before and after the program's introduction, the Massachusetts reforms cut the proportion of the state's residents without insurance by about one-half; as of 2008, only 4.1 percent of the total population (and just 2.1 percent of children) were uninsured. The surveys also showed clear gains in access to health care and reduced financial stress from illness.[26] Critics objected that an expanded public program would result in diminished employer coverage, but there was no such decline (even the minimal $295 assessment may have deterred employers from dropping insurance).[27] What makes these gains in health insurance especially impressive is that they occurred at a time when the number of uninsured was rising elsewhere in the United States.

Although the Massachusetts program achieved its objectives, it did not slow the rate of growth in health-care costs in the state. In that sense it fell short of being comprehensive and guaranteeing long-term stability; a second wave of reform efforts has subsequently focused on cost containment.[28] But the program maintained the support of both parties, business leaders, health-care organizations, and the public at large. As controversial as the individual mandate would later be in the nation as a whole, it did not inspire any organized protest in Massachusetts. According to public opinion surveys, support for the mandate increased over time.[29]

After the Massachusetts reforms were enacted, the Heritage Foundation offered its endorsement. Governor Romney and the legislature, wrote Edmund Haislmaier of Heritage, "have provided their citizens with the tools to achieve what the public really wants: a health system with all the familiar comforts of existing employer group coverage but with the added benefits of portability, choice, and control. Other governors and legislators would be well advised to consider this basic model as a framework for health care reform in their own states."[30]

Some governors did attempt to follow the example of Massachusetts. The most notable was California, where another Republican governor, Arnold Schwarzenegger, introduced an ambitious plan along similar lines. But with a far higher proportion of its residents uninsured and a state government paralyzed by deep fiscal problems and supermajority requirements for legislative action, California was unable to act on health care.[31]

Still, the Romney vision in Massachusetts might well have become the national Republican vision in a different era. The individual mandate— "the ultimate conservative idea" of individual responsibility, as Romney called it—had originated as a Republican proposal. The insurance exchanges were a market framework for reform. A public program for the poor and tax credits for the near poor were what Republicans had called for as an alternative to Medicare in the early 1960s. But, instead, it was the Democrats who carried the Massachusetts model to the national level. To do that, however, they would have to drop some ambitious goals that they had long wanted to achieve. They would have to work within the limits of the American health policy trap and hope that they could overcome its worst effects.

Toward Minimally Invasive Reform

The Democrats' congressional victories in November 2006 triggered a burst of attention to universal health care in the following months. As the new Congress met in January, three new proposals for national reform were announced in Washington, and influential business leaders and interest groups moved to embrace more of a government role in health care. At the beginning of February, one of the candidates for the Democratic presidential nomination, John Edwards, announced his plan for universal coverage, setting an early standard that his rivals sought to match.

The ensuing debate might have reproduced the pattern of the early 1990s, when Democrats contributed to their own defeat by lining up behind different plans and attacking everyone else's plan but their own. To be sure, none of those interested in passing health-care reform wanted to return to those battles, but consensus is never achieved merely by wishing it so. By 2007, however, the range of opinion within the circles that had the attention of Democratic leaders was narrower than it had been in the early 1990s. Key interest groups and advocacy organizations were converging on the same general model of reform, and although the candidates in the Democratic primaries offered their own health-care plans, they all reflected the same basic approach. That framework owed a lot to Republican ideas, particularly to the reforms that Romney had championed in Massachusetts. On the Republican side, though, the candidates for the 2008 presidential nomination, including Romney, rejected that vision as a model for national policy and offered more limited changes, chiefly in the tax treatment of health insurance. The presidential campaign prefigured what would happen after the election: the Democrats came together in rough agreement on health care, while the Republicans united in opposition.

The rapprochement on health reform between liberal advocacy organizations and the major interest groups did not emerge suddenly and spontaneously. It grew out of extended, formal mediation efforts over a period of two and a half years, involving a group of 16 national organizations called the Health Care Coalition for the Uninsured. The coalition's recommendation for a two-stage process for broadening coverage was one of the proposals for national reform announced in January 2007. The coalition supported covering children first—and then adults—by expanding Medicaid and SCHIP for people below the federal poverty line and by giving tax credits for private insurance to those between 100 percent and 300 percent of the poverty level.[32] Though the proposal did not include an individual mandate or insurance exchanges, it followed the same lines as the Massachusetts reforms in extending public coverage for the poor and tax credits for private insurance for the near-poor. The other similarity to Massachusetts was that the coalition focused on coverage, not cost containment.

This effort—the first of two such consensus-building exercises that came to be known as the "strange bedfellows" meetings—included most of the major interest-group organizations representing doctors, hospitals (both nonprofit and for-profit), insurers, and pharmaceutical companies. The signatories ranged from the U.S. Chamber of Commerce, representing employers, to AARP to Families USA, a liberal advocacy group that catalyzed the process. Not all the participants were satisfied. Both the National Association of Manufacturers and the AFL-CIO as well as the Service Employees International Union (SEIU) refused to sign the January 2007 coalition statement. The manufacturers' group objected on fiscal grounds, while the unions did not want to endorse a proposal that left out an employer mandate and a publicly run insurance option.[33]

Nonetheless, the process signaled a growing willingness among old adversaries to join together. Economic changes were having their impact on the health-care industry. Year by year, as premiums rose, millions of additional people were being priced out of health insurance, particularly if they had to buy it on their own. The growing numbers of the uninsured were bad for the business of health care, not just for the insurers, which lost customers, but for the hospitals, doctors, and all other providers depending on third-party payments. The reality was that there was no keeping the government out of health care. Regardless of whether reform passed, Medicaid and Medicare would come to represent a larger source of income for the industry. Even the pharmaceutical companies, which had long resisted Medicare coverage of prescription drugs, now saw advantages from public financing of insurance. To be sure, as in the old days, health-care interest groups could have dug in their heels and said, "No further." But as long as they could protect their interests, it made sense to many of the leaders of the industry to support coverage of the uninsured.

Another reason for the industry's interest in reform was more subtle. The projected growth in Medicare and Medicaid spending made cuts inevitable sooner or later. But if health-care reform itself made those cuts and used the savings to finance coverage of the uninsured, the revenue would come back to the health-care industry. As Chris Jennings, a former Clinton health-policy adviser who was closely involved in the discussions, explains, "Anyone who looked at the budget knew there would be an effort to reduce federal health spending. You could inoculate yourself by embracing savings but having them reinvested in health care."[34]

From the standpoint of the advocates of reform, the immediate value of the strange-bedfellows agreement was to secure support for SCHIP, which Congress had authorized for 10 years in 1997. In their effort not only to reauthorize the program in 2007 but also to expand it to cover more children, the advocacy groups would need the widest possible support to overcome the opposition of the Bush administration. Seventeen Republican senators, including Charles Grassley and Orrin Hatch, did join the Democrats in voting for an expansion of SCHIP with $35 billion in new cigarette taxes, but Bush vetoed the bill on the grounds that it was a step toward a government take-over of health care. After Bush vetoed a second bill, the congressional supporters of children's insurance had to settle for an extension of the program at its current level of funding to March 2009.[35]

Beyond the children's program, the liberals involved in the strange-bedfellows meetings hoped to build trust and alliances with interest groups in order to achieve universal coverage on a mutually acceptable basis. As Jennings recalled, they were now convinced that health-care reform had to minimize disruption to avoid heightening worries not just in the industry but among the well-insured. Playing on those fears was how the opponents of the Clinton plan had turned public opinion against it; a new effort had to assure middle-class Americans that they would be able to keep the insurance they had if that was what they wanted.[36]

That premise was critical to the emerging paradigm for policy—*universal coverage through minimally invasive reform*. A good example of the approach had come in 2005 from the Democrats' most influential think tank, the Center for American Progress. Rather than create "a new system," Jeanne Lambrew, John Podesta, and Teresa Shaw wrote, their plan would build on Medicaid and employer-based insurance, "the two major existing sources of health coverage" for people below age 65. Medicaid would be enlarged to cover people with incomes up to 100 to 150 percent of the federal poverty level, and a new national insurance exchange would offer private insurance "to anyone who lacks access to job-based insurance" and to any employer that wanted to use it. Refundable tax credits would ensure that "nobody pays more than a certain percentage of income (for example,

5–7.5 percent) on health insurance premiums." This was basically the Massachusetts architecture, though it included several other elements aimed at improving "the value of coverage": an emphasis on disease prevention and management, support for research evaluating the effectiveness of different methods of treatment, and investments in information technology. These would all become the standard boilerplate of Democratic proposals. The plan also suggested a 3 to 4 percent value-added tax to finance expanded coverage, though none of the Democratic presidential candidates would adopt that idea.[37]

The commitment to minimally invasive reform ultimately ruled out two other strategies embodied in proposals also announced in January 2007. Both of these plans had genuine appeal as policy to influential figures in progressive circles. But if either of them in their original form had won strong support among Democrats, the party might have been as fragmented as it was in 1993. The eventual marginalization of these proposals was therefore critical to the outcome in 2010.

One of the strategies, best exemplified by legislation introduced originally by Oregon Democratic Senator Ron Wyden, called for moving away from employer-based insurance to a new system in which individuals and families would purchase coverage through state agencies that would organize the private insurance market. Like the Massachusetts reforms, Wyden's Healthy Americans Act included an individual mandate, insurance exchanges, and income-related subsidies for the poor and near-poor. But unlike the Massachusetts reforms or the other minimally invasive proposals, Wyden did not simply add to Medicaid, SCHIP, and employer-provided coverage. He wanted to do away with them in favor of a system in which everyone under age 65 acquired insurance through state-run exchanges. His bill also replaced the existing tax exclusion of employer health insurance contributions with progressive tax credits. People below poverty would have their premiums covered in full, while there would be sliding-scale subsidies for those earning up to four times the poverty level.[38]

In its own way, Wyden's proposal became the best-known exemplar of a strange-bedfellows alliance when Senator Bob Bennett, a conservative Utah Republican, offered to join forces in 2007 and co-sponsor the legislation. (Bennett was later denied renomination by Utah Republicans because of his deviation from orthodoxy in working with Wyden.) The Wyden-Bennett bill then gained about a dozen sponsors, equally split between Republicans and Democrats, and became the darling of journalists who seized on the proposal as evidence that bipartisanship was still possible. Wyden's argument was that Democrats were right about covering everyone and that Republicans were right about giving people lots of private choices, and Wyden-Bennett achieved both aims.

The great hope behind Wyden-Bennett was that it would break the linkage of health insurance with jobs and attract support from both business and labor leaders who recognized the folly of basing insurance on employment. At a press conference previewing the bill in December 2006, Wyden had been flanked by a CEO, Steve Burd of Safeway supermarkets, and a labor leader, SEIU president Andy Stern.[39] In an article in the *Wall Street Journal,* Stern had argued that the employer-based insurance system was collapsing because of "out-of-control costs, a revolutionary global economy and masses of uninsured." Historic changes, Stern wrote, made the system obsolete: "By the time they are 35, young people entering the job market today will already have worked in eight to 12 jobs. . . . In other words, we are rapidly moving from employer-managed work lives to self-managed work lives, in which workers must figure out on their own how to maintain things like health insurance and retirement."[40] But instead of leaving individuals on their own in the existing insurance market, Stern wanted to create a way to cover workers independently of their job. Although he would have preferred a single-payer system, Stern called upon business leaders to meet the challenge of the new era, and he saw Wyden's proposal as one way to do it. In February, Stern would appear with the CEO of Wal-Mart, H. Lee Scott, Jr., to announce another coalition, Better Health Care Together, which aimed to bring business and labor together in pursuit of universal health insurance.[41] And in yet another strange-bedfellows alliance, Stern's SEIU and AARP joined with the Business Roundtable and the National Federation of Independent Business to create Divided We Fail, in support of comprehensive reform of health and retirement programs.[42]

These efforts reflected a desire to escape from ideological straightjackets, but they ended up not amounting to much, at least not in the short run. Neither the Wyden-Bennett bill nor the general idea of breaking the link between jobs and insurance ever gained traction. Explaining the changes that Wyden-Bennett called for, *Washington Post* columnist Ruth Marcus wrote, "The result—as Wyden cheerfully acknowledges—would be to blow up the existing health insurance system."[43] But blowing up the system was not a feasible political strategy when so many people were satisfied with what they had. None of the interest groups would help light the fuse. The bill's chief sponsor in the House, Tennessee Congressman Jim Cooper, later recalled ruefully that no major trade association would endorse Wyden-Bennett.[44] Even the Republican co-sponsors of the bill wouldn't necessarily have voted for it. Although they put their names on the bill, some of them specifically disavowed its main provisions. They seemed to like appearing to be for a bipartisan bill without actually being for it.[45]

The second strategy for health reform that threatened the emerging consensus among Democrats came from the left of the party. Progressive activists still preferred single-payer but were searching for an alternative that had a better chance of winning support. As he had in the early 1990s, Rep. Pete Stark, chair of the health subcommittee of Ways and Means, submitted his AmeriCare bill, requiring employers to provide insurance or pay into a new part of Medicare that would cover their workers as well as others without insurance.[46] In January 2007, the Economic Policy Institute, a liberal organization, presented a plan along the same lines prepared by political scientist Jacob Hacker. Under the proposal, businesses would have to provide insurance or pay 6 percent of payroll; every legal resident otherwise without coverage would then be able to buy into "a new public insurance pool modeled after Medicare," which would offer access "to an affordable Medicare-like plan with free choice of providers or to a selection of comprehensive private plans."[47] The Lewin Group, a respected private firm, estimated that the Medicare-like plan would attract about half the population under age 65.[48]

During the previous decade, as Hacker pointed out, Medicare had controlled costs more effectively than private insurers had. Perhaps for that very reason, the proposal did not win warm applause from the health-care industry. On average, Medicare paid hospitals about 20 percent less than private insurers did; a shift of more than 100 million Americans below age 65 from private insurance to Medicare rates would have dramatically cut the flow of revenue to the industry, probably sending some hospitals into default on their bonds. In its original form, therefore, the proposal was not consistent with the Democrats' interest in minimal disruption.

But while Democratic leaders did not fully embrace the Hacker proposal, it became the basis of an idea that did have legs—the public option, an alternative to private insurance to be offered within the new insurance exchanges. During 2007, a group of progressive activists began putting together an organizing committee to start a new national campaign for universal health insurance, recognizing that they had no realistic chance even of persuading Democratic primary voters to support single-payer. As Roger Hickey of Campaign for a New America explained in a speech to New Jersey Citizens Action in November:

> The good news is that people are ready for big change. But the hard reality, from the point of view of all of us who understand the efficiency and simplicity of a single-payer system, is that our pollsters unanimously tell us that large numbers of Americans are not willing to give up the good private insurance they now have in order to be put into one big health plan run by the government.
>   Pollster Celinda Lake looked at public backing for a single-payer plan— and then compared it with an approach that offers a choice between highly regulated private insurance and a public plan like Medicare. This alternative, called "guaranteed choice," wins 64 percent support to 22 percent for single-payer. And even the hard core progressive part of the population, which Celinda calls the "health justice" constituency, favors "guaranteed choice" over single-payer.[49]

Beginning in January 2007, Hickey and the other activist leaders took Hacker to see the Democratic candidates and their advisers. From the candidates' standpoint, the big problem with the dominant paradigm modeled on Massachusetts was that health insurance exchanges, tax credits, and the individual mandate did not have enthusiastic activist supporters, but single-payer did. If they could incorporate a public option into their plans, they might win over that constituency. Instead of attacking the dominant framework of reform, the left would then be arguing only for a specific provision within it. From a political standpoint, the great function of the public option was to bring the left within the fold.[50]

Making 2008 a Health-Care Election

It was not Obama who put health-care reform into the center of the 2008 presidential race. His two major rivals in the Democratic primaries, John Edwards and Hillary Clinton, each had a better claim to that role. But the focus on health care was not the doing of any of the candidates; they were all responding to the activist constituencies and ultimately the voters in the Democratic primaries. According to the Kaiser health tracking polls, health care was the top domestic issue for voters during 2007, and even when the economy jumped ahead as a concern in February 2008, the proportion that month identifying health care as one of the top two issues was 40 percent among Democrats, compared with only 18 percent among Republicans.[51] Health care mattered to Democratic constituencies and primary voters, and they made it a focus of the campaign.

How that process worked was evident on March 24, 2007, when Obama and the other candidates spoke to a Las Vegas meeting co-sponsored by the Service Employees International Union. According to SEIU's Andy Stern, the union had informed all the candidates invited to speak that they were expected to have a detailed health plan by that time.[52] Obama began by warmly recalling his long ties with SEIU going back to his days as a community organizer in Chicago and pledged that health-care reform would be crucial if he was elected. "I want to be held accountable for getting it done," he said, though he was vague about specifics. Immediately after Obama finished his speech, the moderator turned to what was surely a prearranged question from a woman named Morgan Miller, who pointed out that Obama hadn't yet provided a definite health-care plan. Pressed on the issue and unable to give crisp answers, Obama alluded to a plan that he was "in the process of unveiling."[53] Angry with himself afterward, he told his staff that he had "whiffed" the event for lack of a worked-out proposal, and as a result, according to his campaign manager David Plouffe, health care "shot to the front of the line" in the campaign's decision-making about issues.[54]

By that point, Edwards had already released his plan, staking out a position on the left, though perhaps not as far to the left as his wife Elizabeth—a persistent advocate for single-payer inside his campaign—wanted him to go.[55] The Edwards plan called for state insurance exchanges, an individual

mandate, and the expansion of Medicaid, and in these respects his proposal followed the standard Massachusetts pattern. Edwards, however, also
included a government-run insurance plan as an option within the exchange, as well as a play-or-pay requirement that employers provide coverage or pay 6 percent of payroll. Not shying away from the cost, Edwards
estimated that the program would require an additional $90 billion to $120
billion in federal spending, which he said he would raise by eliminating
the Bush tax cuts for people with over $200,000 a year in income and by
enforcing capital-gains taxes more effectively. Discussing his proposal on
Meet the Press, Edwards presented a description of the public-plan option
that was indicative of the confusion about the idea:

> We're going to create health markets all across the country which will help
> provide some of these efficiencies. One of the choices, by the way, available
> in these health markets is the government plan. So people who like the
> idea of a single-payer insurer health plan, that is actually one of the alter-
> natives that people can choose. They'll be allowed to choose.[56]

As the name "single-payer" plainly indicates, the conception means one
payer. An optional government plan in an insurance exchange which itself
would be optional for employers is not a single-payer. Medicare was originally conceived as a single-payer for the elderly: rather than being optional,
the hospital insurance it provided under Part A was financed by a tax that
every worker had to pay (and the coverage of doctors' bills under Medicare
Part B was so heavily subsidized by general revenues that no competition
with it was possible). After all, the free choice that Medicare was designed
to protect was free choice of doctor, not free choice of insurance company.
But by 2008 Medicare had been turned into a pool with private options,
and choice of health plan was so well entrenched in public expectations
that not even Edwards could resist it.

Prodded by the Las Vegas convention, Obama was the second of the major Democratic candidates to issue a plan. Before the campaign began, his
background and legislative experience gave little evidence of a strong interest in health care. In 2003, while he was still in the Illinois Senate, Obama
had been warmly applauded at an AFL-CIO meeting when he said, "I happen to be a proponent of a single-payer universal health care plan."[57]

However revealing that statement may be of Obama's initial impulses, it did not reflect extensive involvement in health-care legislation or policy. As a U.S. senator, Obama had one of his policy advisers, Karen Kornbluh, set up meetings with health-care experts. But Gruber, who met with the senator toward the end of 2006 in Washington, says Obama did not appear at that time to be very knowledgeable about health policy. "It just wasn't his thing. I just sensed his heart wasn't in it." Later, Gruber said, he was surprised by what "a masterful job" Obama did as president. "I regret thinking he wouldn't."[58]

In late May 2007, two months after the Las Vegas fiasco, Obama finally did "unveil" his plan for health care, promising to provide "affordable, comprehensive and portable health coverage for every American." Like Edwards, Obama proposed expanding Medicaid, establishing an insurance exchange (though he described it as a single national exchange), and creating a "new public insurance program" for uninsured individuals and for small businesses. But Obama declined to endorse an individual mandate; his plan required only that parents sign up their children for coverage. And while saying that employers would have "to contribute a percentage of payroll" toward their employees' insurance, he didn't specify what that percentage would be.[59] To liberals, Obama's plan was a disappointment; writing in the *American Prospect,* Ezra Klein called it "a plan of almosts. It is almost universal, without quite having the mechanisms to ensure nationwide coverage. It almost offers a public insurance option capable of serving as the seed of single-payer, but it is unclear who can enroll in it, and talks with his advisors suggest little enthusiasm or expectation that it will serve as a shining alternative to private insurance."[60]

Obama put the federal cost of the plan at $50 billion to $65 billion per year and, like Edwards, said he would pay for it by eliminating the Bush tax cuts for the highest earners. In his Iowa speech, Obama promised the insured that nothing would change about their health care, except "the amount of money you will spend on premiums. That will be less."[61] In a memo, his advisers estimated the savings for "the typical family" at $2,500, which they broke down into five categories, citing references to show the basis for the estimates in research. But these were not the kind of numbers that the Congressional Budget Office or Medicare actuaries would accept.[62] And even if the savings proved accurate, Obama's promise raised unrealistic expectations. Health-care costs were going up; any savings would be against a rising baseline. Many people also had insurance with pre-existing condition exclusions and other limitations that would no longer be allowed; their coverage would be improved, but not without some increase in premiums. As a candidate, Obama should never have given a number with an exaggerated precision that could come back to haunt him as president. What he could have legitimately said was that premiums would be "less than they otherwise would be for the same coverage," though that might have left people scratching their heads in puzzlement.

In the Democratic primaries, the main concern raised by Obama's plan was that it would fall substantially short of universal coverage—some 15 million people short, according to Gruber's estimate—because Obama called for an insurance mandate only for children. Obama's position was that insurance had to be affordable before he would consider a mandate. In a conference call with his campaign staff, according to Plouffe, Obama said, "Let's attack costs from every angle, provide incentives for small businesses and families to allow them to provide and buy coverage. I am not opposed to a mandate philosophically. But I don't think we should start there. It could be a recourse if coverage goals aren't being met after a period."[63]

At the time the race for the Democratic nomination began, some observers doubted whether Hillary Clinton would highlight health-care reform. They assumed that as the front-runner she would play it safe and that health care would be an issue on which she was vulnerable because of her role in 1993. But at the first meeting of her issues staff in December 2006, Clinton said, "If I can't propose universal coverage, I shouldn't be running," and she asked for a complete review of all the alternatives.[64] That review ended up with a proposal that closely tracked the 2005 Center for American Progress plan, and during 2007 she rolled out her ideas for health care in a series of speeches, culminating in September with a speech on universal coverage. The basics of her "American Health Choices Plan" were also the same as the other major candidates' proposals: expansion of Medicaid to cover all of the poor and the provision of income-related tax credits to enable the near-poor to buy private insurance in a reformed marketplace with an insurance exchange. The tax credits would limit the cost of premiums to no more than 10 percent of income and to lower percentages for those just above poverty. Clinton agreed to include a government-run insurance plan as an option in the exchange, and she paid for expanded coverage, as Edwards and Obama did, by eliminating the Bush tax cuts on the highest earners. Unlike her husband's 1993 plan, Clinton proposed to require only the largest firms to pay for coverage, 99 percent of which already did; the purpose of that limited mandate was mainly to prevent those employers from dropping coverage—it was not a means of expanding it.[65] The theme of "choice" was plainly meant to counter the impressions left from 1993. "If you like your health insurance, you can keep it" was originally her line (later appropriated by Obama). In an interview with the *New York Times* when her proposal was released, Clinton declared, "I'm the decision-maker now. I have a plan that is 100 percent my plan." The implication was that the 1993 Clinton plan was not 100 percent hers, which was, in fact, true.[66]

Unlike Obama, Clinton proposed an individual mandate, and with Edwards soon out of the picture after Iowa, the mandate became a central focus of the race between the two remaining major candidates. Most analysts had expected the nomination to be decided quickly, but instead it stretched on for months, and in one state after another, Obama confronted Clinton in debates that regularly turned to health care. Since Clinton had a thorough mastery of the subject, Obama was at a disadvantage. On health care, he was in the position of an amateur athlete going up against a pro, but sparring with a pro can be excellent preparation for the main event. The debates forced Obama to think about health care and learn how to talk about it, and they may have even changed his mind about the mandate.

Although his campaign advisers deny it, Obama's stance on the mandate had political advantages. It helped to reinforce the idea promoted by the campaign that despite the preconceptions that voters might have about an African American candidate, Obama was actually more of a centrist than Clinton. The contrast fed into commentary tying together the candidates' personalities and their policies, suggesting that Clinton was more controlling and coercive—an uptight, bossy woman—while Obama was more relaxed and easy-going. Obama pressed the point about coercion in a January 2008 debate, saying to Clinton: "If they cannot afford it, then the question is, what are you going to do about it? Are you going to fine them? Are you going to garnish their wages?"[67] The next month, an Obama mailer warned:

The way Hillary Clinton's health care plan covers everyone is to have the government force uninsured people to buy insurance, even if they can't afford it. . . . Punishing families who can't afford health care to begin with just *doesn't make sense*.[68]

And during the Pennsylvania primary an Obama TV ad leveled the accusation again: "What's she not telling you about her health care plan? It forces everyone to buy insurance, even if you can't afford it. And you pay a penalty if you don't."[69] Of course, Clinton's plan included subsidies to make coverage affordable, which Obama's ads didn't mention.

These attacks on Clinton were not a moral highlight of Obama's campaign. While some of his policy advisers dutifully argued that the lack of a mandate wasn't a big deal, their candidate never offered any alternative policy that would have accomplished the purpose of a mandate. And without any alternative, the insurance reforms that Obama favored, such as guaranteed issue and elimination of pre-existing-condition exclusions, would drive up the price of insurance by giving people an incentive to delay purchasing coverage until they were sick. Any system that allows people to buy insurance on the way to the hospital, and then to drop it when they get back home, is bound to be very expensive.

The critical importance of the mandate (or its equivalent) for affordable coverage was clear to the insurance industry, and not long after Obama locked up the nomination, Karen Ignagni, the president of America's Health Insurance Plans, flew out to Obama's campaign headquarters in Chicago to say that the industry would accept a reform plan that included guaranteed issue of policies with no pre-existing-condition exclusions if the legislation also included a mandate that everyone be covered.[70] In other words, the mandate was the price for the industry's cooperation.

At some point that spring or summer, Obama's view of the individual mandate apparently changed, though he said nothing publicly about it. At the beginning of July 2008, Neera Tanden, a long-time adviser to Hillary Clinton, became the Obama campaign's policy director for the general election, and at a meeting on July 2 in Chicago, Tanden wanted to know what Obama thought of the mandate. "I kind of think Hillary was right," he told her. At that meeting, Obama's pollster Joel Benenson and other political advisers were skeptical about whether Obama should emphasize health reform in the general election; "the wisdom of the room was that we shouldn't talk about health care." This would not be the last time that Obama's political advisers suggested he pull back from the issue. But the candidate didn't share that view. According to Tanden, "He said, 'I want to do health care in my first term. And I am not going to be able to do it if I haven't talked about it.'"[71]

But during the campaign he was unable to address the question of the mandate forthrightly, so he never prepared the political ground for it. Indeed, his attacks on Clinton foreshadowed the attacks that would later be made on him after he signed the mandate into law in 2010. On the mandate, Obama would go from a position that was good politics but bad policy during the election to a position that was good policy but bad politics when he was president, without ever figuring out a position that was both good policy and good politics.

Health care was not a salient issue in the Republican primaries, though the candidates each had a position on it. In January 2007, President Bush had proposed to change the tax treatment of health insurance by creating a new standard deduction of $15,000 for families and $7,500 for individuals instead of the unlimited exclusion of employer contributions from taxable income. Several of the Republican candidates offered similar proposals, while John McCain presented a variant: instead of the current unlimited tax exclusion, the federal government would offer tax credits worth up to $2,500 for individuals and up to $5,000 for families. McCain also called for federal legislation to allow insurers to sell policies across state lines. The general thrust of his proposal was to move away from employer-based insurance and state regulation to a largely deregulated, national, individual insurance market.[72]

McCain often described the new tax credits without mentioning that his plan eliminated the current tax exclusion: "Let's give everyone a $5,000 refundable tax credit to go out and get the health insurance of their choice," he declared at one of the presidential debates in October, confusing the individual and family credits and omitting the loss of the existing exclusion.[73] Since many people who benefited from the tax exclusion did not understand it—and even those who did understand it usually had no basis

for calculating how much it was worth to them—McCain's tax-credit proposal must have seemed like an extra federal benefit aimed at increasing
insurance coverage, putting him on an equal footing with Obama.

But replacing the current tax exclusion with a tax credit would have
complex effects, resulting in less coverage for some people and more for
others. In some respects, a flat tax credit would be more equitable. The tax
system would no longer provide a greater benefit to people the higher their
tax bracket or the more expensive their insurance. People who bought insurance on their own would receive as great a tax benefit as did those with
employer-provided insurance. But if employer contributions to health insurance were no longer excluded from taxes, many employers would stop
providing coverage, and millions of workers would then have to buy insurance individually. Although some conservatives liked that prospect, many
voters wouldn't. The administrative costs of insurance in the individual
market are twice as large as in the group market; for the same money, many
people would get worse coverage. Employer coverage has also shielded
workers and their families from the underwriting practices of the individual market, where people who are older or who have pre-existing conditions
are charged higher rates or denied coverage altogether. McCain's proposal
would have forced millions of older and sicker workers into a market where
his tax credit would not have been enough for them to afford insurance or
in some cases to obtain it at all. He called for a high-risk pool for people
denied coverage, but the funds he proposed as subsidies for the pools would
have limited them at best to about 3 million people.[74]

Republicans had talked about changing the tax treatment of health insurance for a long time, but even when they had control of Congress and
the presidency, they had not done anything about it. The proposals may
have only been for show. George H. W. Bush and his son introduced their
proposals late in their presidencies, when they were under pressure to offer some response to rising numbers of uninsured. But ending the special
benefits for employer-provided coverage carried enormous political risks
if, as most analysts agreed, the result would be a substantial decline in
employment benefits. The American health-policy trap ensnared the Republicans too.

Prepare to Launch

As the election was playing out, work was proceeding outside of the political spotlight to lay the groundwork for health-care reform. Some efforts focused on building support among elites and in Congress to win the "inside game" in Washington, while others targeted grass-roots organizations to prepare for the "outside game" in the country at large. No group was coordinating all these efforts, nor did the people involved agree about the substance of reform, but they all anticipated that legislation had a shot if the Democrats won the election, and they wanted to be ready.

In Washington, no one expected that health-care reform could pass without bipartisan cooperation in the Senate, and in June Max Baucus, chair of the Senate Finance Committee, held a public meeting called "Prepare to Launch" at which the committee's members from both parties had some initial discussions. Baucus was plainly taking the leadership in the effort to craft a legislative compromise and move it through the committee that was generally expected to have the greatest influence on the outcome.[75]

Another bipartisan effort in Washington began that spring under the auspices of the Bipartisan Policy Center, established in 2007 by four former Senate majority leaders—Democrats Tom Daschle and George Mitchell and Republicans Howard Baker and Bob Dole. In April 2008 the center set up its Leaders' Project on the State of American Health Care and recruited a former Clinton official, Chris Jennings, and a former Bush official, Mark McClellan, to serve as advisers. The center's reform plan would come out a year later.[76]

The Congressional Budget Office was also getting ready for a new push on health care. After the Democrats took control of Congress in January 2007, economist Peter Orszag had become director of CBO, and in his first year, he saw two big issues, health care and climate, on which the agency needed to "bulk up" and expand its staff. Consequently, over some internal objections, he added 30 health-care specialists, created a new health-care advisory committee, and began work on a survey of more than one hundred options in health policy. In Orszag's view, members of Congress had been justifiably frustrated by the agency's mysterious "scoring" process. They would send a proposal to CBO for an estimate of the cost, and CBO would give them a number—a thumb up or a thumb down—but without much explanation. Instead, CBO would now lay out in advance the projected cost and impact of major policy alternatives. Its mammoth report on health-care options, issued in December 2008, would become a key reference point for both the administration and Congress.[77]

Elsewhere in Washington, in September 2008, the strange-bedfellows group began meeting again with the help of professional mediators, now under the name "Health Reform Dialogue." Subgroups on coverage, cost, and quality of care were established. No formal agreement would come out of this process, but key interest-group and reform leaders thrashed out compromises on specific issues at those sessions, which continued into 2009.

Some participants in the strange-bedfellows coalition, such as Families USA and AARP, were also involved in media and grass-roots activity on behalf of health-care reform. Families USA developed reports highlighting the problems of health care in what were expected to be the battleground states in the coming struggle over health-care reform. It also created a "story bank" with accounts of personal struggles with health insurance and health care. Some of those stories then found their way into news articles and political speeches, providing the color to go along with the grim, gray data about the uninsured.

On the left, critics argued that the previous campaigns for health-care reform, from the Progressive era to the Clinton administration, had been too focused on elites and failed to mobilize the mass public. It was time, they argued, to create a popular movement for health-care reform.[78] That was the aim of Health Care for America Now (HCAN), a coalition launched by progressive organizers in July 2008, bringing together labor unions, Moveon.org, Campaign for a New America, community organizations, and women's, minority, and faith-based groups.

From its beginnings in the offices of the community-organizing group USAction in early 2007, the HCAN coalition was built around a statement of basic principles, which it asked all the member organizations and political candidates to accept. The statement reflected a commitment to equality and solidarity: "A truly inclusive and accessible health care system. . . . A standard for health benefits that covers what people need to keep healthy and to be treated when they are ill. . . . Health coverage through the largest possible pools in order to achieve affordable, quality coverage for the entire population and to share risk fairly." Among the principles was guaranteed choice "of a private insurance plan, including keeping the insurance you have if you like it, or a public insurance plan." Obama and Biden endorsed the statement.[79]

Rather than just concentrate on advertising and media, the coalition set out from its inception to build a network of field organizers throughout the country, capable of mobilizing progressives in individual congressional districts. Each of the groups represented on the executive committee would have to contribute at least $500,000. To raise more substantial funds, the organizing committee approached Atlantic Philanthropies, a foundation whose new president, Gara LaMarche, favored support for public advocacy. Families USA also approached Atlantic with a proposal to fund its national campaign for health-care reform, including the strange-bedfellows process. But after both groups made presentations to Atlantic in February 2008, LaMarche decided to ask his board to put all its support behind HCAN because it would develop a bottom-up, popular movement based on a set of clear principles. HCAN received an initial grant of $10 million from Atlantic and ultimately would raise $51 million from all sources for the fight to pass health-care reform.[80]

Although some members overlapped, the progressives allied with Families USA and those allied with HCAN represented two distinct political orientations in the movement to pass reform. Families USA worked with the private insurers, pharmaceutical companies, and other interest groups in search of common ground, while HCAN took an openly anti-corporate stance. The biggest substantive difference between them came over the public option. Families USA regarded other provisions of the law concerning Medicaid and the affordability subsidies to be more important, while HCAN stressed the public option because it offered an alternative to private insurance, which many of its members regarded as the root of the health system's problems. These differences could have flared into major schisms in the campaign for health-care reform, as they had in the past. But at least during 2008, they were just different shades of opinion within a movement that shared a broad consensus about the structure of reform. That unity was a notable political achievement.

But would it last? On election night, as Obama and the congressional Democrats rolled to victory, there was no way to tell whether they and their supporters would be able to sustain the movement for health reform once they confronted the opposition and their own internal divisions. In fact, there was no certainty that the president-elect would give priority to health-care legislation. Influential voices in Washington and Obama's own inner circle were saying he should put health care aside to deal with the financial crisis and the economy. Just after the election, Orszag had a call from an aide to Obama saying that the president-elect wanted him to join the cabinet as director of the Office of Management and Budget. The caller assured him there would be no need to come out to Chicago because Obama already knew Orszag well enough and was sure that he was the right person for the job. But Orszag wasn't sure he wanted to accept it; as director of CBO, he already held an influential position. There was one thing he wanted to know: Was the president-elect going to go ahead with health-care reform? And he insisted on flying out to Chicago to get the answer to that question from Obama himself.

CHAPTER 7

Breaking Through, 2009–2010

FOR ADVOCATES OF REFORM, THE 2008 election campaign raised hopes of at long last breaking the national impasse on health care. The Democrats were ahead in the polls and promising a comprehensive program, while behind the scenes reformers were meeting with leaders of the major business and health-care interest groups to work out compromises all parties could live with. Although still divided on some key matters, the reformers, interest-group leaders, and the Democrats had nonetheless arrived at a rough consensus on an approach that built on private, employer-provided health coverage and incorporated ideas for insurance exchanges, tax credits, and an individual mandate that a leading Republican, Mitt Romney, had championed. The hope was that legislation along these lines could win some support from Republicans in Congress and avoid the deadly combination of interest-group and ideological opposition that had sunk previous efforts.

Compared with the health-care systems of other democracies or with the plans that liberals had advocated in the past, the proposals now under discussion called for only limited change. Yet while the advocates of reform tried to adopt as mild a remedy as possible, mild is not how anyone would describe the reaction. The remedy was different, but the reaction would be the same. The past was not really past. As in previous conflicts, fear and facts would go to war with each other, and a debate that began with the hope of compromise would end in anger and division.

But history never unfolds the same way. The fall of 2008 brought two developments that heightened the emotional intensity of American politics and created an unanticipated context for the national debate about health care. In rapid succession, the financial system and economy went into free fall and the nation elected Barack Obama, elevating anxiety and hope at the same time.

The electrifying passion of Obama's campaign triggered expectations of a new political era, and the mere fact of a black man's rise to the presidency seemed to confirm it. Even before he took office, Obama was being compared with Abraham Lincoln and John F. Kennedy. Entering the White House in the most severe economic crisis since the Great Depression, the new president drew comparisons with Franklin Delano Roosevelt. Liberals hoped that, like his greatest predecessors, Obama would become—in the language of the historian James McGregor Burns—a "transformational" rather than a "transactional" leader and inaugurate a new framework for politics instead of merely negotiating within the old constraints.[1] The FDR parallel invited a further analogy: Obama's passage of health-care reform would be the equivalent of Roosevelt's enactment of Social Security.

But genuine transformations are few and far between, or they come so slowly that people are hardly aware of them. The very institutions that conservatives wanted to eliminate or curb, from welfare-state programs to the Federal Reserve, cushioned the majority of Americans from the shocks in the economy and prevented the financial crisis from spurring demands for change on a Rooseveltian scale. In the case of health care, progressives who hoped for a transformation were bound to be disappointed. Going into the election, Democrats had already decided to settle for reforms that would be minimally disruptive. But the concessions made by Democrats were of little interest to most Republicans, who responded to what they took to be the broader ideological implications and meaning of the new policies. From their standpoint, regardless of what Democrats said, the proposed changes amounted to a "government take-over" because, in the final analysis, government would take responsibility for seeing that everyone had health care.

The economic crisis didn't just put Americans on edge. By the time the right-wing reaction to health-care reform gained full force—in the summer of 2009—the role of the federal government had, in fact, dramatically increased. Some of that increase actually came under the Bush administration in the form of the Wall Street bailouts and federal take-over of the two mortgage giants Fannie Mae and Freddie Mac. A further increase came with Obama's stimulus program and the bailouts of General Motors and Chrysler. None of these measures would have been adopted under normal circumstances; Democrats had not been hankering for a government take-over of the car industry. But conservatives saw it all as evidence of Obama's "socialism," and the bailouts didn't upset conservatives alone; many other people who were watching their businesses collapse and jobs disappear were furious about government aid to Wall Street and big corporations.

It was in this context that health-care reform took on a significance for both sides that transcended the specifics of the legislation. For Republicans, it would be all about what they saw as an overreaching federal government. And for Democrats it would also be about government. It would become a test of whether after so many failures, government could finally deal with a problem as complex, costly, and emotional as health care. And because the prognosis for their other priorities would suffer if the Democrats failed on health-care reform, it would become a test of nothing less than their ability to govern.

Health Care First

When a political campaign is over, the sorting out of promises into priorities begins. Offered the job of budget director, Peter Orszag flew out to Chicago five days after the election to ask Obama whether he would make health-care reform a priority, and when Obama said he would, Orszag accepted the position. Still, it was unclear even to members of Obama's inner circle whether the president-elect intended to push health care early in his term. Among his economic advisers, Larry Summers wanted to put it off. David Axelrod and other influential senior political advisers were opposed to a big push on reform, just as they had been during the campaign. No one had the ear of the president on health policy more than former Senator Tom Daschle, whom Obama nominated to become secretary of Health and Human Services as well as director of a new White

House Office of Health Reform. Yet, as Daschle writes in his book *Getting It Done,* he was unsure at first whether Obama intended to press health-care reform because the president-elect "did not shut down the talk of a delay. . . . But every time I grew frustrated and asked him whether this was truly a priority for him, his answers were so convincing that they easily put my doubts to rest."[2]

The activists who supported reform were not content to leave the decision to the new administration. On election night, labor leader Andy Stern later recalled, his union's members wore buttons that read "Health Care First," and the next day they began another political campaign, this time to make certain that Obama and the Democratic Congress would follow through on health-care reform.[3]

What was more surprising was the push for reform that came from the chairman of the Senate Finance Committee. Eight days after the election, Max Baucus issued a white paper that began with the striking line, "It is the duty of the next Congress to reform America's health care system." The paper then set out a plan that reflected what was now the standard Democratic model for reform: "a nationwide insurance pool called the Health Insurance Exchange" to ensure access to "affordable, guaranteed coverage" with no pre-existing-condition exclusions, an expansion of Medicaid to cover all of the poor, tax credits to subsidize premiums "for qualifying families and small businesses," and a requirement for individuals to obtain coverage once the exchange was established. The proposal was basically the same as the plan Obama called for during the campaign, except on two points: Baucus included an individual mandate and, as a short-term measure before the exchanges were established, proposed to allow 55- to 64-year-olds to buy into Medicare.[4]

The significance of the white paper lay entirely in who it came from. Baucus had opposed the Clinton health plan in 1994, voted for the Bush tax cuts in 2001, and supported Bush's Medicare prescription-drug legislation in 2003. Many liberals regarded him warily because of his record of cooperation with Republicans. But his early and emphatic support for comprehensive health-care reform in November 2008 sent an unmistakable signal to the new administration, other members of Congress, and private interest groups.

Another auspicious sign for health-care legislation came from the House on November 20, when Henry P. Waxman of California unseated the veteran John P. Dingell of Michigan as chairman of the Energy and Commerce Committee. Although both men were committed to health-care reform, Waxman was widely regarded as the more effective legislator.[5]

Just two days earlier, America's Health Insurance Plans, the industry's main lobby, had publicly announced its support for a system of universal coverage, with guaranteed issue of policies and no pre-existing-condition exclusions, as long as there was an individual mandate, just as Baucus had called for. The group also supported expanding Medicaid to cover all of the poor and subsidies for private coverage up to four times the federal poverty level.[6]

These developments impressed political observers in Washington who were familiar with the role that key congressional committees and the insurance industry had played in derailing previous reform efforts. In late November *Washington Post* columnist David S. Broder wrote that congressional leaders were lining up in favor of reform, and the next month he reported on a meeting in Washington where representatives of the Business Roundtable, the National Federation of Independent Business, America's Health Insurance Plans, and one of the major drug companies all "agreed that major health legislation has a much better chance of passage" than in the early 1990s, an assessment that Broder supported.[7]

The readiness to act of congressional leaders, receptivity to reform of key interest groups, and broad consensus about the architecture of reform must have factored in Obama's post-election calculus about whether to give health care priority. That's not to say that moral and emotional considerations played no role in Obama's decision. The memory of his mother's struggle to deal with health insurance as she was dying from ovarian cancer may well have influenced him. One of Obama's aides said how deeply he thought Obama had been touched by personal stories that he had heard on the campaign trail from people who were battling the health-care system. But health care was only one of many issues that tugged at moral concerns. For any president, the start of a new term offers the best chance for major initiatives because of the losses that the party holding the White House usually sustains in the midterm congressional elections. It would not make sense to waste precious time and political capital on causes with little chance of success, which is how nearly everyone would have described universal health insurance a few years earlier. By the time Obama was elected, however, reformers had already won an unheralded victory. They had changed the conventional wisdom on the odds of passing health-care reform and therefore made it a rational course for a president to pursue.

Obama said he wanted to do big things as president, and according to Daschle, Obama told him shortly after the inauguration that health-care reform was "the most important thing we will ever do" and would be his "legacy" as president.[8] But Obama also wanted to do other important things that ended up not receiving as great a commitment from him. As a candidate he had often spoken about legislation to deal with energy and global warming as a moral imperative, and during one of his debates with McCain, he had rated that issue ahead of health care. "We're going to have to prioritize, just like a family has to prioritize," he had said. "Energy we have to deal with today. . . . Health care is priority number two."[9] In his early months as president, Obama called for Congress to pass both climate and health-care legislation, but it became clear relatively quickly that the odds on a climate and energy bill were worse than on health-care reform. Democrats, environmentalists, and major interest groups concerned with energy had no consensus. Most supporters of climate legislation favored a mandatory, declining cap on carbon emissions, with tradable emission permits ("cap and trade"), but others preferred a carbon tax, and powerful lobbies as well as Democrats from coal-dependent states opposed both alternatives. And since a limit on greenhouse gases was not going to yield improvements that people would see in their own lives in the short run, a climate bill was less likely than health-care legislation to generate support for a second term for Obama.

Finally, Obama had been emphatic in the campaign that his performance as president should be judged by whether he succeeded in enacting health-care reform. It was a standard he had set himself. In discussing the subject, Obama also frequently alluded to the many failed efforts of the past. The very difficulty of achieving health care for all gave it an almost mythical significance; it had become the Everest of social reform. If Obama could climb that mountain, his achievement would reverberate throughout the nation and earn him an honor that had eluded his predecessors.

Obama's appointments reflected his seriousness about getting health-care reform through Congress. None of the academic health-care advisers from the campaign were kept on in a central health-policy role in the administration; instead, Obama turned to people with experience in government, particularly Congress. His initial choices of Daschle and Orszag for the two key cabinet positions relevant to health policy epitomized the overall pattern. So did other choices for senior White House positions, beginning with the selection of Rep. Rahm Emanuel as chief of staff. Obama filled key positions in the White House with long-time aides to Senator Baucus (Jim Messina), Daschle (Pete Rouse and Jeanne Lambrew), Rep. Henry Waxman (Phil Schiliro), Senator Kent Conrad (Lisa Konwinski), and Senator Ted Kennedy (Melody Barnes).[10] In some societies, clans forge alliances through intermarriage. By an analogous principle, Obama "married" into the Democratic Congress by hiring the senior staff of congressional chieftains, including the key players on health-care reform.

The fast startup reformers envisioned suffered a reverse in January when Daschle's cabinet nomination ran into trouble because he had failed to report the free services of a driver as income on his taxes, and the former senator was forced to withdraw. In his place, Obama nominated Kansas Governor Kathleen Sebelius, a former state insurance commissioner, to be secretary of Health and Human Services and chose Nancy-Ann Min DeParle, a former Clinton administration official, to run the health-reform office in the White House. But because Obama conspicuously left the early development of health-care legislation to Congress, the internal decision-making of the White House and cabinet departments did not become the focus of public scrutiny, as it had in the Clinton years. Observers said Obama had learned the lessons of Clinton's mistake in foisting a bill on Capitol Hill, but the circumstances were entirely different. Obama could leave the initial steps to Congress because he and congressional Democrats agreed on the model for reform, and the congressional leadership did not need or want White House intervention at that point.

Letting Congress take the initiative also had distinct political advantages for Obama. Instead of conspicuously reversing himself on the individual mandate, Obama could simply accede to the mandate as the policy chosen by Congress. The president could benefit from not being too closely identified with provisions of the legislation that proved controversial. Eventually, though, he would not be able to stay out of the legislative fray. And despite the distance he kept at first, the opponents would call the law "Obamacare" as they had come to ridicule the Clinton plan as "Hillarycare."

Bipartisanship in One Party

The drive to pass health-care reform in 2009 did not start out on the assumption that it could succeed only with Democratic votes or that it could prevail over the opposition of major interest groups. Democratic leaders expected to strike bargains to pass legislation. During the primaries, Obama had said that he would bring the different groups together around a "big table" to negotiate the issue, and in one debate John Edwards had harrumphed, "Some people argue that we're going to sit at a table with these people and they're going to voluntarily give their power away. I think it is a complete fantasy; it will never happen." Obama responded there was no option except to negotiate with the interest groups: "We want to reduce the power of drug companies and insurance companies and so forth, but the notion that they will have no say-so at all in anything is just not realistic."[11] In fact, Obama and the congressional Democrats would be able to reach deals with critical interest groups. One group, however, wasn't interested in a deal—the Republicans.

At the beginning, it looked like health-care reform would face a greater challenge in the Senate than in the House. Although the Democrats had done exceptionally well in 2008 Senate races, they did not come out of the election with the 60-vote supermajority needed to break a filibuster. Their caucus initially numbered 58, counting two independents, and one of those independents was Joe Lieberman, who had endorsed McCain. To keep Lieberman from bolting to the GOP, Senate Majority Leader Harry Reid ruled out any reprisals against the Connecticut senator. At best that still left the Democrats two votes short of the 60-vote threshold. As 2009 began, they could not have anticipated that they would later reach that threshold thanks to the defection of Pennsylvania Republican Senator Arlen Specter in March and the seating of Democrat Al Franken on July 30 after the recounts and litigation in his Minnesota race were finally resolved.

To protect themselves against the risk of a Senate filibuster, the Democrats passed a budget resolution in early 2009 that gave them the option of enacting health-care reform through the budget-reconciliation process, which requires only a simple majority. That recourse, however, would open the measure to rules challenges and limit the changes they could make on a permanent basis. It would also face opposition not just from Republicans, but even from within the Democratic caucus in the Senate because it would reduce the leverage of moderate and conservative Democrats. But if necessary, it was there as a fall-back. In the end, it turned out to be critical for passing the legislation in a completely unexpected way.

The search for bipartisan support had advantages beyond whatever Republican votes it might net. Even a few Republican votes for the bill would provide political cover for Democrats from states that went for McCain. Some extra Republican votes for the legislation would also reduce the ability of any individual senator to extract special-interest concessions. And the effort to work with the Republicans fulfilled Obama's promise of an open-minded, inclusive process.

In that light, it seemed fortunate for the Democrats that they had two accomplished coalition-builders chairing the Senate committees with jurisdiction over health policy. Kennedy had co-sponsored dozens of bills with Republicans in the Health, Education, Labor, and Pensions (HELP) committee, and Baucus had worked closely with Republicans on Finance, especially the ranking Republican, Grassley of Iowa. But in May 2008, Kennedy had been diagnosed with a brain tumor and would be unable to continue either as chairman or as a bridge-builder. So the burden of finding support among Republicans fell primarily to Baucus, who had a tradition of bipartisan comity in Finance working in his favor. When Grassley chaired Finance, Baucus had helped him on Medicare prescription drugs; it was not unreasonable to expect Grassley to reciprocate.

Substantively, Baucus and the Democrats were starting off from a position that hardly appeared irreconcilable with Republican views. The roots of the Democratic approach lay in earlier Republican proposals. Not only were Romney's reforms in Massachusetts the immediate precedent and model for the Democrats; the idea of providing tax credits for private insurance dated back to proposals that Republicans had offered in the late

1940s as alternatives to national health insurance and to proposals they
had made in the 1960s as alternatives to Medicare. The approach Democrats supported in 2009 more closely resembled the legislation Richard
Nixon submitted in the early 1970s than what Ted Kennedy originally advocated. The individual mandate had been introduced as a conservative
idea in the 1990s, when it became the core of the Senate Republican alternative to the Clinton plan.

As part of the effort to widen the coalition for reform, Obama convened a
meeting on March 5, 2009, in the East Room of the White House with more
than 50 members of Congress and more than 80 interest-group representatives. At least publicly, all sides professed an interest in being constructive.
"Max Baucus and I have a pretty good record of working out bipartisan
things," Senator Grassley said, recalling that they had worked out agreements on all but two bills during the previous eight years in Finance. (One
of those, the reauthorization and expansion of the Children's Health Insurance Program, had finally been passed and signed by Obama the previous
month after two vetoes by Bush—but in the end, Grassley voted against the
bill because Democrats added a provision allowing states to lift a ban on
covering children of legal immigrants who had been in the country less
than five years.) The leaders of major interest groups offered their support
for reform, albeit in general terms. Speaking for America's Health Insurance Plans, Karen Ignagni stood up to say, "You have our commitment to
play, to contribute, and to help pass health care reform this year."[12] President
Obama had another public, feel-good occasion on May 11, when he announced that six major health-care industry groups had voluntarily agreed
to steps that would take 1.5 percent off the growth rate in costs—potentially
worth $2 trillion in savings over 10 years, except that it was unenforceable.[13]

The hard bargaining was taking place behind closed doors. The White
House and Senate Finance Committee made two notable deals with the
health-care industry—one with the pharmaceutical companies, the other
with the major hospital associations. Both agreements would cause trouble
for Obama and the Democrats, though in different ways.

Like other providers of health-care goods and services, the drug companies and hospitals stood to benefit from the extension of coverage to the
uninsured and improvements in coverage for people with limited policies.

The demand for prescription drugs would increase, and hospitals would get paid for treating patients who otherwise would leave unpaid bills. The Senate Finance Committee added an economist to its staff specifically to estimate how big the gains for each industry would be. Since the aim of reform was not to enrich the drug companies or the hospitals, Baucus and the Democrats wanted the industry representatives to agree to measures that would, in effect, give back part of their gains and help control costs over the long run. The industries naturally wanted to limit those measures.

The lobbying group for the drug industry—the Pharmaceutical Research and Manufacturers of America, known as PhRMA—was particularly concerned about the risks it faced because many Democrats, including Obama, had called for two measures that the industry regarded as dire threats: direct federal negotiations with the manufacturers over prices paid under Medicare for prescription drugs and approval for the importing of drugs from Canada and Europe, where they were sold at lower prices than in the United States. In the hope of locking down an agreement to block these and other policies, the drug makers came in early during 2009 to talk with Baucus and the White House. On the basis of his committee's estimates of the prospective gains to the pharmaceutical industry, Baucus was looking for $100 billion in cost restraint over 10 years.[14]

PhRMA's president Billy Tauzin, a former Louisiana congressman who had switched from the Democrats to the Republicans after the 1994 Republican take-over of Congress, boasted in private meetings that the association had a $200 million war chest, which he said it could use to run TV ads either to support health-care reform or to oppose it, depending on whether negotiations worked out. "PhRMA would be the worst enemy to have," one of the interlocutors in private discussions later said, not just because of the advertising the drug industry could run, but because of the scale and sophistication of its lobbying and its connections with members of Congress.

Senior members of both the administration and Congress believed an agreement was essential to avoid the kind of ad blitz that PhRMA could mount. That seemed to be one of the lessons of 1994. For many in Washington, the diverse reasons for the failure of the Clinton plan had congealed into the legend of Harry and Louise, the idea that one lobby, the health insurers, had single-handedly defeated health-care reform with a massive advertising campaign.

In a series of meetings between March and June with PhRMA representatives, Baucus and senior White House staff agreed to the terms of a deal. PhRMA got what it wanted: the legislation would not include direct negotiations over Medicare prices, importation of cheap drugs from abroad, or several other measures the industry opposed. In return, PhRMA would provide $80 billion of cost savings on drugs and pay for an advertising campaign in support of reform. The cost savings would come in two forms: rebates on drugs purchased under the Medicaid program and discounts on drugs that seniors purchased out of pocket when they entered the gap ("donut hole") in Medicare prescription drug coverage. The PhRMA deal, however, turned out to have another cost when it finally became public later that year—a political cost to Obama's image and reputation, not just among his opponents, but among many independents and progressives, who saw it as an example of the president caving in to the special interests he said he would resist.

The deal with the hospital associations did not cause the same indignation, though it also later became a political problem. Avoiding more stringent cost-control measures, the hospitals agreed to accept payment reductions that would save the government $155 billion over 10 years, an amount the hospitals could accept because of the additional revenue that expanded health insurance would bring. The legislation would be written so that the payment reductions were contingent on the expansion of coverage.[15] The savings, however, came through reduced updates to Medicare rates, which Republicans would portray as cuts in Medicare and use as evidence that health-care reform would hurt the elderly.

If Obama and the Democrats had been in a stronger position politically, they could have insisted on stronger cost containment and avoided making as large concessions to PhRMA and the hospitals as they did. But the institutions of American government (especially the need for 60 votes in the Senate) and the polarization between the parties were going to make it hard to pass any bill. Reform needed interest-group allies: there would be no way to pass it if the entire health-care industry went into all-out opposition. So Obama went back on campaign promises about how he would govern. At an August 2008 town meeting in Virginia, in the course of one of his riffs about negotiating around a "big table," Obama had said that the doctors, nurses, insurers, and drug companies would "get a seat at the table, they just won't be able to buy every chair. But what we will do is, we'll have the negotiations televised on C-SPAN, so that people can see who is making arguments on behalf of their constituents, and who are making arguments on behalf of the drug companies or the insurance companies."[16] That part did turn out to be a fantasy.

On Capitol Hill in early 2009, the Senate took the lead in drafting health-care legislation. In April Kennedy and Baucus sent a letter to the president promising to work on complementary bills that could be easily merged after their committees marked them up (reviewed and amended them) in June.[17] Obama wanted them to work expeditiously, with the aim of having both the House and Senate pass their bills before the August congressional recess. With Kennedy's health worsening that spring, Senator Christopher Dodd of Connecticut took over as chair of the HELP committee, while Kennedy's staff remained and drafted the bill's central provisions. It was partly through Kennedy's staff that the Massachusetts reforms and the private consensus-building efforts had a direct influence on the federal legislation. The original HELP draft took some of its language directly from the Massachusetts statute, and beginning in late 2008, Kennedy's staff held regular meetings with representatives of major health-care, labor, and business groups to discuss the critical choices Congress would have to make. The participants in these "workhorse meetings" overlapped with the strange-bedfellows sessions already in progress. A Senate staffer later recalled how "astonished" he was in one of the first workhorse meetings at the "general consensus" on major features of the law, such as expanding Medicaid up to 100 percent or 133 percent of the federal poverty level. The representatives of the American Federation of Labor, America's Health Insurance Plans, and other groups were in agreement. "I was sitting there, 'Oh my God, we've just settled on a scheme that will cover just about everybody.' Once you had the basic elements—expansion of Medicaid, insurance reform, the mandate, subsidies—all the rest fell into place. One thing led to another." But this consensus with the stakeholder groups did not translate into bipartisan support. When the HELP committee began to mark up the bill on June 17, the

Republicans savaged it on the basis of a preliminary and incomplete analysis of its cost, and when the committee approved the bill on July 15, the vote was on straight party lines.

According to Republican sources, the Democrats on HELP never seriously consulted them in writing the committee's bill, but the story was different in Finance, where Baucus made a "good-faith" effort to involve the Republicans in drafting the legislation. On June 17, Baucus convened the first of a series of meetings with a subgroup of the committee that originally included four Republicans (Grassley, Olympia Snowe of Maine, Orrin Hatch of Utah, and Mike Enzi of Wyoming) as well as two other Democrats (Conrad of North Dakota and Jeff Bingaman of New Mexico). If there was any hope for bipartisanship, it rested with this group.

In the House, meanwhile, the Democratic leadership worked out an unusual collaborative process among the three committees with jurisdiction over health care. Instead of marching off in different directions, the chairmen of Ways and Means, Education and Labor, and Energy and Commerce agreed to develop a common bill to present to their committees, and during the spring they had large, combined meetings to formulate the legislation. It quickly became apparent that they would have no Republican support. When Rob Andrews, chair of the health subcommittee of Education and Labor, approached Republicans who he thought might be open to working on the bill, he found that none of them would support any of the potential means of financing coverage of the uninsured. The Democrats, however, had enough votes in the House to pass the legislation on their own—if they could hold the right and left flanks of their party together. The 2006 and 2008 elections had brought in a substantial number of Democrats from swing districts who were wary of endangering their popularity back home by voting for a costly bill with a big federal role. But the Democrats in the House also included about 60 progressives who would have preferred a single-payer system and believed they had already conceded enough by settling for a public-insurance option in the exchange.

Two developments, both originating in the Energy and Commerce Committee, complicated and slowed the House's progress on health-care reform. First, Waxman decided to give priority to a climate bill calling for a cap-and-trade system. After difficult negotiations, the bill passed his committee in

May and narrowly won approval on the House floor in June. But the legislation never went anywhere in the Senate, and it aggravated relations between the House leadership and Democrats in swing districts, who resented being asked to take a tough—and ultimately fruitless—vote that jeopardized their chances for reelection. The climate legislation also became one of a long series of House-approved bills that died in the Senate and caused rising friction between Democrats in the two chambers.

The second development slowing health-care reform in the House came as a result of resistance by centrist and conservative Democrats to the liberal cast of the health-care bill being developed under the House leadership. In May, 45 members of the Blue Dog Caucus signed a letter protesting their exclusion from the drafting process controlled by the chairmen of the health-related committees and Speaker Pelosi and praising "the collaborative approach being taken by our Senate colleagues."[18] The control of the health-care bill reflected the new distribution of power in the Democratic caucus. Through most of the twentieth century, southern Democrats in safe seats accumulated seniority, became chairmen of the key committees, and either blocked health-insurance legislation or gave it a relatively conservative stamp. But with the regional shift in American politics, the Democrats with safe seats and seniority tended to come from the Northeast and Pacific coast. Of the three chairs of the committees concerned with health, two came from California (Waxman and George Miller) and one from New York (Charles B. Rangel). Of the chairs of the subcommittees concerned with health, two came from New Jersey (Andrews and Frank Pallone) and one from California (Pete Stark). Democrats from predominantly white districts in the South were more at risk of defeat in Republican wave elections (as in 1994) and consequently lacked the seniority and power their predecessors once had.

Nonetheless, the Democrats did not have enough votes to pass the health-care legislation without support from a significant number of the 58 members of the moderate-to-conservative Blue Dog Caucus. While both the Ways and Means and the Education and Labor committees were sure to approve the health-care bill, the trouble would come in Energy and Commerce, where seven of the Blue Dogs threatened to join with the Republicans to vote down the legislation. In 1994, with John Dingell as chair, the committee had been unable to act on health-care reform because of opposition from centrist and conservative Democrats. Now it was Waxman's turn to overcome the same obstacle.

Although the Blue Dogs said they shared the aim of covering all Americans, they objected to several aspects of the "tri-committee" draft finally released by the House leadership in June. Under the bill, Americans who received coverage through a national insurance exchange would be able to sign up for a public plan run by the Department of Health and Human Services that would compete with private insurers, offer several policies ranging in comprehensiveness, and pay hospitals, doctors, and other providers Medicare rates plus 5 percent. Reflecting the views of providers in their districts, particularly in rural areas, the Blue Dogs objected that Medicare payments, even with the additional 5 percent, were so far below private-insurance rates that they would threaten the availability of services. Likewise, the Blue Dogs saw a threat to small business from the employer mandate in the bill, which would require firms either to provide coverage to their workers directly (paying 65 percent of premiums for families and a slightly higher share for individuals) or "contribute" 8 percent of the average salary toward the purchase of coverage through the exchange. In addition, the Blue Dogs insisted that the total federal cost of the legislation be reduced below $1 trillion over 10 years (at that point, the tab was running about $1.5 trillion). These demands were in tension with one another: eliminating the public option or raising its payment rates would increase the legislation's cost, not reduce it.

When the conflict with Blue Dogs came to a head in late July, Waxman succeeded where Dingell had failed in 1994 and worked out a deal to get the bill through his committee. The agreement preserved a public insurance option, but instead of paying "Medicare plus five," the public plan from the start would pay rates that it would negotiate with providers (in the earlier draft, the public plan would have moved to negotiated rates after three years). Employers with an annual payroll under $500,000 would be exempt from any requirement to pay for coverage, and the legislation would include a provision for an independent board to contain Medicare costs. Other changes, the Blue Dogs were assured, would reduce the total cost below $1 trillion. Not all the moderate and conservative Democrats were ready to support the bill. Some of them particularly objected to the tax increase for people earning more than $350,000 a year, which at that point was how the House proposed to raise much of the revenue to finance the legislation. Another group was not satisfied that the bill prevented public funds from being used to pay for abortions. With these and other issues still unresolved, the House would be unable to vote on a final bill before the August recess.[19]

The Senate Finance Committee was also running into difficulties and delays. On July 22, Hatch dropped out of the negotiations, while the six remaining senators continued to go point by point through the details of the legislation. The members of the Gang of Six (as the group became known) illustrated to an extreme degree one of the institutional differences between the House and Senate. While the committee chairmen drafting the House bill came from California, New York, and New Jersey, the senators in the Gang of Six represented Montana, New Mexico, North Dakota, Maine, Iowa, and Wyoming—states that in total, as the liberal blogger Matt Yglesias pointed out, accounted for just 2.74 percent of the nation's population and did not include any of the nation's 50 largest metropolitan areas.[20] Yet, for a while, the fate of health-care reform seemed to hang entirely on their discussions.

With the benefit of hindsight, critics would later accuse Baucus of unnecessarily stringing out negotiations with the Republicans. As of midsummer, though, an agreement still looked possible, and with Senator Kennedy's health deteriorating, the Democrats might lose their sixtieth vote any day (Massachusetts law at that point did not provide for a temporary appointee by the governor). The discussions in Finance had narrowed the issues under consideration; by July 30, the cost was down to $900 billion over 10 years, according to a preliminary CBO estimate. "Quantifiably, we're on the edge," Grassley told the *Washington Post* in one of several statements he made in late July and early August suggesting an agreement was in reach.[21] Altogether, the bipartisan group in Finance would meet 31 times for an average of about two hours, and many of the features ultimately included in the legislation emerged from those sessions.[22] These compromises with the Republicans also served to win over the most conservative members of the Democratic caucus, such as Lieberman and

Senator Ben Nelson of Nebraska. But Grassley was always a long shot despite his reassurances. While Snowe might vote for the bill on her own, Grassley had consistently said he wouldn't do so unless a significant number of Republican senators joined him. That criterion might have been satisfied if the Republican caucus had included as many moderates as it had in the early 1990s. Outside of Congress, former Republican Senate majority leaders Bob Dole and Howard Baker joined with Daschle in the Bipartisan Policy Center's proposal for health-care reform, which bore a strong resemblance to the Senate Finance bill.[23] But as a result of the party's ideological shift and the pressures from the right on Republicans in office, Grassley would have to stick his neck out, which he was not willing to do. Running for reelection the next year, he stood the risk of being "primaried" from the right. Obama not only was in continual contact with Baucus throughout this period but also talked directly with Grassley. In one conversation, Grassley asked the president to give a public signal that a government insurance plan was not essential. Obama then asked Grassley if he got every concession he was asking for, would he support the bill? "Probably not," Grassley said, and when pressed, he explained, "Because I'd have to have a number of Republicans."[24] He was not about to become a new profile in courage. With no agreement in Finance, the search for a way forward in the Senate would have to continue in September after members of Congress went home for the August recess.

Democrats had already been adjusting to the probability that health-care reform would have to pass without Republican votes if it was to pass at all. At a breakfast with reporters in late June, Rahm Emanuel had insisted: "This will be bipartisan; there will be ideas from both parties. . . . Whether Republicans decide to vote for things they promoted will be up to them."[25] In another era, the kind of bill that Baucus was drafting could have been a bipartisan compromise. Unfortunately for the Democrats, it was a compromise with a Republican Party that no longer existed.

Reaction and Resolve

"If we're able to stop Obama on this, it will be his Waterloo. It will break him," Senator Jim DeMint of South Carolina said in a conference call on heath care with conservative activists on July 17. DeMint was looking ahead to the August congressional recess, and he predicted that after members of Congress returned home and felt the wrath of their constituents about the health-care legislation, they would "come back in September afraid to vote against the American people."[26]

All the necessary elements for a right-wing counterattack against the Democrats' reform effort came together that summer—rallying cries and rhetoric, financing and organization, strategy and tactics. The counterattack took the Democrats by surprise and, for a time, it dominated the news and eroded support for reform. But the distortions and sheer belligerence on the right produced a reaction too, engaging many progressives who had stood on the sidelines and stiffening the resolve of both the president and congressional Democrats.

Just the day before DeMint predicted a summer of rage, the conservative writer Betsy McCaughey declared on a radio show that she had read the health-care bill pending in the House and discovered that "Congress would make it mandatory—absolutely require—that every five years people in Medicare have a required counseling session that will tell them how to end their life sooner."[27] In 1994, McCaughey had gained national prominence by falsely charging that the Clinton health plan would prohibit people from paying for any doctor's services other than those covered by the government. Now she was reclaiming the national spotlight the one way she knew how. The supposedly "mandatory" requirement that Medicare beneficiaries have a counseling session telling them how to end their lives was actually a provision to pay physicians if their patients voluntarily sought counseling about living wills, hospice care, and other end-of-life services. The provision had originated in a stand-alone bill co-sponsored by Representatives Earl Blumenauer, an Oregon Democrat, and Charles Boustany, a Republican physician from Louisiana. In the Senate, the Georgia Republican and prominent pro-life advocate Johnny Isakson had proposed a similar bill in 2007, the Medicare End-of-Life Planning Act.

Nevertheless, McCaughey's charge ricocheted through the conservative media, and on July 23, Rep. John Boehner, the Republican leader in the House, said, "This provision may start us down a treacherous path toward government-encouraged euthanasia." Another Republican congressman,

Louie Gohmert of Texas, said the Democrats' bill would "absolutely kill senior citizens. They'll put them on lists and force them to die early because they won't get the treatment as early as they need." Rep. Virginia Foxx of North Carolina declared that the elderly would be "put to death by their government."[28] On August 7, former Alaska governor Sarah Palin hit upon the phrase that indelibly implanted McCaughey's charge in the public mind. In a post on Facebook, Palin said that seniors and the disabled "will have to stand in front of Obama's 'death panel' so his bureaucrats can decide, based on a subjective judgment of their 'level of productivity in society,' whether they are worthy of health care."[29]

In an interview just after Palin's "death panel" charge, Senator Isakson told Ezra Klein of the *Washington Post,* "How someone could take an end of life directive or a living will as that is nuts. You're putting the authority in the individual rather than the government. I don't know how that got so mixed up."[30] It was hardly an inadvertent mix-up. The concept of the "death panel" brilliantly exemplified the kind of rhetoric that the Republican political consultant and wordsmith Frank Luntz had recommended in May in a report on the "language of healthcare." Republicans, Luntz advised, should stop talking about "the free market, tax incentives, or competition" and focus instead on how "politicians," "bureaucrats," and "Washington" would deny Americans medical care. It was "essential," Luntz wrote, "that *'deny'* and *'denial'* enter the conservative lexicon immediately because it is at the core of what scares Americans most about a government takeover of healthcare." A "government takeover" was exactly how Republicans should describe what Democrats wanted to do. "Takeovers are like coups—they both lead to dictators and a loss of freedom." After testing "40 distinct messages," Luntz reported that "nothing turns people against what the Democrats are trying to do more immediately and intensely than the specter of having to wait for tests and treatment thanks to a government takeover of healthcare by nameless, faceless bureaucrats."[31]

The script that Luntz recommended was not new; it was how conservatives had fought Truman's national health insurance plan, Medicare, and the 1993 Clinton health plan. The Democrats' proposals had changed— they were now proposing to give tax credits that people could use to purchase private coverage through insurance exchanges—but it didn't matter. "Imagine waking up one day and all your medical decisions are made by a central national board," ran one of the first right-wing ads against the Democrats' proposed reforms. "Bureaucrats decide the treatments you receive, the drugs you take, even the doctors you see."[32]

The man issuing the warning in that advertisement was Rick Scott, who earlier in 2009 had founded and funded a group called Conservatives for Patients' Rights, one of several organizations set up to oppose the Democrats' health legislation. Scott had a checkered history. Once the CEO of Columbia/HCA Healthcare—the largest for-profit hospital chain in the country—he had been ousted by his board in 1997 in the wake of a federal indictment of the company for Medicare fraud, which ultimately led it to pay $1.7 billion in fines. (In 2010 he would be elected governor of Florida.) According to the news site Politico, Scott "seeded" Conservatives for Patients' Rights with $5 million of his own money and said the group would spend "up to $20 million" to fight the Democrats' reforms.[33]

Other conservative groups with wealthy and powerful backers also began focusing on the health-care battle in 2009. Americans for Prosperity—established in 2003 by Charles and David H. Koch, the billionaire owners of the oil, chemical, and paper-products conglomerate Koch Industries—spun off Patients United Now to organize demonstrations against health-care reform.[34] A third organization, FreedomWorks, led by former Republican Majority Leader Dick Armey, helped to create the Tea Party Patriots, which then also became one of the primary organizers of protests against the Democrats' health legislation. It was the "Tea Party Patriots Health Care Freedom Kick Off Conference Call," arranged with Scott's group, that provided the occasion for Senator DeMint's prediction of a wave of protest during the August congressional recess.[35]

By July 17, the planning for the recess was well under way. The previous month, the national coordinator of the Tea Party Patriots had read a memo by a FreedomWorks volunteer in Connecticut laying out a tactic that their members might find useful. "Rocking the Town Halls: Best Practices" described how with only about 30 people "spread out among the crowd of about 150 people in the hall," the tea partiers in Fairfield County, Connecticut, had shaken up a meeting by the local Democratic congressman. "You need to rock-the-boat early in the Rep's presentation. Watch for an opportunity to yell out and challenge the Rep's statements early," the memo's author, Robert MacGuffie, advised. "The goal is to rattle him."[36]

During the first week of August, Democrats returning from Washington to their districts were unprepared for what was waiting for them. Americans for Prosperity, Conservatives for Patients' Rights, and other groups in the Health Care Freedom Coalition had obtained schedules of town meetings, emailed the times and locations to their supporters, and arranged for buses to bring them there. When the congressmen began to speak, they were interrupted, hooted, and booed and, as YouTube videos of the events show, could often hardly make themselves heard above the hubbub. On August 6, for example, 1,500 people came to a venue seating only 250 for a town hall meeting in Tampa with Representatives Betty Reed and Kathy Castor, who were drowned out by catcalls. According to the *St. Petersburg Times,* Fox TV host Glenn Beck's 912 Project had drawn his followers to the event. "Tyranny! Tyranny! Tyranny!" "Forty-million illegals! Forty million illegals!" people shouted as Castor struggled to speak.[37]

That same day the 83-year-old Michigan Rep. John Dingell showed up for a town hall in the Detroit suburb of Romulus to face a crowd of about 225 people, of whom probably no more than 40 were his supporters. One demonstrator, applauded by others, held aloft a poster showing Obama morphing into Hitler. Right at the start, a man wheeled his disabled son to the front and demanded to know why Dingell wanted to take away his child's health care, and when Dingell (whose own crutches leaned against the wall behind him) said that was not true, the man kept repeating "liar" until he was finally escorted away. In support of Dingell, the Michigan Universal Health Care Access Network had arranged for a woman with disabilities who had lost her health insurance to be there to tell her story. She was heckled ("I shouldn't have to pay for your health care," one protester yelled) and, after she was finished, a large man bent over to warn her, "They're going to euthanize you."[38]

By early in the second week of August, Organizing for America—the grass-roots organization created for Obama's presidential campaign—was coordinating rapid response with the progressive coalition Health Care for America Now (HCAN). According to Richard Kirsch, HCAN's national campaign manager, the Democrats' supporters soon began outnumbering

conservative protesters. But by then the storyline had already been established in the media. Irate citizens were erupting at the Democrats' town
halls, telling them to their faces they didn't want them to pass their health-
care legislation.

It didn't help the Democrats that the news about the White House deal
with the pharmaceutical industry broke that month after House Democrats, who were never party to the negotiations, included a provision in
their bill for direct negotiations with the industry over Medicare prescription drug prices. PhRMA's representatives then told the press about its
agreement with the White House, which confirmed it.[39] Unlike the death-
panel story, this one was true, but it suggested that there were indeed secret aspects to health-care reform. The news about the PhRMA deal also fit
into the conservative populist view of the Wall Street and auto-industry
bailouts. The sequence of developments during 2008 and 2009 had helped
to shape the context in which health-care reform was received. "Health
care was a big issue, yes, and it took up most of the questions at the town
meetings," Senator Grassley said. "But it seemed to me it was the straw
that broke the camel's back. People were bringing up the stimulus bill not
doing any good and [costing] $800 billion. Or the Federal Reserve shovel-
ing $2 trillion out of an airplane and not seeing it does any good. And the
nationalization of banks and [General Motors]."[40]

The confrontations at the town meetings in August produced a surge in
news coverage about health-care reform, and it was not the coverage Democrats wanted. They were frustrated that when they had quiet, civil conversations with constituents, it wasn't news. When Obama went to answer
questions at a town meeting in New Hampshire and there were no erup-
tions, Fox News broke away as anchor Trace Gallagher said, "Any contentious questions, anybody yelling, we'll bring it to you."[41] Fox not only
highlighted the shouting; its anchors congratulated the shouters and
urged others to join them. The media and the right-wing protesters were
feeding off each other. On August 11, the Tea Party Patriots national coordinator emailed her list, "We have a media request for an event this week
that will have lots of energy and lots of anger. This is for CNBC."[42] In a
media-drenched society, people can be counted on to perform for the cameras. And with YouTube, they didn't even need the news media to show up;

a video showing a besieged and flummoxed Democratic congressman could go viral and serve the same purpose.

The counterattack worked, to a degree. On the basis of a content analysis of news stories, the Project for Excellence in Journalism found, "In the crucial battle over the words and themes that can help define a policy debate, opponents of the health care bill seemed to enjoy considerably more success than the supporters."[43] By mid-August, according to a Pew poll, 86 percent of Americans said they had heard the claim that health-care reform legislation "includes the creation of so called 'death panels' "; an NBC poll at the time found that 45 percent of the public—and 75 percent of Fox News viewers—believed the legislation would give the government power to cut off care for the elderly.[44]

But August had another side. The right-wing attacks fired up the left too. In an account of the month's skirmishes, Kirsch writes that after a "disastrous" August 2 town meeting in Philadelphia, the director of Pennsylvania HCAN Marc Stier saw "what every great organizer recognizes: the opposition always presents the greatest opportunities to build power." The right-wing mobilization was a wake-up call to progressives, who had been warily following the legislation in Washington but after seeing the uprising on the right "knew in their gut they had to fight back." Just as important, according to Kirsch, once Democratic members of Congress came under attack, they asked for help from HCAN in bringing supporters to their town hall meetings. The result was to bring the congressional Democrats closer to the progressive base.[45] Even some of the steadfastly neutral news media decided they couldn't just report the death-panel scare as a fact and had to make clear that it was untrue.

The summer of 2009 brought another change: some sectors of business decided to fight the White House on health-care reform. "K Street [the business lobbying community in Washington] is a three-billion-dollar weathervane," Grover Norquist, a central figure in conservative circles, told the *New Yorker*'s Jane Mayer in 2010. "When Obama was strong, the Chamber of Commerce said, 'We can work with the Obama Administration.' But that changed when thousands of people went into the street and 'terrorized' congressmen. August is what changed it."[46]

Though it was not known publicly at the time, August was the month when a check for $86.2 million went from America's Health Insurance Plans (AHIP) to the Chamber of Commerce to mount a campaign against the health-care legislation. That was no small sum; it was greater than the Chamber's entire budget for the preceding year.[47]

But this was not the whole story. According to a member of AHIP's board, the money that went to the Chamber did not come from AHIP itself, and even members of its board were not informed of the transaction. The funds came from the Big Five for-profit insurers (Aetna, CIGNA, Humana, United-Healthcare, and WellPoint), which were using AHIP to pass along the money to the Chamber to run a campaign that AHIP itself would not run.

The health insurance industry was not as homogenous as many of its critics believed. As of the early 1990s, three separate groups had represented insurers in Washington: the Health Insurance Association of America, which represented the for-profit indemnity insurers and ran the "Harry and Louise" ads; the American Managed Care and Review Association, made up of for-profit managed-care plans; and the relatively liberal Group Health Association of America, representing the nonprofit HMOs. By 2004, all three had combined to form AHIP to provide the industry with more unified representation—that is, when it was unified.

Although many people supposed that AHIP supported the health-care legislation in Congress, it had endorsed only general principles. In 2006, according to AHIP's president Karen Ignagni, the association began reexamining its position on health-care reform. Recognizing that costs were going up unsustainably, the insurers decided to participate constructively in discussions with other stakeholders and to undertake an extensive internal analysis of policy alternatives. That internal process led to AHIP's endorsement in late 2008 of principles for comprehensive reform, including universal coverage and cost containment. The insurers would accept guaranteed issue of policies with no pre-existing-condition exclusions if the government required everyone to be covered and provided subsidies to low-income people so they could afford to pay for it.[48]

But while the AHIP board voted unanimously for this position, not all the member companies were behind it, according to one insurance company president. The Big Five for-profit insurers were not well represented on the policy committee that formulated the position. The business they know how to do, as this executive explained, is "a business of risk selection," and under a system of guaranteed issue with no rating by health status—the system envisioned for the insurance exchanges—the for-profit insurers would not be able to do business the way they had always done it. As a result, the Big Five were uneasy with AHIP's position from the start. Moreover, as the legislation took shape in 2009, "there was something for every insurance company to hate." The insurers didn't only dislike the public option; they were unhappy about many other provisions even in the bill being developed by Baucus.

Unlike the pharmaceutical and hospital industries, the insurers never made a deal with the Senate Finance Committee or the White House. AHIP's board could never agree on a list of a few things it wanted in return for which it would promise to support the legislation. If there was ever a chance for such a deal, it was out of the question after the news of the White House deal with PhRMA leaked in early August. It was also in mid-summer that relations between the Democrats and the insurance industry deteriorated sharply. At a news conference on July 22, Obama said of the insurers, "Right now, at the time when everybody's getting hammered, they're making record profits and premiums are going up."[49] At least publicly, Ignagni resisted replying in kind.[50] Others in the industry, however, were ready to go to war. In August one of the Big Five, UnitedHealthcare, encouraged its employees to join the Tea Party groups fighting reform.[51] Progressive organizations then responded by organizing protests against the private insurers. Yet AHIP did not take a position against the legislation. Still hoping to influence the outcome, it focused its criticism on specific provisions.

Despite the Chamber's ad campaign, employers did not generally mobilize to oppose the Democrats' health-care reform efforts in the summer of 2009 as they had in February 1994, when the Clinton effort was devastated by an abrupt shift of business lobbies to the opposition. Big business stayed relatively aloof from the battle. In 2009, as Helen Darling, director of the National Business Group on Health, says, the financial crisis led big business to be "focused on other things."[52] The health-care legislation did not impinge strongly on the interests of large employers. Although the reforms might require them to make some adjustments in benefits, the changes would be relatively minor. The Business Roundtable was blandly support-ive of reform. Even the Chamber's competitor in small-business advocacy, the National Federation of Independent Business, which had vehemently opposed the Clinton plan, started out in 2007 in general sympathy with the reforms, though after a change in leadership in early 2009, NFIB shifted to the opposition. Still, employers were not a decisive force in the debate. Ideological politics trumped interest-group politics in 2009.

But amid all the attacks on the Democrats' legislation, public anxieties were growing. The monthly Kaiser tracking polls showed a steady rise in the proportion of Americans who were worried that health-care reform would make their families worse off. As of February 2009, only 11 percent expected reform would have a negative personal impact; by July that figure was up to 21 percent, and in August it jumped to 31 percent (as against 36 percent who expected their families to be better off, and 27 percent who thought reform would have no effect on them).[53] Inside the White House, Obama was hearing the bad news about the trends, and Rahm Emanuel and Vice President Joe Biden were urging him to give up on comprehen-sive reform and call for a more modest program.[54] But Obama not only re-solved to go ahead; in September and again in the new year, the president took charge of the effort to steady the health-care initiative and prevent it from careening off the tracks.

Obama and the Rollercoaster to Reform

Senator Kennedy's death on August 25 brought a raucous month to a somber close and served as a reminder, if any were needed, of the long struggle to achieve health care for all that he and so many others had been pursuing. In the wake of the summer's developments, Obama faced two separate challenges: reverse the conservative onslaught in public debate and overcome the remaining obstacles to action in Congress, particularly in the Senate, where the bipartisan negotiations were stalled. To turn things around, the president would give an address to a joint session of Congress on September 9, possibly releasing at that time the health-care bill that, unknown to the public, the White House had been preparing in the event of a legislative impasse.

By September, some Democrats were concerned that in ceding the initiative on health care to Congress, Obama had overreacted to the Clinton experience. Although the president was actively involved in the health-care negotiations—and DeParle, Sebelius, Emanuel, and others represented the White House in discussions on Capitol Hill—the picture presented to the public suggested that the legislation was being determined entirely by Congress. Yet the congressional leaders were not nearly as popular as Obama was, and the congressional process was complex and uninspiring. As the study of media coverage by the Project for Excellence in Journalism later found, the health-care legislation tended to fare better in public opinion "when Obama actively carried the ball."[55] One clear advantage from holding back in the early phases, though, was that Obama could take the ball and seize the nation's attention when the "game" demanded it.

Regaining control of the debate would not be easy. Despite impressions to the contrary, presidential speeches rarely succeed in shifting public opinion, and the ability of presidents to command a national audience has declined dramatically.[56] In the 1960s and '70s, nearly half the households in the country would watch a prime-time presidential TV appearance. In those days, most Americans had only a few channels to choose from, and the networks often all agreed to broadcast a president's speech at the same time. But with the explosion in the number of channels in the 1980s, the TV audience splintered, and presidents had to compete with entertainment. By 1995, one of Bill Clinton's news conferences drew only 6.5 percent of households.[57] Obama started out with comparatively high ratings. According to Nielsen data, 31 percent of TV homes watched his first press conference on February 9, but that share dropped to 16 percent by his fifth, on July 22, when he talked about health-care reform.[58] The ratings for Obama's speeches to joint sessions of Congress followed the same trajectory, though they started at a higher point. Fifty-two million people watched his first address in February, but on September 9, the audience for his health-care address was down to 32 million.[59] Even so, no other figure in American politics could have drawn as many people, and Obama took full advantage of the occasion to give an exceptionally effective speech.

After a month of fear and anger, the president needed to restate the moral case for health-care reform. A few months earlier, in June, when Obama addressed the American Medical Association, he had told his speechwriters to focus on cost containment, and in the speech itself he had mentioned the uninsured only toward the end. Members of the administration at that time often talked about "bending the cost curve," a concept that was sure to warm the heart of every accountant. Standing before Congress, however, Obama put the problems of the uninsured up front, and toward the end he quoted from a letter that Senator Kennedy had asked to have delivered after his death. "What we face," Kennedy had written, "is above all a moral issue; at stake are not just the details of policy, but fundamental principles of social justice and the character of our country."[60]

But Obama did not spend a lot of time spelling out the problems of health care. "We know we must reform this system," he said. "The question is how." And then, unlike Clinton 16 years earlier, Obama gave a clear, succinct account of how the reforms would work in practice in an attempt to overcome the misinformation that had swamped public discussion in the previous month.

Many political consultants believe it is an error for a political leader to repeat false charges made by opponents on the grounds that repetition only reinforces those accusations in the public mind. But Obama disagrees with that view—so says one of his speechwriters—and in his address to Congress he rebutted several of the charges leveled against the health-care legislation. After pronouncing the death-panel scare "a lie, plain and simple," the president denied that the reforms would extend insurance to illegal immigrants—and just at that point a Republican, Rep. Joe Wilson of South Carolina, brought the flavor of the town halls to the floor of Congress by shouting, "You lie."

While that moment predictably became a focus of attention, hardly anyone seemed to notice something more important in the speech: Obama kept referring to "my plan" and "my proposal." Most of the audience must have assumed that he was taking ownership of the reforms in a general way, which he was doing. But when Obama said, for example, that "the plan I'm proposing will cost around $900 billion over ten years," he was actually referring to a specific plan developed in the White House. Right up until the speech, Orszag assumed that the bill they had been working on and costing out would be released that evening. Wouldn't the press insist on seeing Obama's plan? But expecting that it would just create more controversy, other advisers to the president opposed a release (a vague sketch was posted online instead). And, to Orszag's surprise, when no bill was forthcoming, there was no chorus of demands to see it.[61]

Obama's speech stopped the decline in public support for health-care reform registered in the previous months. According to the Kaiser Foundation tracking polls, the proportion of Americans saying they expected their families to be better off if health reform passed increased by six percentage points in one month, up to 42 percent.[62] The speech also introduced one new policy idea. Recognizing that it would take years to establish the new insurance exchanges and carry out other long-term reforms, Obama called for a short-term fund—a subsidized high-risk pool—to provide coverage for at least some people denied insurance because of pre-existing conditions.

But if there was one bombshell in the speech from the standpoint of Democrats in Congress, it was the $900 billion figure for the legislation's cost. "We were furious," says one of Nancy Pelosi's top advisers. The House had been trying to get the cost under $1 trillion, and now it seemed that Obama had moved the goalpost $100 billion further back. (Later, the White House clarified that $900 billion was not a "gross" but a "net" figure, though exactly what that meant was ambiguous.) The president had also said, "Most of these costs will be paid for with money already being spent—but spent badly—in the existing health care system. The plan will not add to our deficit." That reflected the financing strategy that Baucus was following in the Senate Finance Committee, where the idea was to find most of the money for reform from within the health-care system, without the tax increase on the highest earners in the House bill. That approach would lead Baucus and the president to support a new tax on high-cost ("Cadillac") health insurance plans, which would become another source of conflict among Democrats in the final months of the legislative battle.

Baucus had set a September 15 deadline for the Gang of Six negotiations. Although Grassley made a new counterproposal in early September, Democrats had given up on him, particularly after he had sent out a fund-raising letter in August asking for "support in helping me defeat 'Obama-care.'"[63]

After the last meeting of the Gang of Six ended with no agreement, Baucus released his own bill, which included many of the provisions negotiated with the bipartisan group. By this point, however, he could hope for the support of only one Republican, Olympia Snowe, who did vote with the Democrats when the committee passed the bill 14 to 9 on October 13. But Snowe made it clear she still had reservations and might change her mind when the legislation reached the Senate floor.

As the House and Senate moved toward final bills, the Democrats in each chamber became embroiled in conflict over two emotionally charged issues that many of those pressing for health-care reform had hoped to avoid altogether. In the House, the issue was abortion. In the Senate, it was the public option. In both cases, liberals in Congress were forced to make what seemed to them at the time to be major concessions in order to pass the legislation, dismaying many of their supporters and creating a new problem for the Democrats—loss of support on the left.

In the House, Speaker Pelosi was now fully in charge of decisions about the health-care legislation. Beginning in August, her office had merged the bills coming out of the three committees that had marked up the original "tri-com" draft, and during September and October the Speaker resolved a series of issues raised by the members of the Democratic caucus as they met in groups to review each aspect of the bill. Endorsements by both the AMA and AARP boosted prospects for passage, but as of the beginning of November, the leadership was still short of votes, and Pelosi found herself with no alternative except to address the concerns of a group of anti-abortion Democrats led by Rep. Bart Stupak of Michigan.

Beginning with the Hyde Amendment in 1976, Congress had barred the use of federal dollars to pay for abortions, except in cases of rape, incest, or a threat to the life of the mother. Democrats generally agreed on maintaining this principle; they just disagreed on what maintenance of the principle meant. Under current law, private insurance plans could cover abortion, and many of them did (the exact proportion was unclear because of conflicting survey data). Most supporters of reproductive rights believed that private insurance plans offered through the new exchanges should be able to continue to cover abortions as long as they segregated the federal subsidies they received from the private share of premiums and used only the private dollars to pay for abortions. The U.S. Conference of Catholic Bishops regarded this separation as a sham; if an insurance plan covered abortion and received federal subsidies, the federal government would be promoting abortion. In line with that view, Stupak's amendment not only prohibited abortion coverage in the public-insurance option; it also barred private insurance plans in the exchange from covering abortion if their subscribers received any federal subsidy. Since many of those using the exchange would receive tax credits for part of the premiums, insurance plans in the exchange would not be able to cover abortions (and some women who previously did have such coverage would lose it). The Stupak amendment allowed insurers to offer abortion coverage in an unsubsidized supplemental policy. But pro-choice advocates expected that few people would buy abortion coverage on its own (which would make it more expensive for the few who did buy it) and that insurers consequently might not even offer it.[64]

On the night before the floor vote, Pelosi tried to negotiate a compromise with Stupak and pro-choice Democratic women in the House, but when that effort failed, she acceded to Stupak's demand for a separate vote on his amendment. Because of her own credentials as a pro-choice advocate, Pelosi was able to give way without losing other liberal Democrats on the overall legislation. On Saturday, November 7, the Stupak amendment passed, and so did the health-care reform bill, 220 to 215, with 39 Democrats, most of them Blue Dogs, voting against the bill, and one lone Republican, from New Orleans, voting for it.

In the Senate, the Majority Leader Harry Reid had the parallel responsibilities of merging committee bills and assembling the votes—in this case, 60—necessary for passage. Reid generally deferred to the committees, and on the health-care legislation, he accepted the work of the HELP and Finance Committees insofar as they did not conflict with each other. That deference to the committees resulted, for example, in HELP's liberal public-health provisions becoming part of the final Senate bill. But where the two bills differed, Reid had to choose between them or work out a compromise, bearing in mind the need for 60 votes. A critical factor in his decision was that he now had the possibility of finding those votes entirely in his own caucus. On September 25, after the Massachusetts state legislature passed a statute authorizing a temporary replacement for Senator Kennedy, Governor Deval Patrick had appointed Paul G. Kirk, a lawyer who had once chaired the Democratic National Committee. Since Kennedy had been too ill to vote in the month before his death, this was actually the first time the Democratic caucus in 2009 had 60 senators capable of voting. The window for the Democrats to pass health-care reform on their own—the strategy that Reid adopted instead of pursuing Snowe, who seemed continually to raise new objections—would last only until January.

Throughout the 2009 debate, the public-insurance option had taken on high symbolic importance for both the left and right, and in the final stages it became the central focus of conflict in the Senate. While the HELP bill included a public option, the Finance bill did not. When the public option came up in the Finance Committee in late September, Baucus had said, "No one has been able to show me how we can count up to 60 votes with a public option. I want a bill that can become law."[65] So he had voted against it in committee, going along instead with a provision aiding nonprofit insurance cooperatives, an idea proposed by Senator Conrad of North Dakota, where agricultural and other co-ops have historically played an important role.

For progressives, however, the public option really meant a federally run insurance plan, and they regarded it as a litmus test of worthwhile health-care reform, even though the idea had already been drastically downgraded. The original promise of "guaranteed choice" was to give everyone with private insurance the option of enrolling in a public plan, but the public option in the bills under consideration would have been available only to the individuals and small groups buying insurance through the exchanges. Originally, the public plan would have had lower costs because it would have paid hospitals and physicians at Medicare rates (or Medicare rates plus 5 percent), which were on average 20 percent to 30 percent lower than private insurance rates—but that possibility had been quashed in both the House and Senate. The politics of the public option were more complicated than most people understood. Progressives saw the insurance industry as the force behind all the opposition, but the insurers weren't alone; the hospitals and other provider groups were also opposed. And that wasn't all. The ratio of Medicare to private insurance rates varied regionally; Democrats from states where Medicare payments were especially low opposed a public option keyed to Medicare rates. That was ultimately what killed a Medicare-like public option, according to one of Pelosi's aides. Although a public plan with Medicare rates would have saved the federal government far more money, it could never have passed the House.

But without the benefit of paying low Medicare rates, the public option might not be cheaper than private insurance, nor would it necessarily attract a large enrollment. According to the Congressional Budget Office, the public option would enroll less than 2 percent of the population and probably have higher premiums than those of private plans.[66] The problem was adverse selection: the public plan would likely end up with disproportionate numbers of enrollees with high costs. To be sure, all plans in the exchange would be required to take all prospective enrollees, but private insurers have long experience designing and marketing plans to attract healthy people. In contrast, a public plan would likely abstain from those practices; indeed, many advocates favored it in the belief that it would be a better choice for people with chronic illnesses and disabilities. And although risk-adjusted payments in the exchanges were intended to compensate plans with sicker enrollees, those methods were unlikely to offset 100 percent of their extra costs. A public option would also lead private insurers to resist strong risk-adjustment procedures so they could use the public plan as a dumping ground for the unprofitable sick in the classic way that private hospitals and other providers have used public institutions.

Despite its likely marginal significance, the public option overshadowed other aspects of health-care reform for many progressives. Although the Senate bill now put the reforms off until January 2014, neither the liberals in Congress nor progressive organizations made an issue of the delay. Nor was there much concern about the possibility of a backlash against the individual mandate, though polls revealed it to be the one distinctly unpopular aspect of the reform legislation. Like the right, the left saw the public option as a stealth single-payer plan—even though it might well have ended up as the high-cost option and an example for the conservative case that government is incompetent.

Not wishing to be the executioner of the public option, Senator Reid included it in his merged bill, though he knew a government insurance plan of the kind progressives wanted did not have 60 votes. He then convened a group of ten Democratic senators, evenly representing liberals and centrists, to find a compromise. This new Gang of Ten proposed three ideas in lieu of the public option. The Office of Personnel Management, which ran the federal employees' health benefit system, would negotiate two national private insurance plans, one of which had to be nonprofit, to be offered in every state's exchange. Private insurance plans would be required to spend at least 85 percent of their revenue on medical care for large groups and 80 percent for individuals and small groups. And people aged 55 to 64 would be allowed to buy into Medicare. The Medicare buy-in, proposed by Clinton in the late 1990s and endorsed by Gore and Lieberman in their 2000 campaign, had enthusiastic backing from the advocates of the public option, who saw it as a step toward "Medicare for all." But opening up Medicare to 55- to 64-year-olds raised the same opposition as a public plan based on Medicare rates; even some liberal Democrats from states with low Medicare payments were opposed to the idea. Lieberman spared them the embarrassment of killing a proposal that so many progressives wanted. Since August, he had been expressing doubts about the entire health-care bill, and given his record, he might well have voted against it. Now he said that the Medicare buy-in had all the "infirmities" of the public option, and Reid got his vote by agreeing to kill both alternatives.

To most people who had been following the legislation, it had seemed clear for a long time that the public option would not survive the Senate. The one advantage for the Democrats in keeping it alive was to use it as a bargaining chip at a crucial moment, and it had served that purpose with Lieberman. But because progressives had turned it into a measure of the legislation's value, the inevitable sacrifice of the public option demoralized the progressive base. On December 15, in the wake of the news that both the public option and Medicare buy-in had been abandoned, former Vermont Governor Howard Dean said Democrats should "kill the bill," and the next day, on ABC's *Good Morning America,* he charged that the legislation was "a bigger bailout for the insurance industry than [the bailout of] AIG."[67] Taking their cue from Dean, several prominent progressives in the media such as MSNBC host Keith Olbermann also called for killing the bill and starting over, which would have meant no legislation at all. If just one progressive senator such as Dean's fellow Vermonter, Independent Bernie Sanders, had followed that advice, Obama's effort to pass reform would have ended up like Clinton's, with nothing to show.

Reid's task in reaching 60 votes in the Senate was, if anything, more daunting than Pelosi's in reaching 218 votes in the House. With 258 members in her caucus, Pelosi could allow up to 40 defections, but Reid could not afford a single one. As a result, the final hold-outs had enormous bargaining leverage, which was just the problem that Democrats had been hoping to avoid by getting extra Republican votes. The deals that Reid made with individual senators reflected the position he was in. In what proved the single greatest embarrassment, Reid agreed to give Nelson special treatment for Nebraska on Medicaid. The legislation generally provided that the federal government would pay 100 percent of the cost of expanded Medicaid eligibility for the first years, gradually declining to 90 percent. Reid agreed to keep the federal share for Nebraska at 100 percent. To pass the Medicare prescription drug bill in 2003, Republicans had made deals that Karl Rove described as "the kind of horse-trading that has always been part of politics."[68] Now Republicans portrayed the Democrats' horse-trading as being emblematic of the thorough corruption of health-care reform. Nelson's "Cornhusker kickback" got more attention than any other aspect of the Senate bill (though in the end it never made it into law).

The giveaways in Medicare in 1965—cost-based reimbursement for hospitals and usual and customary fees for doctors—were of far greater fiscal consequence than the concessions to individual states in the health-care legislation in 2010. But Obama had promised a different kind of politics, and the "sausage-making" in Congress was politics as it had always been. Congressional politics had changed, however, in one respect. The final votes on the Affordable Care Act were on straight party lines, 60 to 40, with not a single member of either party crossing the divide. No one in Congress could recall a major piece of national legislation on which the party divisions in the Senate had been so absolute and the tenor of the debate had been so bitter.[69] The air in the Senate was thick with accusations of corruption and tyranny when the final votes on the legislation were cast on

December 24, 2009, the first time in 114 years that the Senate had voted on Christmas Eve.

Even though House and Senate had passed separate health-care bills, there was no guarantee of legislation. The two houses are sometimes unable to resolve their differences, and the differences in this case were substantial. The House had a public option; the Senate did not. The House had the Stupak amendment; the Senate did not. The House generally vested more power in the federal government, the Senate in the states. For example, the House had a single, national insurance exchange (though states could establish their own if they submitted an acceptable proposal), while the Senate had state-based insurance exchanges (unless the states failed to establish acceptable exchanges, in which case the federal government would step in). The House bill called for the startup of reforms on January 1, 2013, the Senate a year later. Unlike the House, the Senate provided for an Independent Payment Advisory Board, whose cost-containment recommendations for Medicare would become effective unless Congress overruled it. The House raised much of the revenue for health-care reform through higher income taxes on individuals earning more than $500,000 and couples earning more than $1 million, while the Senate taxed high-cost health insurance plans—and just as the House's income-tax increase was unacceptable to the Senate, so the Senate's tax on high-cost plans was unacceptable to the House.

The negotiations were especially difficult because the Democratic leaders in both houses did not have room to make concessions that would endanger what were only razor-thin majorities in the first place. A concession to the House on the public option would cost the votes of Lieberman and Nelson and probably bring down the bill when it went back to the Senate. But if the House simply gave way to the Senate on every issue, Pelosi would face a revolt from the progressives in her caucus.

A further complication was that in early January the labor unions went ballistic over the Senate's tax on high-cost insurance plans. The AFL-CIO called for members of unions to deluge Congress and the White House with telephone calls, and union leaders fumed over the betrayal of the president and the Democrats on the taxation of health benefits. Obama was now strongly committed to the tax, but he was flexible on the specifics and sought to accommodate labor's concerns. During the middle of January, non-stop negotiating sessions took place at the White House, and the outlines of a deal began to take shape. The House would give in on the public option, while the Senate would give in on a national insurance exchange. Obama would get his way on the tax on high-cost plans, but the tax would be deferred for several years and kick in at a higher threshold. These negotiations, however, never reached a conclusion—and might never have reached a settlement that would have retained the support of all 60 Democrats in the Senate and 218 in the House.

But the Democrats did have a way around this problem. The House could approve the Senate bill and then vote to modify it with a second, budget-reconciliation measure, which would then need only a simple majority in the Senate, thereby dispensing with the need to satisfy Lieberman, Nelson, and some other centrists. Although the House would have to accept all the provisions of the Senate bill that were not relevant to the budget, there would be more flexibility on everything that the Senate parliamentarian would judge to be budget-relevant. Under the circumstances, this was the best route for the House to modify the Senate bill. But House Democrats ruled out this option until independent events compelled the Democrats to adopt it.

Massachusetts had one more role to play in the health-care saga. The state had provided the model for reforms in 2006. Its senior senator, Ted Kennedy, had helped to move those reforms to the national level, and when he died, the state legislature's decision to authorize the governor to appoint a temporary replacement had given the Democrats their sixtieth vote. But on January 19, 2010, Massachusetts seemed to cancel out all its prior actions when the state's voters went to the polls in a special election to fill Kennedy's seat and chose a Republican, State Senator Scott Brown, over a Democratic candidate, Massachusetts Attorney General Martha Coakley, who had thought she could coast to victory and had waged a weak and inept campaign.

The election immediately set off a panic among Democrats about the health-care legislation. Brown's victory did show serious voter discontent with the Democrats. But regarding health care, the panic was not rational.

Massachusetts already had most of the reforms that the federal law would introduce; there was no state for which the federal law meant less change. A poll taken immediately after the election found that of those who said they voted, 68 percent supported the Massachusetts health reforms (and that included more than half who had voted for Brown).[70] Brown himself voted for the Massachusetts legislation when he was in the state senate, though he pledged to fight the federal law. "Why would we subsidize and why would we pay more for something we already have? It makes no sense," Brown told Fox News.[71] This was not an argument that could have been made anywhere but Massachusetts (and only to Massachusetts voters who never expected to move to another state). The Massachusetts election also took place at the height of liberal and union disappointment over the failure of the public option, the passage of the Stupak amendment, and the prospective tax on high-cost health plans. Nationally, the Kaiser tracking polls showed the country evenly split on the legislation, but the proportion saying they expected their families would be worse off under reform had jumped from 24 percent in November to 33 percent in January.[72] People assumed that all of the disaffection was coming from conservatives who opposed the reforms altogether, but the opposition was partly coming from progressives who wanted the reforms to be more liberal, not less.

In the glow of Brown's victory, conservative commentators confidently predicted that the health-care legislation was dead, and on the morning after, even some liberal members of Congress dressed for the funeral.[73] Within the White House the same voices that had been calling for retreat in August advised Obama again to agree to a slimmed-down program. For a few days, the president gave no clear indication of what he wanted to do, and his own speechwriters were unsure what direction he wanted them to take. Some panicky Democratic members of Congress suggested that instead of one big measure, they pass a series of little bills, each of which would be framed so as to be popular and thus hard for Republicans to oppose—an attractive political idea, except that the individual steps, such as banning pre-existing-condition exclusions, were impractical apart from the wider changes. These suggestions predictably came to nothing.

When the dust settled and heads cleared, the president and the congressional leadership agreed that they were too close to the finish line to give up. Although Pelosi insisted that the members of her caucus would never vote for the Senate bill, that is exactly what they would have to do before revising it in a follow-up reconciliation measure. For a while, this approach was confused with the idea of passing the entire reform through reconciliation, which would have run into the same problems that made it a bad choice from the beginning. Limited to budget-relevant matters, a reconciliation measure could not establish the insurance exchanges or much of the other institutional architecture of reform. But because the Senate had already passed the institutional changes in its December bill, those provisions did not need to be passed again. When Democrats had adopted the budget resolution early in 2009 and provided for the use of reconciliation for health-care reform, they had not imagined combining a reconciliation bill with regular legislation. But that unanticipated combination, which could never have been planned, turned out to be essential for the final settlement.

Several developments in February gave the Democrats a boost. The news that a California insurer had raised some of its rates by 39 percent provided Obama with potent evidence of the need for reform. The president also succeeded in temporarily cooling down partisan passions. After dealing adroitly with House Republicans when he spoke to a meeting of theirs in Baltimore on January 29, he proposed a bipartisan summit to discuss health-care reform in front of the cameras. Finally, Obama was fulfilling his promise of a televised meeting around a "big table." The discussion did not yield any big surprises, but it enabled the president to listen to the congressional Republicans' criticism and answer it; afterwards, he made a show of accepting some of their suggestions in a revised plan that substantially reflected the agreements the Democrats had negotiated in January, which would be incorporated into the reconciliation bill. Most important, the summit gave the bruised House Democrats time to work through all their options and come to the conclusion that they had to vote for the Senate bill and then amend it immediately with a reconciliation measure that a majority of the Senate had agreed in advance to pass.

The reconciliation measure made the Senate bill more progressive. It raised the affordability subsidies for low-income people buying coverage through the new exchanges. While eliminating the special provision for Nebraska, it increased support for the states' expansion of Medicaid. It provided a $250 rebate for the elderly who had entered the "donut hole" in prescription drug coverage, and it filled the donut hole over the next decade by building on the drug companies' 50 percent discount on brand-name drugs beginning in 2011 to provide 75 percent coverage for both brand-name and generic drugs by 2020.

Perhaps the most important changes in the reconciliation measure involved the revenue provisions. The Senate bill's tax on high-cost plans was postponed to 2018, and the thresholds were raised to $10,200 for single coverage and $27,500 for family coverage. To make up for the lost revenue, the reconciliation bill extended an increase in the Medicare payroll tax that Reid had introduced to investment income for individuals with income above $200,000 and couples earning more than $250,000. That way of increasing upper-income taxes had the effect of both fortifying the Medicare trust fund and reducing the deficit (a two-fer that Republicans complained was unfair but, in fact, reflects the structure of the unified federal budget). As the House prepared to vote, the CBO put a ten-year price tag on the health-care legislation of $940 billion and projected that it would reduce the deficit by $138 billion over that period.[74]

The drama had one scene left. Before the House voted on the Senate bill, a half-dozen Democrats led by Rep. Stupak threatened to withhold support because the Senate's language on abortion was not as iron-clad as the House's. But Stupak, who was a strong supporter of the legislation in other respects, agreed to go along when the president issued an executive order reaffirming the Hyde Amendment. With that agreement, Pelosi had her majority.

On their way to the Capitol for the final vote on March 21, the House Democrats passed through a crowd of Tea Party supporters, who jeered and spat on them, and during the debate, conservatives massed outside the House chamber and chanted "Kill the bill" as Republicans appeared on a balcony to denounce the proceedings inside. As the long debate came to a close, the sides rehearsed their standard lines. While Democrats saw themselves as extending the tradition of Social Security and Medicare, Republicans pictured the legislation as freedom's darkest hour. One Republican shouted "baby killer," later claiming that he was hurling the epithet not personally at Stupak but at the bill itself. On the final vote, 219 to

212, not a single Republican joined the Democrats. Two days later, the president signed the Patient Protection and Affordable Care Act, and on March 25, both the House and Senate enacted the follow-up reconciliation measure. Health-care reform was now law.

Why Health-Care Reform Passed (and Climate Legislation Didn't)

For many Democrats, climate legislation and health-care reform were both moral imperatives. Each cause had an iconic leader—Kennedy for health care, Gore for climate—who had endorsed Obama in the primaries and handed off the torch to him. "America, this is our moment," Obama had said in a victory speech at the end of his primary campaign. "We will be able to look back and tell our children that this was the moment when we began to provide care for the sick . . . when the rise of the oceans began to slow and our planet began to heal."[75]

If Obama had been blocked on both fronts, however, it would not have been surprising. Never easy in the United States, large-scale reform has become especially difficult because of the routine use of the filibuster and the increased distance between the parties. On both health care and climate, the Republicans in Congress gave Obama no cooperation. It took every vote the Democrats had in the Senate, during the short time they had 60, to pass the main health-care legislation. And though the cap-and-trade bill passed the House, it could not surmount the barriers in the Senate because of the opposition of senators from coal-dependent states. The odds on climate legislation were bleak from the start: environmentalists had not won over energy interests to the extent that health-care reformers had won support among the physicians, hospitals, drug companies, and even insurers. But passing health-care reform turned out to be more difficult than the White House or congressional leaders anticipated, and those difficulties indirectly prejudiced the outcome on climate.

Environmental and health-care policy and politics have evolved in similar ways since the 1970s. In both areas, reformers have adopted a market model partly in the hope of gaining support from conservatives.

Environmentalists have moved from a reliance on regulation and litigation to an embrace of markets in emissions permits, while health-care reformers have moved from support of a government insurance plan to an embrace of private coverage, tax credits, and insurance exchanges. In both cases, the idea has been to design a well-functioning, efficient market to accomplish public purposes. But in 2009 the political pay-off didn't materialize; the moderate Republicans who were the hope for bipartisan alliances had nearly vanished from Congress, and the few congressional Republicans open to working with Democrats retreated when they heard rumblings at their party's base and faced the prospect of conservative primary challenges. As a result, the ideas that were supposed to bridge party differences had no support except in the Democratic Party.

After Obama became president, the climate and health-care bills became rivals for legislative priority. Although the House passed climate legislation before health-care reform, the climate bill stalled in the Senate. According to journalist Eric Pooley, when leaders of the U.S. Climate Action Partnership came to the White House in late spring 2009, Rahm Emanuel told them, "We want to do this climate bill, but *success breeds success*. We need to put points on the board. . . . If the climate bill bogs down, we move on. We've got health care."[76] By the next year, the chances of the climate bill had been damaged by the wear-and-tear of the health-care battle. "The long and brutal health-care fight had caused a rift in the White House over legislative strategy," the *New Yorker*'s Ryan Lizza reports. On one side, the former congressional aides who occupied senior White House positions said Obama had to get involved in the bargaining, as he had on health care. "The other group, led by David Axelrod, believed that being closely associated with the messiness of congressional horse-trading was destroying Obama's reputation." By the time the Senate took up cap-and-trade in 2010, according to Lizza, "Axelrod's side was ascendant." The president and senators hoping to pass climate legislation did come up with a compromise, but one of its key elements—an expansion of off-shore drilling in exchange for support of cap-and-trade—proved to be ill-timed when the Deepwater Horizon oil rig in the Gulf of Mexico exploded on April 20, 2010. As Lizza writes, "The White House's 'grand bargain' of oil drilling in exchange for a cap on carbon had backfired spectacularly."[77]

The early optimism about the health-care battle was not entirely misguided. Democrats had seen a chance to pass legislation because the major interest groups in health care would go along with reform on the minimally invasive model—and that proved correct. It was because the interest groups were comfortable with the framework of reform that they didn't launch an all-out campaign to defeat it, and the White House and Baucus were able to close the deals with the pharmaceutical companies and the hospitals. In this respect, the Democrats' embrace of private coverage, tax credits, and insurance exchanges was successful. They gave themselves the chance to pass legislation, though that also limited the kind of legislation they could pass.

Adopting this approach did not, however, avoid a bitter and prolonged fight with the ideological and partisan opposition. Historically, health-care interest groups had helped to shape the conservative view of a public health insurance program. When Ronald Reagan recorded his speech against Medicare in 1961, he was doing it on behalf of a campaign paid for and organized by the American Medical Association. But the AMA was no longer necessary to finance and coordinate the opposition; the case against "socialized medicine" had taken on a life of its own. Conservatives could now even use the original arguments against Medicare to appeal to the elderly on the grounds that "socialized medicine" would threaten Medicare (even though the new program, with its reliance on private insurance, was not as "socialized" as Medicare had been). The death-panel hysteria and the campaign of fear against reform also found receptive ears because of the high anxieties following the financial crisis. The campaign particularly found a home in the larger Tea Party movement, made up almost entirely of middle-aged and older whites—people who, by and large, already enjoyed protection against health-care costs, believed they had earned it, and did not want to pay for anyone else's. This was the how the American health-policy trap worked. Some of the well-protected literally screamed and shouted at the prospect of change.

But in March 2010, the trap did not work as it always had. By that time, although the political costs of health-care reform were clear, the president and Democratic congressional leaders were too invested to give up. Health-care reform would probably not yield the political benefits they had originally expected, but failure would leave them in even worse shape. If they couldn't pass health-care reform, what could they do? And if they couldn't stand up to the right-wing hysteria and Republican intransigence, what did that say about their own character? As the final decision arrived, health-care reform became a statement about the Democrats' identity and purpose. They knew there was trouble ahead, but they were exuberant about defying it.

CHAPTER 8

The Affordable Care Act as Public Philosophy

It was big—the most ambitious effort in recent decades to reorganize a major institution on a basis that agrees more closely with principles of justice and efficiency. Yet it was also comparatively limited—compared, that is, with the health-care systems of other democracies or with the ideal remedies that many reluctant supporters of the legislation would have preferred.

This is the puzzle of the Affordable Care Act. It calls for major changes, but it is also notable for what it leaves unchanged. After four decades of rising inequality and insecurity, it provides a major boost to the living standards of low-wage workers and their families and increases economic protections for the middle class. The central thrust of the law is to change how health insurance works and to make it affordable, though it also includes measures to improve the quality of medical care and control its cost. But the law does not substantially alter how medical care is organized, and it may not change the long-term trajectory of health spending. Most Americans with secure, employment-based insurance will see little difference in their own coverage or health care.

Legislation is rarely a straight-forward statement of moral and political philosophy; compromises are in the nature of representative government, and the Affordable Care Act concedes far more to the status quo than many of its supporters would have liked. Nevertheless, it reflects a series of moral choices about how health insurance and health care should work and what rights and obligations individuals should have.

The legislation rewrites the rules of the insurance market. Under the old rules, insurers in most states have been free to deny coverage to people they deem too great a risk and to charge however much they want based on health, age, or other characteristics. Many people have been denied coverage of conditions that predated their policies, and many have had their policies rescinded when they became ill. The old rules of the market gave insurers an incentive to design every aspect of their business so as to avoid individuals with high health costs. While large and mid-size employers have mostly shielded their employees and dependents from the worst of these problems, people working for small businesses or buying insurance on their own have felt the brunt of the system's limitations and faced high prices for spotty coverage. The system guaranteed that millions of people would be left without any protection, and as health-care costs rose in relation to median income, the share of the population with private insurance inevitably fell.

To create a market with different incentives, the Affordable Care Act introduces new rules for insurers as well as new requirements and subsidies for individuals. The new rules require insurers to issue policies and renew them for all legal applicants, and they prohibit the companies from refusing to cover pre-existing conditions or charging according to an individual's health. While insurers can vary premiums by age and tobacco use, they can do so only within limits. To prevent people from taking advantage of the system by purchasing insurance only when they get sick, the law requires individuals to maintain a minimum level of coverage. And to increase the number with insurance and enable low-income people to comply with the mandate, the law (as originally written) extends eligibility for Medicaid to all citizens with incomes under or near the federal poverty line and subsidizes private insurance for both citizens and legal immigrants earning up to four times the poverty level. According to projections by the Congressional Budget Office at the time the law passed, it would extend coverage to about 32 million people, roughly half through Medicaid and half through added private insurance, raising the insured share of the population to about 94 percent.[1]

The law's central organizational innovation—the establishment of insurance exchanges—is aimed at reducing costs and improving access to coverage for people who buy insurance individually or through small groups.

The exchanges play a critical role in restructuring and policing those markets. To discourage insurers from cherry-picking the healthy, the law requires them to pay into a risk-adjustment fund if they enroll a relatively healthy, low-cost population; conversely, the fund compensates insurers if they sign up a more costly group of subscribers. In other words, although the system prevents individuals from being charged according to their risk, it pays insurers on that basis.

There is much else in the law.[2] But rather than plunge into all the details, the following discussion presents the law's provisions as they bear upon some central problems of public philosophy: fairness and equality, responsibility and freedom, federalism and finance, and the scope of concern for health and health care in the public household.

Fairness and Equality

The Affordable Care Act restructures health insurance so as to achieve for all Americans the aims it has been serving only for some—to provide access to health care and protection against the risk of being bankrupted by medical costs. Unlike Britain's National Health Service, the legislation does not make health care free at the point of service; unlike Canada's national health insurance system, it does not make health insurance a right. It seeks the more limited goal of making health care and health insurance "affordable."

In a liberal, capitalist society, the fundamental choice about health care and health insurance is whether or not they should be treated as ordinary commodities. If they are, they will be available only to those who can pay for them at the market price. A competitive market for insurance should drive rates toward their actuarially fair value, which means that insurers will ask individuals and groups to pay premiums in line with the risks they represent. The healthy will pay less than average, while individuals with a record of illness or disability will be charged hefty rates or may find no insurer willing to offer them coverage. Even at an average price, many low-income people will not be able to afford health insurance and therefore will not receive the medical care they need. Those effects are to be expected if health care and insurance are treated as ordinary commodities.

If, in contrast, health care and insurance are considered services that at some level the community has an obligation to provide to all its members— as it does for education—other principles apply. The costs of insurance should then be spread over the healthy and sick alike to avoid imposing burdens on the sick that effectively bar them from access to medical care. Instead of being actuarially fair, the price of insurance should reflect a norm of shared responsibility (or "solidarity," as the Europeans call it). On that same principle, the poor should receive subsidized access to insurance or to health care directly.

To say that there is some shared responsibility for health costs is not, however, tantamount to saying that all costs should be shared or that government should ensure that services are equal in all respects. The moral interest in ensuring care for the sick does not require shared responsibility for services such as cosmetic surgery or amenities such as private hospital rooms. Practical considerations—for example, the "moral hazard" that insurance may increase overall costs—may also dictate limits in the sharing of risk.

Few people advocate treating medical care purely as a commodity or spreading across the community the cost of all possible medical services. Rather, the debate lies among a series of intermediate possibilities. In the United States, the two rival conceptions of equity in insurance—actuarial fairness and shared responsibility—govern different parts of the health-care system. Depending on state law, private insurance approximates the norm of actuarially fair pricing (and would approximate it more closely in a deregulated market), while Medicare, Medicaid, and other public programs reflect a norm of shared responsibility. In addition, the various private and public systems of coverage differ in scope of benefits and levels of payment to providers and therefore in effective access to services. Consequently, even for the insured population, the system is multi-tiered and unequal. Federal law recognizes only one right of all persons to essential health care—a right to receive emergency medical services. Hospitals generally finance those and other services to the low-income uninsured by shifting the costs to insured patients—a hidden transfer that the American public has apparently preferred to being openly taxed for the same purpose. Nonetheless, many of the uninsured (and underinsured) face medical bills that drive them into bankruptcy, and their limited access to medical treatment takes a toll in lost lives and diminished well-being.

The Affordable Care Act attempts to extend shared responsibility without entirely banishing actuarial fairness, and it makes the health-insurance system more inclusive without flattening its tiered and unequal structure.[3] Rather than superseding Medicaid as earlier reform proposals had sought to do, the law extends Medicaid (and CHIP) to cover all those with incomes up to 133 percent of the poverty level (actually 138 percent because of how income is counted). That income level serves as the boundary dividing public from private coverage for the civilian population under 65 years of age. But because private insurance has become so expensive, the law also provides subsidies to pay a share of premiums for people with incomes between 133 percent and 400 percent of the poverty line (which, as of 2013, includes individuals earning between $14,860 and $44,680). The subsidies come in the form of tax credits, graduated by income. For example, the credits limit the cost of premiums to between 3 and 4 percent of income for people whose income lies between 133 percent and 150 percent of poverty. The higher the income of an individual or family, the greater the share they are expected to pay: the subsidies will keep the cost of premiums to between 8.05 percent and 9.5 percent of income for people with incomes ranging from 250 percent to 400 percent of poverty. The credits are refundable, which means even those who do not owe taxes will be eligible to receive them, and they can be advanced during the year when premiums are due, not merely paid out after the tax year is over.

People receiving premium credits will be free to buy any insurance plan in the exchange, but the subsidies will be keyed to a plan near the low-cost end. To give the different levels of coverage memorable names, Congress adopted the color code used in Massachusetts. At the low end are the bronze plans, which cover 60 percent of the average estimated benefit costs ("actuarial value"); then come the silver plans at 70 percent, gold at 80 percent, and platinum at 90 percent. No matter which plan an individual selects, the subsidies are calculated on the basis of the second-lowest-cost silver plan in their area.

In addition, people with incomes below 250 percent of poverty will get some help with deductibles and co-payments, and that assistance will effectively bump up the value of their coverage. For example, those with incomes between 150 percent and 200 percent of the poverty line will receive cost-sharing subsidies that increase the actuarial value of the benchmark plan from 70 percent to 87 percent.

To make health care more affordable for everyone, not just the poor, the law also includes several protections against ruinous costs. It bans lifetime and "unreasonable" annual limits on coverage, and it caps patient cost-sharing at the levels set by federal law for a tax-advantaged, high-deductible plan and health-savings account ($5,950 for individual and $11,900 for family coverage as of 2010). Subsidies reduce these caps the closer an individual's income is to the poverty level. Nonetheless, the total cost of premiums, deductibles, and co-payments can still run up to about one-fifth of income for people near the level where subsidies phase out (400 percent of poverty). So while the law will reduce financial stress from illness, it will not eliminate it—though without the law, there would be no limits at all on financial burdens.

Two issues—insurance rates for young versus old and the coverage of immigrants—illustrate how the Affordable Care Act tries to balance competing concerns about fairness.

How much should insurers be able to vary rates depending on age? Actuarial fairness calls for as wide a gap in rates as variations in the health costs of the young and old justify, while completely shared responsibility calls for no gap at all. In the unreformed health-insurance market, older adults may pay as much as 11 times what young adults are charged. Under "pure" community rating, that ratio would be one to one: a 60-year-old and a 20-year-old would pay the same price for health insurance.

The law adopts a middle ground ("modified" community rating), limiting differences in rates to a three-to-one ratio between old and young. Appealing to the norm of actuarial fairness, the libertarian Cato Institute attacks "Obamacare" as a "bad deal for young adults" because it "would drive premiums down for 55-year-olds but would drive them up for 25-year-olds—who are then implicitly subsidizing older adults."[4] Taking the opposite view, some on the left criticize the three-to-one ratio as creating unacceptable financial burdens for older adults.

The impact of age rating is largely limited, however, to people with incomes over 400 percent of poverty who buy insurance independently of any group. The age-rating limits do not apply to coverage provided directly by employers, who generally do not ask older workers to pay more than younger ones for health insurance. In the exchanges, the premium credits for people with incomes below 400 percent of poverty will largely nullify the impact of different age-rating ratios. For example, according to estimates by the Urban Institute, more than 80 percent of the 25- to 34-year-olds getting non-group coverage will qualify for subsidies; the limit on age rating to a three-to-one ratio mainly affects the more affluent young who have greater ability to pay.

To be sure, some affluent, healthy young adults buying insurance in the exchange will pay more than they would if there were no limits on age rating. But if they lose their job or their income falls, they too may benefit from the law's subsidies—and assuming they live to become middle-aged, even those who were healthy and prosperous when they were young may stand to benefit from limits on age rating later in life when fortune as well as youth may have deserted them. "Shared responsibility" can also be described as enlightened self-interest.

In its criticism of the Affordable Care Act, the Cato Institute ignores what a bad deal the unreformed market is for young adults, who often work at entry-level jobs with no health insurance benefits. According to the U.S. Census Bureau, as of 2009, 30 percent of 18- to 24-year-olds and 29 percent of 25- to 34-year-olds were uninsured.[5] The legislation establishes insurance exchanges where young adults can buy subsidized coverage more cheaply, and it requires insurers to allow young adults to remain on their parents' insurance policies up to age 26. To make coverage attractive to other young people, the law requires the exchanges to offer a high-deductible young-adult plan covering only catastrophic costs. The Massachusetts Health Connector introduced a similar option, one of the reasons the state's reforms cut the number of uninsured young adults by 60 percent.[6]

The three-to-one age-rating ratio is not without problems. At that level, some regions with high medical costs will have significant numbers of 55- to 64-year-olds with incomes just above four times the poverty level for whom the cheapest plan in the exchange will exceed 8 or 9 percent of income. But for every move downward in the age-rating ratio, there would be higher premiums for the young and an increase in young people remaining uninsured. There is no perfect solution to this problem.

Immigrants raise another difficult set of issues: How widely should the circle of shared responsibility be drawn? Should it include only citizens? Citizens plus legal immigrants? Or all persons regardless of whether they have a legal right to be in the United States? Hospitals have an obligation to provide emergency care to all persons, but neither Clinton in 1993 nor Obama 16 years later proposed extending a right to subsidized coverage to illegal immigrants. During Obama's speech to Congress in September 2009, Rep. Joe Wilson shouted, "You lie," when the president insisted that the reforms would not cover illegal immigrants. On this score, the legislation is plain enough: illegal immigrants are eligible for neither Medicaid nor any subsidies for private insurance. They cannot even make unsubsidized use of the insurance exchanges. In fact, some illegal immigrant workers who now receive health insurance directly from their employers will lose that coverage if their employers shift coverage to the exchange. To the disappointment of immigrant groups, the law also does not change the exclusion from Medicaid of legal immigrants with less than five years of residency in the United States.

The Affordable Care Act does, however, extend premium and cost-sharing subsidies in the exchanges to legal immigrants regardless of years of residency. In addition, all immigrants, legal and illegal, will benefit from the expansion of community health centers, which are projected to double in capacity with the additional funds authorized under the law.[7] In sum, while new immigrants continue to be barred from getting free care under Medicaid, all legal immigrants acquire the same rights as citizens in the purchase of subsidized private insurance. And though illegal immigrants receive no rights to insurance coverage, the law provides support to the clinics that provide them charity care. By reducing the number of uninsured, the law should also improve the financing of hospitals in low-income areas, including immigrant communities. The presence in the United States of 11 million people with no legal rights is for many reasons an untenable situation, which only general reforms of immigration can address.[8] In the absence of that legislation, the Affordable Care Act strikes a reasonable compromise.

Responsibility and Freedom

On first glance, the differences between conservatives and liberals over the Affordable Care Act seem to fit into an easily understood pattern. According to the conventional view, conservatives object to "Obamacare," especially the individual mandate, because they care more about freedom, while liberals support the legislation because they care more about equality.

The trouble with that interpretation is that it implicitly accepts a shriveled conception of freedom, and it ignores the awkward fact that conservatives originally introduced and supported the individual mandate, the very provision that has raised the most objections as an infringement on individual rights.

Health itself is matter of personal freedom. To be ill and debilitated is to be less free. To be made destitute by sickness, and therefore dependent on others, is also to be less free. Illness cannot be avoided, but social arrangements can increase our freedom by providing access to care and preventing illness from destroying our means of independence.

For some conservatives, however, freedom means only freedom from government, which taken to the extreme means freedom from any constraint that law imposes. But because there are no rights without a government to protect them, freedom is impossible without the framework of law that the state upholds. The legitimate basis for concern about government is an interest in being free from arbitrary and capricious power. But that same interest should also motivate a concern about private power, such as the power of an insurance company, insofar as it is arbitrary and unreasonable. A law that constrains that power may also increase individual freedom.

The history of modern liberal democracies has seen a progressively broader understanding of what an equal right to freedom means. The original concern with civil liberty and limits on arbitrary power evolved in the late eighteenth and nineteenth centuries into a more democratic interest in a right to political liberty and an equal share in the government. The twentieth century saw a further expansion: a concern for limiting excessive private power (as in private monopolies) and guaranteeing a right to the basic requirements of human development and security necessary to ensure equal opportunity and personal dignity.[9]

On one right to human development—a right to education—Americans have had no trouble taking that additional step. Social Security was more contentious, though most Americans now recognize that by preserving their independence in old age and disability, Social Security also contributes to their ability to live a free life. Health care is the American anomaly. Every cousin to the United States in the democratic family of nations sees health care as one of the requirements of human development and security that a good society must meet for all its citizens. The Affordable Care Act is America's effort to fulfill that obligation.

All rights imply responsibilities—and not just in the logical sense that every right imposes a correlative obligation on another party (an individual's right to a fair trial implies the government's obligation to provide one). Rather, publicly recognized rights imply publicly assumed responsibilities. Of what use is the right to political liberty if people do not assume the responsibilities of citizenship? Similarly, a right to the requirements of human development has no real meaning unless people recognize obligations to one another, mutually and through their government, to ensure that the conditions exist that make it possible for every person to have the opportunity for success in life.[10]

The Affordable Care Act creates both rights and responsibilities in its measured efforts to ensure access to health care. Asked in his second debate with McCain in 2008 whether health care is a right, a privilege, or a responsibility, Obama said that "it should be a right for every American."[11] But the legislation he signed as president does not actually establish a general right to health care or to health insurance. Instead, it creates a series of individual rights in relation to private insurance—for example, a right against arbitrary rescissions and unreasonable limits of coverage. It also creates a right to federally subsidized coverage for people who otherwise would not be able to afford it. And to make the system workable, it calls for what the law itself terms "shared responsibility," referring primarily to obligations of individuals and employers to pay for insurance.

From Truman to Clinton, Democrats sought to require employers to pay most of the cost of insurance through payroll taxes or a minimum percentage of premiums, but the Affordable Care Act imposes only limited employer responsibilities. The main obligation of employers—applicable only to firms that have more than 50 workers—is either to provide a minimum standard of coverage or to pay a penalty of $2,000 per employee (counting only those above 30) if any of the employees receive premium credits.[12] Rather than being a primary means of financing the subsidies, this is mainly intended as a deterrent to firms that might otherwise drop coverage. The Affordable Care Act also includes some subsidies to small businesses that cover their workers. An analysis by the Rand Corporation estimates that the law will result in a net increase in the number of employees being offered health insurance, which is consistent with the pattern in Massachusetts after the state enacted its reforms.[13]

The most controversial responsibility imposed by the law is the requirement that individuals maintain a minimum standard of health coverage. That minimum is set at the "bronze" level (60 percent of actuarial value), which can be satisfied with a high-deductible plan, the form of insurance that many conservatives favor. The law also provides exemptions from the mandate on a number of grounds, including religious objections and financial hardship. The hardship exemption applies to all those with an income below the threshold for filing federal income taxes and anyone who would have to pay more than 8 percent of income for the least expensive, subsidized plan in the exchange (these will mainly be older people with incomes near or just above four times the poverty level). Penalties for not insuring are to be paid as part of income taxes, though they are not backed up with sanctions as other taxes are. As of 2016, the fine will be $695 per person (up to a maximum of $2,085 per family) or 2.5 percent of taxable income above the filing threshold, whichever is greater, but the fines are lower for the first two years—just $95 or 1.0 percent of taxable income in 2014 and $325 or 2.0 percent of taxable income in 2015.

The rationale for the mandate is that it is necessary to carry out other reforms that the public overwhelmingly approves. If the legislation banned pre-existing-condition exclusions but included no mandate or an equivalent measure, healthy people would rationally refuse to buy coverage until they got sick. But no system of health insurance is workable unless the healthy as well as the sick contribute. Some states with no mandate have required insurers to issue policies for individuals at community rates, and the predictable result is high premiums that deter many relatively healthy people from obtaining coverage. Insurance companies opposed any national legislation without a mandate for fear that they would be blamed for the high rates they would have to charge. To some on the left, the mandate therefore seemed merely a special-interest concession, but a purely governmental insurance system would suffer from the same problems if it had no mandate while offering guaranteed coverage at community rates with no pre-existing-condition exclusions.

Even the traditional insurance system, as some conservatives have argued, is an invitation to free-riding. In a 1994 article laying out the conservative case for the individual mandate, Robert E. Moffitt of the Heritage Foundation argued that everybody else was already paying for the uninsured in two ways: through taxes and through insurance rates that reflect costs for uncompensated care shifted to insured patients by hospitals and other providers: "So, we already have a mandate," Moffitt wrote. "But it is both inefficient and unfair." The libertarian argument against a mandate, he insisted, "misses the practical point" that some people, "even with the availability of tax credits to offset their costs," will "take advantage of their fellow citizens by not protecting themselves or their families, with the full knowledge that if they do incur a catastrophic illness . . . we will, after all is said and done, take care of them and pay all of the bills. They will be correct in this assessment. But the rest of us should realize that we are thus being victimized by deliberate irresponsibility."[14] Curbing irresponsibility was the rationale that Mitt Romney invoked in justifying Massachusetts' individual mandate, a policy that he and others at the time saw as fundamentally conservative.

In coming to this conclusion, conservatives were saying, in effect, that rather than being an arbitrary imposition of governmental power, the individual mandate was well-grounded in rational concerns of public policy. When 20 Republican senators in the early 1990s supported federal legislation with an individual mandate, none expressed a concern that it might be an excessive or unconstitutional use of federal authority. At the time when the mandate was the Republican alternative, no one doubted that it came within the authority to regulate interstate commerce.

The conservative pedigree of the individual mandate may have led many Democrats to expect that it would enjoy public acceptance as well as bipartisan support and unanimous judicial approval. During the debate over the health-care legislation, however, public opinion surveys showed it to face considerable opposition.[15] To be sure, many people did not grasp that some of the provisions they wanted, like banning exclusions of pre-existing conditions, were tied to the mandate. Many people also did not understand the new system of subsidized coverage in the exchanges or did not trust that government subsidies would be adequate. What they knew was that health insurance was too expensive, and what they heard was that the government was going to force them to buy it. To some people who have trouble paying for insurance, the mandate sent a punitive message about a program that was intended to help them.

For fear of a backlash, Congress was unwilling to back up the mandate with sanctions. If people without insurance fail to pay the fines they owe, the Affordable Care Act does not authorize criminal penalties, the garnishing of wages, or liens against property. To obtain compliance, Congress is mainly counting on a general willingness to follow the law and perhaps some confusion about potential sanctions because the fines are paid as part of federal income taxes. (The one way the government can enforce a fine is to withhold a tax refund.) In Massachusetts, the public did overwhelmingly comply with the individual mandate, but the state started out with a relatively small uninsured population and its legislation enjoyed overwhelming bipartisan and business support. In other states with much larger numbers of uninsured and elite-led opposition to the law, the mandate may not yield the same results.

While the Affordable Care Act was under debate, Congress gave no attention to alternatives to the mandate that could achieve the same purposes without generating as much opposition. The mandate's central purpose is to deter people from opportunistically dipping into the insurance funds when they are sick and refusing to contribute when they are healthy, but there are other ways to bring about that result. For example, in an alternative that I proposed before the legislation passed, the government could allow individuals to opt out of the new insurance system, without a penalty, by signing a form on their tax return acknowledging that they would then be ineligible for federal health insurance subsidies for a fixed period— say, five years. During that time, if they had second thoughts and decided to buy health insurance, they would have no guarantee that they could find a policy or that it would cover pre-existing conditions. In other words, they would face a market much like the one that existed before the law.[16]

An individual opt-out would provide an escape valve for people who, rationally or not, see the mandate as a threat. With this added provision, people without coverage through a group or Medicaid would have three basic choices. They could use the new insurance exchanges to buy guaranteed coverage, receiving subsidies if their incomes were within four times the poverty level. They could take the five-year opt-out. Or they could do neither and pay the annual penalties, but those penalties would be increased and backed up with enforceable sanctions. With both an opt-out and stiffer penalties, the law could be both more libertarian and more tough-minded, and it might achieve as high compliance as the mandate Congress adopted, which is, in fact, a mandate in name only.

There are also other alternatives to the mandate, such as raising premiums for individuals who fail to sign up for coverage during the initial open-enrollment period. The Affordable Care Act could have given the states an open-ended menu of options to curb free-riding, which might have included the mandate, the five-year opt-out, and rising premiums for people who failed to sign up at the beginning. A state that followed the example of Massachusetts and enacted a mandate would have done so under state law, eliminating any constitutional challenge that could be brought into federal court. If states tested out different policies, they could have also served their classic function as laboratories of democracy—one of the advantages of a federal system.

Federalism and Finance

As a federal republic, the United States divides authority between the national government and the states, but it does not divide it consistently on the basis of general principles.

In the abstract, there is a good argument for keeping decisions at no higher level of government than is necessary (a principle sometimes called "subsidiarity"), which might argue for leaving health care entirely to the states. But history complicates theory. The United States developed out of radically different social systems in the South and the North, and while the South invoked states' rights in defending slavery and later Jim Crow, federal intervention was crucial in efforts to achieve equality from the Emancipation Proclamation to the civil rights movement. Even now, in economic and social policy, states in the South (and Southwest) show the influence of their traditions. Compared with the rest of the country, they continue to provide the least support for the living standards, including the health care, of their low-income population. In Louisiana, for example, unemployed parents have had to earn less than $2,400 (11 percent of the federal poverty line) to qualify for Medicaid.[17] In practice, therefore, turning health policy entirely over to the states means denying access to medical care and insurance protection for millions of the poor and near-poor in the South and Southwest.

Throughout the country, most states still face two kinds of barriers to ensuring universal coverage: federal laws, particularly ERISA, limiting the states' authority to regulate employee benefit plans, and requirements in state constitutions for annually balanced budgets. During recessions, as private health insurance shrinks and Medicaid enrollment surges, states see their revenues drop and are forced to cut back Medicaid just at the point when more people need it. In contrast, as a purely federal program, Medicare has greater stability over the business cycle.

These considerations have led to a characteristic political divide in the politics of federalism, with liberals usually favoring a greater role in health policy for the federal government and conservatives a greater role for the states. But the general pattern doesn't apply to every issue. For example, Republican proposals to allow health insurance to be sold across state lines would undermine state regulation of the insurance market; similarly, Republican proposals for federal legislation on medical malpractice would override state liability laws. If Democrats had shown a consistent preference for federal power, they would have covered the uninsured by extending Medicare.

Instead, the Affordable Care Act builds on Medicaid, which the states run, and the law calls for the states also to establish the new insurance exchanges, with the Department of Health and Human Services serving as a back-stop in case a state fails to act. Yet the federal government pays for almost all the costs of expanded Medicaid eligibility and all of the subsidies for private insurance in the exchanges. In short, the Affordable Care Act tries to correct the historic regional inequalities in health care by providing money and rules. The money goes to cover most of the uninsured (insofar as the states agree to expand Medicaid); the rules require the pooling of risk in the individual and small-group insurance markets, which then limits the cost of subsidies needed to help people afford that coverage.

By splitting operational and financial responsibility, the Affordable Care Act may invite problems. The states do not have a direct budgetary incentive to keep down premiums in the exchange; if a state runs its exchange incompetently and premiums for silver plans are high, the federal government pays the additional cost of subsidies.

The states fare better financially under the Affordable Care Act than under earlier health programs with mixed federal and state support. Under Medicaid, the federal share has averaged 57 percent of total costs. Under the Affordable Care Act, the federal government pays for 100 percent of the cost of newly eligible Medicaid beneficiaries for the first three years, phasing down to 90 percent in 2020 and thereafter. As of 2015, the law also increases the federal match for CHIP by 23 percentage points, up to a maximum of 100 percent. According to an Urban Institute analysis, the Affordable Care Act will yield between $41 billion and $132 billion in net savings for state budgets from 2014 to 2019. The states will face additional costs for Medicaid, in part because of the costs for previously eligible beneficiaries who will sign up in larger numbers as a result of the individual mandate. But the states will also experience lower expenditures as a result of savings on uncompensated hospital care, lower outlays for mental health and behavioral services covered by private insurance, and reduced spending for some Medicaid beneficiaries whose coverage can be shifted into the exchanges, where subsidies are entirely federal.[18]

The law will affect different states in different ways. States that have funded more generous health programs on their own will likely see greater budgetary relief; for example, if a state previously offered Medicaid coverage to adults earning more than 133 percent of poverty, it can move those beneficiaries into the exchange and off the state's budget. But, in a perverse twist, the Affordable Care Act rewards states that have had the most limited Medicaid eligibility because the federal match for newly eligible beneficiaries is higher than for those who were previously eligible. Ironically, the very states that have resisted the law—the red states, with historically low Medicaid eligibility and large uninsured populations—stand to see the greatest influx of federal revenue into their health-care systems. If ideology did not trump self-interest, these states would be the Affordable Care Act's biggest fans.

Many state officials, however, see the law as a source not of new revenue but of new constraints. That response partly reflects a flaw in Medicaid's original matching formula that the Affordable Care Act failed to correct. Under the formula, the federal government pays a larger share of a state's costs the lower its per capita income, which is a measure of the state's capacity to raise revenue on its own. But while the federal share varies across states, it does not vary according to economic conditions that affect a state's fiscal capacity. That limitation becomes apparent during recessions. The cyclical pressures in Medicaid could be greatly relieved by a trigger increasing the federal match when unemployment in a state hits thresholds indicating economic stress.[19] Under the economic stimulus program passed in 2009, Congress temporarily did increase the federal Medicaid match, but not beyond 2011; the Affordable Care Act then required the states to maintain eligibility for most classes of beneficiaries until 2014. The failure to sustain additional federal support in the interim has colored state officials' response to the long-term reforms. Medicaid has become the single biggest item in state budgets. A permanent recession-related adjustment to the federal share of Medicaid would go a long way toward assuring state officials that they can manage Medicaid (and their state's finances) through hard times.

Although the Affordable Care Act imposes constraints on the states, it also provides them with resources and flexibility to adapt the program to local conditions. State Medicaid programs have already evolved in diverse ways. While making eligibility rules more uniform, the Affordable Care Act leaves the states with flexibility in organizing Medicaid and supports new options such as a Basic Health Program for people with incomes up to twice the poverty level (an alternative to subsidizing private insurance in the exchange for those with incomes between 133 percent and 200 percent of poverty).[20]

The law also provides for general waivers for the states as of 2017. Under that provision, states could opt out of any of the law's specific provisions as long as they provide as comprehensive coverage to as many people as the law would otherwise insure, at no greater cost to the federal government. An amendment proposed by Senators Ron Wyden and Scott Brown—and endorsed by President Obama—would move up the date for those waivers to 2014. If Congress passes the Wyden-Brown amendment or a similar proposal, the health-care reforms set in motion by the Affordable Care Act would likely take even more varied forms than the law already allows. The advantage of that approach is the potential to learn from diversity and experimentation; the danger is that states with deeply ingrained inequalities in health care will perpetuate their old patterns.

Unlike the expansions of Medicaid that began in the 1980s, the Affordable Care Act did not pass the costs of expanded health coverage along to the states. Congress did the heavy lifting by providing the funds. In the past, how to pay for health-care reform has often seemed to be a politically insoluble problem. Congress repealed the Medicare Catastrophic Act in 1989 largely because the elderly considered the surtax that financed the program to be illegitimate—and, indeed, by burdening the elderly alone, the surtax did violate the norms previously established for financing Social Security and Medicare. Taking a different approach in passing the State Children's Health Insurance Program in 1997, Congress increased tobacco taxes, a levy with wide legitimacy because it reduces smoking and improves public health. As these cases illustrate, the normative aspect of public finance may be critical. No aspect of government is more political than taxes and spending in the raw who-gets-what sense. But no aspect of government is a better reflection of its working philosophy, even though politicians may not fully articulate the premises of their decisions.

In their decisions about the financing of the Affordable Care Act, congressional Democrats and the president were operating on the basis of several implicit principles. The first was a distributive principle—ability to pay. Much of the money for expanded coverage would come from the uninsured themselves, who would be required to carry coverage and pay a gradually increasing share of costs as their income rises above the poverty level. The idea of "affordable" care implies an ability-to-pay standard. In addition, during the 2008 campaign, Obama said he would finance his health plan by eliminating the Bush tax cuts for people earning more than $250,000. The legislation was not ultimately paid for that way, though it did include an increase in Medicare taxes on people at the top income level. Drawing from the uninsured, who would benefit directly, and from people with the highest incomes, who have reaped the biggest economic gains in recent decades, reflected a judgment about what would count as a fair distribution of burdens.

A second implicit principle reflected wide agreement among Democrats (and many others) that the United States already spends enough of its national income on health care and that health-care reform should at least be partly financed from within the system—that is, by trimming other health expenditures and taking back from insurers and providers some of the profits that expanded coverage would allow them to make. To be sure, health expenditures would rise in the short run because more people would be insured, but well-drawn legislation would increasingly offset those costs with savings in other areas.

Finally, the president and congressional Democrats committed themselves not only to pay for health-care reform, but to use it to reduce the federal deficit.

These three principles reflected a belief among Democrats about how the legislation ought to realize the general goals of distributive justice, allocative efficiency, and long-term fiscal balance. But working out the specifics was not easy. The idea of financing health-care reform by eliminating the Bush tax cuts for top earners fell by the wayside even before Obama took office because of opposition to raising taxes in the midst of a severe recession. As an alternative, the president in early 2009 proposed to raise some of the revenue for health care by limiting how much people in the highest income bracket could deduct for charitable donations, but Congress quickly killed that idea too. The final House bill did raise income taxes on top earners, but that proposal died at the hands of the Senate. What survived was the Senate's provision for an increase in the Medicare tax rate of 0.9 percent on earnings over $200,000 for individual taxpayers and $250,000 for married couples. In the final wrangling over the budget-reconciliation bill, Congress further increased the Medicare tax on the top brackets by extending it to income from interests, dividends, and capital gains.

Much of the effort to pay for reform with savings from "within the system" involved Medicare as well, though it did not require cuts in the program's legislated benefits. Private Medicare Advantage plans were receiving $1,100 more per enrollee than it would have cost had their beneficiaries remained in traditional Medicare.[21] The Affordable Care Act changes the formula to reduce these overpayments and reward plans for quality of care. In response, some private plans may cut extra benefits they offer their enrollees, but these are not benefits generally available to Medicare beneficiaries, and it is hard to see why the plans should be overpaid even if they use some of that excess to give bonus benefits to their members. In addition, as per the agreement with the major hospital associations, the Affordable Care Act reduces future updates in Medicare payments, reflecting the hospitals' increased revenues from broader insurance coverage. The law also cuts the extra payments to hospitals that historically have had large numbers of uninsured patients because that burden should decline as coverage expands. Finally, the legislation includes a series of clawback taxes on insurers, pharmaceutical companies, and medical-device manufacturers to recapture part of the gains they are projected to make from expanded coverage.

The most controversial aspect of the financing is the excise tax on high-cost, employer-sponsored health insurance plans, known as the "Cadillac tax." As of 2018, plans costing more than $10,200 for individuals and $27,500 for families will be subject to a 40 percent tax on the amount over those thresholds (which will be adjusted upward for employees in high-risk occupations and for early retirees age 55 and older). The excise tax was a substitute for the more straight-forward policy of limiting the tax exclusion of employer contributions. That exclusion has long been the target of criticism on both distributive and allocative grounds: it provides the biggest subsidies to higher-income employees with the most generous insurance, and it contributes to America's inflated health spending by obscuring the true costs. Nixon and Clinton considered limiting the exclusion, but each rejected the idea because of political opposition. The opponents (and the media) equate capping the exclusion with "taxing health benefits," as if the full value would be taxed. To make the cap understandable, it needed to be reframed.

Since the tax exclusion is on the margin roughly a 40 percent subsidy to high-end employer health-insurance contributions, a 40 percent excise tax on a level above a given threshold is effectively the same as capping the exclusion. But taxing high-end insurance plans is more palatable than taxing individual health benefits. The excise tax is projected to raise only a small share of the revenue for the Affordable Care Act before 2020 because it becomes effective at high initial thresholds and only in 2018. But those thresholds are indexed to the consumer price index, not to medical inflation, so the tax is projected to raise a considerable amount in the following decade. Analysts do not expect that the excise tax itself will generate most of the revenue; rather, employers will respond to the tax by cutting the cost of health coverage and paying workers higher (taxable) wages. The excise tax is critical to the hope not just for long-run fiscal balance, but for changing the underlying dynamics of the health-care system that have generated such high costs in the first place.

Surprisingly, financing did not turn out to be the intractable political problem for health-care reform that it might have been. The Democrats found ways to pay for the governmental costs of the Affordable Care Act without any general tax increase. But that did not mean they had finally dealt with the larger problem posed by rising health costs.

Health and the Public Household

At the crux of many disagreements about health policy are two contrasting conceptions of health insurance. Conservatives tend to see health insurance as being the same as other forms of insurance and therefore appropriate only for large and unexpected costs, not for costs that are routine or small enough to be paid out of pocket as ordinary expenses. In this view, insurance inherently creates moral hazard (that is, it invites additional spending), so coverage—particularly government-mandated coverage—should be limited to high-cost services.

The opposite view, usually upheld by liberals, conceives of health insurance as being a form of prepayment for medical care and insists that limiting coverage to catastrophic costs creates perverse incentives favoring technologically intensive services to the neglect of primary care and prevention. One of the aims of reform, in this view, should be to promote primary and preventive services precisely to lessen the reliance on high-tech care that accounts for the largest costs in the system.

In practice, these two views lead to different positions on appropriate levels of cost-sharing and the definition of essential health benefits. At a more abstract level, the dispute is about the scope of the "public household," by which I mean not just government itself but the whole sphere of pooled risk, whether those risks are shared through taxes or insurance.

On this seemingly intractable dispute, the Affordable Care Act says to conservatives and liberals, "You're both right," though about different things.

In three critical provisions, the legislation reflects the conservative view of cost-sharing. The first is the benchmark plan to which subsidies are pegged in the insurance exchange; that benchmark is set at the second-lowest cost plan at the silver level, 70 percent of actuarial value. (The program reduces cost-sharing, however, the closer people come to the poverty line.) Second, the minimum coverage needed to satisfy the mandate is set at only the bronze level, 60 percent of actuarial value. And, third, the excise tax on high-cost plans will lead companies to pare back the most generous health benefits, imposing higher deductibles and co-payments to keep down premiums and avoid the tax. These are all significant departures from earlier Democratic proposals from Kennedy to Clinton, which called for more limited cost-sharing.

The Affordable Care Act does, however, uphold the liberal view on the scope of benefits, which cover the full range of medical services in a mainstream insurance policy. Although the law does not spell out the "essential health benefits" in detail (leaving that responsibility to the secretary of Health and Human Services), it does specifically provide for preventive services. In this respect, it is also a departure from historic practices. When health insurance first developed in the United States in the 1930s, it covered hospital and later major medical bills. Insurance had nothing to do with preventive services or public health. And when Congress enacted Medicare in 1965, it did not make preventive and public-health services part of the legislation.[22]

Culminating a long shift in thinking, however, the Affordable Care Act incorporates preventive care into health insurance and seeks to promote public health through provisions aimed at reducing obesity and smoking and encouraging participation in wellness programs.

New private insurance policies—that is, all plans except "grandfathered" ones in existence at the time the law was signed—will have to cover all of the cost of a list of preventive services that have met standards for effectiveness set by the U.S. Preventive Services Task Force. (Clinical preventive services include immunizations, screening tests, and counseling; insurers will now have to cover the services to which the task force has given a grade of A or B.) The law also provides for Medicare to cover the cost of those preventive services as well as an annual wellness visit without any deductible or co-payment. In addition, the federal government will increase matching funds for states that offer the approved preventive services in their Medicaid programs. And it will require Medicaid coverage of smoking-cessation services for pregnant women.

The government has long supported evaluations of preventive services. Established in 1984, the U.S. Preventive Services Task Force is a federally sponsored council of private-sector scientists and health-care practitioners that evaluates the effectiveness of clinical preventive services. A second group, the Task Force on Community Preventive Services, evaluates public-health measures such as tobacco regulations. Besides providing additional funds for both groups, the law establishes a Prevention and Public Health Investment Fund to support increased training of primary-care providers, scientific research on prevention, public-health education, and other purposes.

At the same time, the Affordable Care Act seeks to raise the cost of unhealthy practices. Although it prohibits insurers from charging higher premiums based on an individual's health risks, it allows them to charge a smoker as much as 50 percent more than a nonsmoker. It also permits employers to increase rewards for participation in wellness and disease-prevention programs from 20 percent to 30 percent of the costs of insurance premiums. The law's 10 percent tax on tanning salons falls into the same category of incentives. Since tanning has been linked to skin cancer, the tax is a way both to promote healthier behavior and to recover from tanning salons medical costs that they generate. Congress did not, however, enact a tax on sugared beverages that some public-health advocates have proposed as a means of fighting obesity. But the law does require restaurant chains to provide calorie counts on their menus and make other nutritional information available. By reducing the price for preventive services, raising the price for unhealthy practices, and providing better information about everyday decisions, the government is trying to change the health-care consumer's menu in a larger sense.

Although there are questions about the cost-effectiveness of some clinical preventive measures, the law targets that spending toward services shown to be beneficial by the balance of scientific evidence. But it may be politically difficult to limit preventive spending where the evidence is weak. At a volatile point in the health-reform debate, the Preventive Services Task Force recommended that mammograms should not be routine for women in their forties. Instead, the task force stated, "The decision to start regular, biennial screening mammography before the age of 50 years should be an individual one and take patient context into account, including the patient's values regarding specific benefits and harms."[23] That recommendation set off a storm of outrage from many people who mistakenly interpreted the decision as evidence of health-care rationing. In fact, the task force recommendation considered only benefits and risks to the patient (the risks having to do with the cumulative effect of radiation); costs were not a factor. Nevertheless, Congress decided to grandfather the old standard for mammograms so that insurers would continue to pay for them for women in their forties. But it is true that when the task force gives a grade of C to preventive tests, insurers would ordinarily not have to pay for them. If there are rules for required insurance coverage of preventive care, there must also be limits to the requirements, and scientific evidence is indispensable to drawing those lines.

The combined move toward both the conservative position on patient cost-sharing and the liberal position on preventive care illustrates the absence of any single theory of cost containment in the Affordable Care Act, unless it's an open-ended empiricism and political pragmatism—proceeding on the available data, testing out alternatives, developing better information, and trying to make more intelligent policy as far as political constraints allow.

Besides the excise tax and the emphasis on preventive care, the cost-containment measures of the Affordable Care Act can be thought of as falling in three areas. On costs related to administration and insurance, the legislation takes a relatively aggressive stance. Overhead and profits have accounted for nearly 30 cents of every dollar in premiums for individually purchased insurance.[24] The law limits that share to 20 cents, and it imposes a limit of 15 cents per premium dollar in the group-insurance market. By eliminating the whole process of evaluating individual applicants' medical history and potential risk and by simplifying insurance options, putting them online, and making them more transparent, insurance exchanges should cut overhead dramatically—as long as the political system can resist pressure from insurance brokers and other intermediaries to maintain the status quo. In a related measure, the federal government is providing aid to the states to review insurance rate increases over 10 percent. The law's efforts to accelerate the use of electronic medical records and spur new health-information technology are also in part geared toward reducing the system's overhead.

Congress was far more tentative, however, in trying to limit costs related to clinical decisions. The legislation supports a new non-profit Patient-Centered Outcomes Research Institute to sponsor research comparing the clinical effectiveness of different treatments. But the law bars use of the findings as mandates or guidelines for coverage or payment. Eventually, though, evidence about results must have some weight in such decisions, for if we cannot say no to paying for services that are clinically ineffective, we will surely have no choice but to limit services that are clinically valuable.

In a third area—policies affecting the payment and organization of providers—the law emphasizes experimentation and pilot programs. The experimental path to cost containment is not entirely new. One of the most successful experiments in Medicare's history was the waiver for New Jersey that led to the national adoption of prospective payment for hospital care. The Affordable Care Act authorizes a pilot program in Medicare to take a further step, bundling together all the payments associated with an episode of care—inpatient and outpatient hospital treatment as well as physician services—from three days before hospitalization to 30 days after. The law also calls for initial steps in Medicare toward paying for value rather than volume by rewarding hospitals and other providers for getting treatment right the first time, avoiding complications, and having the best outcomes. In another measure aimed at improving quality as well as controlling cost, the legislation authorizes the establishment of "account-able care organizations" to provide medical care to a defined population through providers that agree to be held accountable for their performance. There is also money for states to test alternatives to the current system of malpractice litigation.

On policies affecting payment and organization, the legislation might well have gone further. It is not as though knowledge about how to control payment is in short supply; systems of rate regulation and global budgeting have successfully controlled costs in other countries, and rate regulation is popular in the United States.[25] The obstacles to effective cost containment have been political. Despite the Reagan administration's success with pro-spective hospital payment, Republicans oppose price and budget regula-tion on ideological grounds. And because Democrats needed support from physicians, hospitals, pharmaceutical companies, and other health-care interest groups to pass health-care reform, the Affordable Care Act did not include stronger cost-control measures such as the budget caps in the Clinton plan. The skewed payment scale that overpays procedure-oriented medical specialties was off-limits in the reform debate. In many parts of the country, hospitals and other providers now form overpowering combi-nations that are driving up costs, but addressing these problems, as Robert Berenson writes, "would have conflicted with the Democratic political nar-rative that identified the insurance companies as the health-care villains and the providers as the good guys."[26] The experiments with bundling payment, value-based purchasing, and other initiatives are all aimed at finding ways around the political barriers, especially by combining cost control with quality-improvement measures. If the same method that cuts costs can also be shown to improve results for patients, it will plainly have wider acceptance.

But even if pilot programs identify successful models, political obstacles may still stand in the way of scaling them up and carrying them out na-tionally. In an effort to overcome those obstacles, the law establishes an Independent Payment Advisory Board, which beginning in 2014 will rec-ommend ways to reduce Medicare spending in any year when the growth rate exceeds the average of the increases in the consumer price index and the price index for medical care. The board is greatly limited in its authority: it can recommend changes in payment methods and rates, but not in benefits, and even regarding payment, it has no authority in regard to hospitals until 2020. Although the board's recommendations can be overridden by Congress, they become law if Congress fails to act. The board can also propose changes in private health insurance, but these do not have any legal force. Together with the insurance exchanges, the board could become a critical new institutional counterweight against pressures for higher spending.

The emphasis on new experiments and new institutions is both a virtue and a limitation of the Affordable Care Act. The virtue is that the experiments may lead to better means of improving quality and cutting costs, and the institutions may put that knowledge to work. The limitation is that the official projections of costs by government actuaries and economists cannot assume the experiments and institutions will succeed, and their prudent assumptions may undermine the will to carry out the law.

The caution of the actuaries is apparent in the difference between the official forecast of the law's impact on national health expenditures (total public and private health spending) and a forecast by economists associated with the Commonwealth Foundation. According to the official forecast, the annual growth rate over the decade ending in 2019 will be 0.2 percentage points higher than pre-reform estimates.[27] According to the Commonwealth Foundation study, the growth rate will be 0.6 percentage points lower. Commonwealth's estimate reflects greater projected savings from the insurance exchanges as well as from various payment innovations and the advent of the Independent Payment Advisory Board.[28] But even accepting the more pessimistic official forecast, by 2019 national health expenditures as a share of GDP will run only three-tenths of a percentage point higher than projected before the legislation, and because of the increased number of insured, the costs per insured person will fall by more than $1,000. Looked at another way, national health expenditures in 2019 will be about 1 percent higher than they would have been in the absence of reform.[29]

Saving that 1 percent doesn't seem like an adequate justification for denying medical care and insurance protection to 32 million people. Underlying the legislation was a moral judgment that those who have been excluded from a minimum standard of protection should not be held hostage to the adoption of a comprehensive, sure-fire method for containing national health expenditures. The Affordable Care Act does pay for the governmental costs of expanded coverage; it also offsets at least some of the impact of broader coverage on total health spending—and if the experiments and institutions the law establishes pay off, it will have more than offset those added expenditures. That was a reasonable basis for moving ahead. In the long run, failing to rein in costs will imperil the effort to ensure coverage for all Americans. But those costs should be controlled in a fair way, not merely at the expense of the weakest in American society.

The great sacrifice in passing the Affordable Care Act was not in cost containment but in complexity. The structure of the subsidy system, the working of the new insurance exchanges, the rationale for the individual mandate, the relationship between the federal government and the states, the financing provisions—all these aspects of the law can be explained, but they are complicated, in part because they are trying to mesh with a system that is already complex and to do it in a responsible way. At the time the Affordable Care Act passed, many liberals as well as conservatives denigrated it. Rarely has a big reform been so widely dismissed as too small even by many of those who supported it. But the legislation is not just far-reaching; despite all the political pressures, it upholds a high moral standard. The challenge should be to follow through on the avenues for cost containment and quality improvement that the legislation opens up.

But first the law has to survive.

CHAPTER 9

Reform's Uncertain Fate

THANKS TO THE INCREASED POLARIZATION between America's two major parties, swings in power may now result in greater swings in policy. After passing the Affordable Care Act on party-line votes in March 2010, Democrats faced the risk that Republicans would try to repeal it or roll it back whenever the voters returned them to power. The law was also at risk of being overturned by the conservative majority on the Supreme Court, though Democrats were at first not concerned about that possibility. Enacting legislation—"getting it done," in Tom Daschle's phrase—had been a struggle, and now preventing it from being undone would be just as difficult.

Through most of the twentieth century, the political system's strong gravitational forces kept national policy from lurching first one way and then the other. Both of the major parties were ideologically mixed coalitions tethered to the center; shifts in control of Congress or the White House, or both, did not usually amount to a wholesale reversal in the direction of government. If the Republicans had won the 1936 election, perhaps they would have repealed Social Security and other programs that Roosevelt had introduced, but the Democrats held power long enough to consolidate the New Deal. When Eisenhower was elected in 1952, Republicans made no effort to undo those programs. Much the same happened during the 1960s. Although Nixon's election in 1968 brought about the end of some Great Society initiatives, his administration's domestic policies were remarkably liberal. The overwhelming pattern from 1933 to the 1970s was continuity, tilting in a liberal direction.

Since then American politics has been a tug-of-war. Expecting the advent of a new, long-lasting political majority, observers have sometimes trumpeted a big electoral victory by one of the parties as evidence of a definitive realignment. Yet neither side has been able to achieve the kind of durable power that Republicans had from the Civil War to the early twentieth century or that Democrats had during the decades of the New Deal coalition. In some instances, one party's advances have done more to stir up its opponents than its own supporters. Bill Clinton and Barack Obama, the two great hopes for a new Democratic era, both had that experience. With Ronald Reagan in 1980 and Newt Gingrich in 1994, Republicans won victories that were touted as revolutionary in their time, but on both occasions the Democrats retained power in another branch of government, and the presence of moderates in the Republicans' own ranks, particularly in the Senate, tempered more radical impulses in their party. As a result, neither Reagan nor Gingrich went as far in reversing New Deal institutions as many conservatives hoped.

Still, the tug-of-war decades have brought important changes in national policy. On the whole, liberals have gained ground on issues relating to tolerance, culture, and equal rights, while conservatives have gained the edge on issues relating to taxation and the economy. In some respects, social equality has advanced (for example, with regard to gays) even as economic inequality has become more extreme.

These developments have shaped the political context of the struggle over health-care reform. The great lost opportunity to resolve the issue on a bipartisan basis came under Nixon just as the era of New Deal liberalism was closing in the early 1970s. In the wake of that missed chance, the development of health care reflected the wider trend toward greater economic inequality as medical costs grew more rapidly than median incomes and the number of uninsured rose. But neither party could escape from the policy trap the nation had created for itself—an increasingly expensive and complicated health-care system that nonetheless satisfied enough people as to make it deeply resistant to change. Democrats were unable to carry out their agenda for comprehensive reform, while Republicans could not undo federal health entitlements and in some respects agreed to extend them.

In his 2008 campaign, Obama offered the hope of transcending the nation's bitter partisan divisions, and in another era, the approach to health-care reform that he and the Democrats adopted—with its clear debt to Romney's reforms in Massachusetts—might have won significant Republican support. But in national politics, Republicans had no interest in joining Democrats to extend coverage to the uninsured. Bill Kristol's claim during the debate over the Clinton health plan that Republicans would do better by rejecting any compromise had seemingly been vindicated in 1994, and that view now dominated the party. In Congress, the number of centrist Republicans had dwindled, and the far right held the surviving moderates in check, threatening primary challenges against any incumbent who cooperated with the Democrats. So the ink was hardly dry on the Affordable Care Act when it came under attack from Republicans determined to reverse it.

The Politics of Slow Implementation, 2010–2011

After a law establishes a new program, the next steps are usually a bureaucratic process of policy implementation. But the Affordable Care Act presented challenges far beyond those of ordinary legislation or even such historic undertakings as the establishment of Social Security and Medicare. With the main provisions of the law not scheduled to go into effect until 2014, Republicans had two elections to wrest back political control and cancel the expansion of coverage. Unlike Social Security and Medicare, the Affordable Care Act depended on cooperation by the states, but Republican governors and legislators opposed the law, and Republican attorneys general filed suits challenging its constitutionality. The conventional model of policy implementation hardly describes the obstacles that health-care reform confronted. To survive, it had to be defended legally and carried out politically, not just implemented in the usual sense.[1]

Many of the law's backers believed that the normal process of implementing the Affordable Care Act would strengthen it politically. The law's good works would soften the opposition, and the more its provisions went into effect, the more they would be woven into the fabric of institutions. At first, these hopes of building political support proved to be illusory. By delaying the most important benefits of the law for nearly four years, the Democrats guaranteed that confusion and uncertainty about the reforms would persist.

In the months after Congress acted, the administration went diligently to work writing the rules needed to carry out the legislation and making the initial grants to state governments for planning the insurance exchanges and other innovations. The urgent focus was the "early deliverables," as the president's top health care adviser, Nancy-Ann DeParle, referred to the short-term reforms intended to serve as a bridge to 2014.[2] In September 2010, six months after the law's passage, several changes in private-insurance regulation became effective, including the elimination of lifetime limits on coverage, a ban on pre-existing-condition exclusions for children, and the extension of coverage up to age 26 of adult children under their parents' policies. The law also called for several forms of relief on insurance rates to go into effect within the first year, including tax credits for small businesses and a reinsurance program for companies that cover early retirees. In addition, the law set up a transitional Preexisting Condition Insurance Plan to enable at least some people deemed uninsurable to buy coverage before 2014 through subsidized high-risk pools.

The Obama administration did a creditable job working with the insurance industry and state governments to implement these reforms, though there were problems. Applying the immediate changes in insurance rules to all existing plans before the larger reforms scheduled for 2014 would have disrupted the market, depriving some people of even the inadequate protection they had. Consequently, the administration decided to give waivers to many plans with deficiencies, even to "mini-med" plans that in some instances offer only up to $2,000 coverage in medical bills. Waivers went to more than 1,000 mini-med plans, with 2.6 million enrollees.[3] The ban on pre-existing-condition exclusions for children did not apply to "grandfathered" plans (that is, insurance that was in effect when the law was signed), and insurers could restrict child-only policies to limited open-enrollment periods.[4] The Pre-Existing Condition Insurance Plan was expected to cover up to 350,000 people, but the program enrolled only 12,000 after a year (and just 94,000 by the end of 2012). Although the premiums were subsidized, they were still too high for the vast majority of the roughly 4 million people with pre-existing conditions who might have qualified.[5] These short-term measures were intended as down payments on reform, and though they did provide tangible benefits, they were too small to make much of a political impact in the first year.

The response to the federal reforms by state political leaders depended largely on their party and ideology. Progressively minded Democrats in the states saw the Affordable Care Act as an opportunity to achieve goals they had long sought. They welcomed the financing for expanded coverage and the legal authority for restructuring the market that would come in 2014, as well as the more immediate aid to bolster insurance regulation, review insurance rates, and provide consumer assistance (for example, to help people in appealing denials of claims). The states could use the Affordable Care Act as a floor and build on it, strengthening the provision of care and developing alternative forms of coverage (including in the case of Connecticut a state-run public option and later in Vermont a single-payer proposal).[6] In Republican-led states, in contrast, political leaders responded with blistering denunciations of the federal law and typically took no action on the major choices regarding insurance exchanges and other issues, expecting that the law might be repealed by a new Congress and president or overturned in the courts.

Rather than becoming more supportive of health-care reform, public opinion remained sharply divided in the period leading up to the fall 2010 election. From 2009 to 2010, public attitudes toward the Democrats' proposed reforms followed much the same course as they had between 1993 and 1994. After an early honeymoon period, support eroded, though there remained more backing for the elements of reform than for the whole—a pattern that public-opinion analysts described as "liking the pieces, not the package."[7] Surveys in the fall of 2010 continued to show support for the pieces—except for the individual mandate—but not the law in its entirety. In October 2010, according to the tracking surveys conducted for the Kaiser Family Foundation, the public was almost equally split between "favorable" and "unfavorable" views of the legislation; roughly equal numbers said health-care reform would make their families better off (31 percent), make them worse off (29 percent), and have no effect (32 percent).[8] Several polls showed more opposition to the legislation than support for it, but some of the opponents thought it didn't go far enough. For example, in a CNN poll in August 2010, 40 percent said they were in favor of the law, while 54 percent were opposed—but the opponents broke down into 41 percent who thought the law was "too liberal" and 13 percent who thought it was "not liberal enough." Together, the supporters of reform and those who wanted it to go further made up a majority. CNN polls in March and December had almost identical results.[9] But supporters and opponents of the law varied in their intensity of feeling. In a September Associated Press poll, respondents had a choice between "strongly" or "somewhat" favoring or opposing the law. Among the opponents, two-thirds "strongly" opposed it, but among the supporters, just one-third "strongly" supported it.[10]

Public opinion about health-care reform followed partisan lines. Some political scientists argue that growing polarization in American politics is an elite phenomenon and that public opinion on controversial issues has continued to be bunched in the center.[11] While that pattern applies to some issues, health care is not one of them. Democrats and Republicans differed sharply from the beginning to the end of the health-care debate. When asked about nine possible priorities for the new Obama administration, Democrats ranked health care second and Republicans ranked it seventh; when the law passed, a survey found 75 percent of Democrats for it and 80 percent of Republicans against. At the time of the November 2010 election, two-thirds of Democrats said they wanted the legislation maintained or expanded, while eight of 10 Republicans wanted it fully or partially repealed.[12]

Emotionally, the two sides were not equivalent. Asked about their reaction to the health-care law in the October Kaiser survey, the leading reactions among the Republicans were disappointment (80 percent) and anger (58 percent). Among Democrats, 67 percent described themselves as "pleased," only 53 percent as "enthusiastic," and 40 percent as "confused."[13] The two parties' congressional candidates in swing districts also showed a similar disparity. In a study of campaign websites in 29 House districts that rated toss-ups, the political analyst Nate Silver found that all but one of the Republicans highlighted health care, as did 23 of the 29

Democrats. But while Republicans made clarion calls to repeal the law, "most Democrats—whether they voted for the bill or against it—suggested that it had been a reasonable start and had worthy goals, but that it required further tinkering."[14] In short, Republicans were clear and passionate and Democrats were ambivalent.

The fall 2010 election brought the Republicans a huge comeback victory, though the health-care legislation was not the only or even the principal issue at the time. According to the Kaiser tracking survey immediately after the election, voters ranked health care fourth, with only 17 percent mentioning it as a top consideration in response to an open-ended question.[15] But the Affordable Care Act probably did contribute to Democratic losses.

In 2010, Democrats were expected to lose ground in Congress, particularly in the House, because of the distressed economy and the large number of House seats (48) held by Democrats in districts that McCain had won two years earlier. As of early September, the standard political-science models for congressional midterms, based on economic indicators or a combination of economic and public-opinion measures such as the president's approval rating, predicted that the Democrats would lose from 30 to 50 seats.[16] In November, they lost 63—the most in a midterm election since 1938—although in the Senate they kept their majority and held their losses slightly below expectations as several incumbents, including Harry Reid, narrowly won their races.

The higher-than-expected losses for House Democrats suggest that some other factors may have contributed to the outcome. The impact of the Affordable Care Act is impossible to isolate with any certainty since it is unclear what Congress would have done if it had devoted time and effort to other issues or passed a different health-care bill. In addition, the faltering economy and other policies, such as the bailouts of banks and big corporations, may have influenced the strength of the reaction against health-care reform among those who opposed the administration. Still, Democratic incumbents, especially in swing districts, appear to have lost votes by supporting the administration's priorities, including health care.[17] And relative to expectations based on previous presidential voting in their districts, incumbent Democrats who voted against the Affordable Care Act outperformed those who voted for it, though not necessarily by enough to win re-election. Of the 34 Democrats who voted against the health-care legislation in March, 17 lost anyway and four did not run again.[18]

The gap in intensity of feeling between opponents and supporters of the legislation and resulting differences in turnout may help explain why the health-care legislation hurt the Democrats. According to the monthly Kaiser tracking survey, the voters in 2010 were more unfavorable to the legislation than the public as a whole, and the 17 percent of voters who ranked health care as a top issue were especially hostile to the law and likely to favor the Republicans.[19]

One reason the electoral map turned red in 2010 was that the electorate turned gray; the elderly went to the polls in droves to vote Republican, while young people stayed home. Older voters typically do make up a larger share of voters in midterm than in presidential-year elections, but seniors' share of the electorate in 2010 was four points higher than in 2006. The contrast between 2008 and 2010 was stark. In 2008, voters 65 years of age and older had actually represented a smaller share of the total (16 percent) than did voters aged 18 to 29 (18 percent). But in 2010, old voters outnumbered the young by more than two to one—23 percent compared with 10 percent. While the young still favored Democrats, the old swung massively to the Republicans, voting for them by a 21-point margin, 59 percent to 38 percent (compared with a roughly even split of seniors' votes in 2006).[20]

The demographic shift in turnout seems to have been critical for the role that health care played in the election. No age group was more opposed to the Affordable Care Act than the elderly. Indeed, in some polls, they were the only age group opposed to the law; a Gallup poll in June 2010 found 60 percent of seniors saying the adoption of reform was a "bad thing," while 57 percent of 18- to 29-year-olds and a plurality of other age groups said it was a "good thing."[21] Beginning with Sarah Palin's "death panel" scare, Republicans and conservative organizations played on the fears of the elderly that health-care reform would hurt them and during the campaign ran ads accusing the Democrats of cutting Medicare.

This was not the first time that the elderly have reacted sharply against new health-care legislation. Their opposition to the Medicare Catastrophic program led to its repeal in 1989, and seniors opposed the Republicans'

Medicare prescription drug program when it was passed in 2003. The elderly may be particularly susceptible to anxiety and fear about any change in policy that affects their health care. The "death-panel" scare persisted among seniors despite every effort to dispel it. The Affordable Care Act had the support of AARP and included benefits for the elderly, but polls indicated that those benefits made little impression. Commenting on a tracking survey from July 2010, Drew Altman, president of the Kaiser Family Foundation, noted, "Fifty percent [of seniors] said the law cut benefits previously provided to all people on Medicare when it does not, and another 16% didn't know. Only 33% knew that it eliminated co-pays and deductibles for many preventive services under Medicare, 26% that it provided bonus payments to doctors who provide primary care services under Medicare and 14% that it would extend the life of the Medicare Trust Fund (by twelve years according to government estimates)." Just half knew the law would fill the "donut hole" in the prescription-drug benefit.[22]

Republicans had been trying for years to use health-care issues to turn the elderly into a GOP constituency. Passing the 2003 prescription-drug legislation did not achieve the desired effect, but opposing "Obamacare" did. For Democrats, the response of the elderly to the Affordable Care Act came as a definitive rebuke to the hope that Medicare would help pave the way for a plan to cover all Americans because the program would be popular among seniors. Seniors do approve of Medicare; in fact, they are the age group most satisfied with their health insurance.[23] But they have also become the age group most resistant to a universal program. In 2008, a national survey by the Harvard School of Public Health and Harris Interactive asked whether the health-care system would be better, worse, or about the same if the United States had "socialized medicine," and among those who said they understood the term, there was a striking difference by age. Fifty-five percent of the youngest group—18 to 34 years old—said socialized medicine would be better, while 30 percent said it would be worse. Among the 35- to 64-year-olds, 45 percent said it would be better, while 38 percent said it would be worse. Just one age group had a majority against socialized medicine—the one age group that, according to conservatives' definition of the term, has socialized medicine: 57 percent of people over age 65 said it would be worse, while only 30 percent thought it would be better.[24]

The Affordable Care Act was not socialized medicine; it was an effort to fill in the holes of the existing insurance system with a minimum of disruption to established institutions and the protected public. But much of the protected public could never be won over to a program that they perceived as primarily benefiting the poor and minorities. The Democrats had also created a huge political problem for themselves by delaying the major benefits of the legislation for four years, mainly to be able to show that it would reduce the deficit. Despite that effort, surveys indicated that an overwhelming majority of the public believed that the official budget estimates showed the legislation would increase the deficit. In the September 2010 Associated Press poll, for example, 65 percent thought that the official estimate was that the law would raise the deficit, while only 19 percent thought it would reduce it.[25]

After the 2010 election, Republicans were in a stronger position to obstruct the implementation of the Affordable Care Act at the state as well as the federal level. They now controlled both the legislative and executive branches in 20 states, compared with nine earlier, and the newly elected Republicans included Tea Party supporters who opposed any cooperation in implementing the federal law, including bills to establish insurance exchanges under state control.

In national politics, repealing the Affordable Care Act was only the beginning of the Republican health-care agenda. In 2011, as in 1995, congressional Republicans proposed to turn Medicaid into a block grant and Medicare into a voucher. These changes would have effectively eliminated the entitlement of the elderly, disabled, and poor to specific health-care benefits under federal law. While making the Bush tax cuts permanent and further cutting the tax rate on the top bracket from 35 percent to 25 percent—levels not seen since 1931—the budget plan introduced by Paul Ryan and adopted by the Republican House on April 15, 2011, focused its cuts in spending on federal health programs. Beginning in 2013, the plan would have reduced Medicaid spending by $700 billion over the next decade by providing the states with block grants slated to increase only according to a state's population and the general consumer price index, not according to health-care costs or the population in need of services. Since Medicaid coverage is 20 percent less costly than private insurance for adults and 27 percent less costly for children, the states were unlikely to achieve substantial savings without limiting the numbers eligible for the program.[26] Unless states raised taxes to replace lost federal revenue, the federal cuts would have been virtually certain to result in the loss of health care by many of the poor.

The changes in Medicare under the GOP budget would have been historic. In 2022, the plan would have ended the traditional Medicare program for people turning 65 and begun raising the age of eligibility to 67, gradually terminating coverage of 65- and 66-year-olds. Instead of qualifying for benefits under the public Medicare program, eligible seniors would have shopped for private insurance with a "premium support" whose value would increase only with the consumer price index. According to the Congressional Budget Office, "a typical beneficiary would spend more for health care under the proposal" for two reasons. First, "private plans would cost more than traditional Medicare," which CBO estimated to be 11 percent cheaper, and, second, "the government's contribution would grow more slowly than health care costs, leaving more for beneficiaries to pay." According to CBO's estimates, the typical 65-year-old in 2022 would have paid twice as much a year out of pocket under the GOP budget than under current Medicare—$12,500 compared with $6,150.[27]

The Obama administration and Senate Democrats thwarted most efforts by the Republican House to roll back the Affordable Care Act, but they did yield on several secondary aspects of the law. The most important of these concessions was the cancellation of a new system of public, long-term care insurance that was supposed to be funded entirely by voluntary premiums. Known as the Community Living Assistance Services and Supports (CLASS) Act, the program was suspended by the Obama administration in October 2011 on the grounds that it was financially unworkable. (Congress eventually repealed it entirely as part of the larger fiscal settlement adopted at the end of 2012.) In another concession, Democrats agreed to stiffen penalties on individuals whose income by the end of a year no longer justified health-insurance subsidies they received earlier that year. Funds for public health and community health centers were cut. The 2011 fiscal negotiations also led to the elimination of a free-choice voucher program, championed by Oregon Senator Ron Wyden, which would have allowed 300,000 employees to choose one of the plans in the new exchanges rather than the coverage offered on their job if their employer's coverage would have cost them between 8 and 9.8 percent of their income. Wyden had seen that provision as a "bridge" to a new system in which employees were free to choose their own plans instead of being restricted to the coverage offered by their company, but employers opposed it.[28]

In his budget battles with Republicans, however, Obama held the line on all the main elements of the Affordable Care Act. At a fundraiser in Chicago on April 14, 2011, unaware there was a live CBS microphone in the room, Obama described his negotiations: "I said [to the Republicans], 'Let me tell you something. I spent a year and a half getting health care passed. I had to take that issue across the country and I paid significant political costs to get it done. The notion that I'm going to let you guys undo that in a six-month spending bill?' I said, 'You want to repeal health care? Go at it. We'll have that debate. You're not going to be able to do that by nickel-and-diming me in the budget.'"[29]

The Supreme Court Rules

During the national debate about the Affordable Care Act, the legislation seemed to die a thousand deaths. Pundits and politicians said health-care reform was finished after the right-wing town hall revolts during the summer of 2009. They said it was teetering on the brink of collapse when anti-abortion Democrats revolted in the House that fall and again when senators Joe Lieberman and Ben Nelson were withholding their support that December. The law was pronounced dead when Republican Scott Brown won the special Senate election in Massachusetts in January 2010, depriving Democrats of a crucial sixtieth vote.

To the consternation of its detractors, the Affordable Care Act survived all those near-death experiences, only to face yet another fateful test and moment of dire predictions when challenges to its constitutionality came before the Supreme Court in March 2012. The law's opponents were seeking to overturn the entire act on the grounds that two provisions—the individual mandate and the expansion of Medicaid—were unconstitutional.

Two years earlier, legal experts had given these challenges almost no chance of success, and even as the cases made their way through the federal courts, it seemed unlikely the law as a whole would be overturned. Of the four appellate courts to consider the challenges, only one struck down the mandate, and even it left the rest of the law standing. Two conservative appellate judges, Laurence Silberman and Jeffrey Sutton, upheld the mandate; no appellate court overturned the Medicaid expansion. At oral argument in the Supreme Court on March 27, however, the conservative justices seemed to accept the challengers' arguments on the mandate; observers took particular note that the conservative thought most likely to uphold the law, Justice Anthony Kennedy, showed little sympathy with the government's case. Immediately afterward some leading journalists predicted that the Court would rule against the government; by the time the announcement of the ruling approached in late June, the prevailing opinion had so changed from two years earlier that the betting market Intrade pegged the odds of the Court overturning the law at 80 percent. But when the decision was finally announced, it took nearly everyone by surprise. In a five-to-four ruling, the Court upheld the mandate, but it was Chief Justice John Roberts, not Kennedy, who sided with the liberals, and he did so on an unexpected basis. In another surprise, the Court declared by a seven-to-two margin that one aspect of the Medicaid expansion was unconstitutional: the federal government could not withhold funds for the existing Medicaid program if a state refused to enlarge it. But the rest of the law stood, and although the Court had effectively made the Medicaid expansion voluntary for the states, the decision was generally interpreted as a victory for the law's supporters.

The conservative effort to overturn the individual mandate through the courts represented an abrupt ideological reversal. Conservatives had supported the mandate for years, and in all that time none of them had questioned its constitutionality. Federal authority to establish a government insurance program such as Medicare was unambiguous; it seemed implausible that conservative judges would declare unconstitutional a measure that preserved private insurance, especially a measure conservatives had proposed in the first place. As late as June 2009, Republican senator Charles Grassley could refer to "a bipartisan consensus to have individual mandates."[30] But only months later, as conservative lawyers invented a new theory about the commerce clause, Grassley and other prominent Republicans who had previously endorsed the mandate began saying it was unconstitutional.

The debate over the constitutionality of the individual mandate primarily focused on whether it was justified under Congress's power to "regulate Commerce with foreign Nations, and among the several States" and to take all "necessary and proper" measures in the use of that authority. Since the 1930s, the Supreme Court had given the commerce clause an expansive interpretation in decisions about the constitutionally of federal economic regulation. In a famous 1942 case, *Wickard v. Filburn,* the Court had even held that under the commerce clause the government could prohibit a farmer from growing wheat to feed his own family and livestock when doing so would exceed his federal acreage allotment, thereby affecting interstate commerce.[31] In 2005, far from reversing *Wickard,* the Court had reaffirmed it in a decision, joined by Antonin Scalia, upholding a federal law banning the cultivation of marijuana for personal consumption.[32] In two other decisions, the conservative justices on the Court had limited the commerce clause to what they saw as strictly economic matters. In 1995, the Court overturned a federal ban on possessing a firearm in a school zone on the grounds that the presence of guns around schools had no substantial relation to commerce, and in 2000 the justices struck down a law providing a private right of action for victims of gender-motivated violence on the grounds that gender-motivated crimes are not an economic activity and do not substantially affect commerce. According to well-established precedent, however, insurance is an economic activity that Congress has authority to regulate. In congressional testimony in February 2011, Charles Fried, solicitor general in the Reagan administration, summed up the case for the constitutionality of the individual mandate: "Insurance is commerce. Health insurance is undoubtedly commerce. Congress has the authority to regulate commerce, and that means that Congress may prescribe, in Chief Justice Marshall's words, a rule for commerce. The health insurance mandate is a rule for commerce and in any event it is a necessary and proper part of the regulation of health insurance that Congress chose to enact."[33]

The new conservative case against the mandate—or the "minimum coverage" requirement—was that it went beyond previous rules because it regulated inactivity rather than activity. Fried and others insisted that nothing in the Constitution supported that distinction as a basis for limiting application of the commerce clause. But almost immediately after oral argument on the mandate began, Justice Kennedy challenged the government's attorney, Solicitor General Donald Verrilli, Jr.: "Can you create commerce in order to regulate it?"[34] The implication was that the mandate was dragooning individuals into the market rather than regulating existing market activity. Later that morning Kennedy suggested that the requirement to carry a minimum level of health insurance represented an "unprecedented" change in the relation of the individual and the federal government.[35] That challenge raised a series of questions: Was the mandate without precedent? Were the individuals subject to it inactive in the market, and what was the relevant definition of the market—health insurance, health care, or commercial activity in general? What principles limited the government's authority to mandate purchases?

The appellate judges and Supreme Court justices who said the mandate was constitutional insisted that there was no shortage of precedents for it. The law upheld in *Wickard,* they observed, required a farmer to go into the market to buy wheat. Environmental laws require car owners to purchase pollution control devices even though they aren't otherwise active in that specific market. The verb "to regulate" was defined in the eighteenth century, and still means, "to direct." In 1790, as Harvard law professor Einer Elhauge points out, Congress (including 20 of the Constitution's framers) voted to require ship owners to buy medical insurance for their sailors, and six years later Congress passed an individual mandate requiring seamen to pay for hospital insurance. Elhauge argues that the constitutional basis for these requirements, never challenged at the time, can be found only in the commerce clause.[36]

The Supreme Court has upheld economic regulation on employers and others on the ground that they are generally active in commerce without requiring the government to establish that they are active in the specific markets related to the regulations. Safety regulations apply regardless of whether people are in the market for safety equipment. Since the mandate in the Affordable Care Act applied only to people with enough income to file income taxes and are therefore clearly active in commerce, the issue might have ended there. But in defending the mandate, Solicitor General Verrilli accepted the premise that the relevant market had to be more narrowly defined; he sought to define it as the health-care market and argued that everyone is sooner or later in that market, though they cannot anticipate when sickness or injury will strike. (The law exempts from the mandate people with religious objections to medical care.) Indeed, Verrilli noted that those challenging the mandate acknowledged it would be constitutional if Congress imposed it at the point an individual enters the market to seek medical treatment; the question, Verrilli said, was therefore one of "timing," and because as a practical matter insurance may be purchased at a reasonable price only in advance of illness, Congress had reasonably determined to establish the requirement prospectively.[37] Health insurance, in the government's view, is only a means of paying for health care; people without insurance, far from abstaining from commerce, leave unpaid bills at hospitals, which are then passed on to taxpayers and others with insurance. The lawyers opposing the mandate insisted that health care and health insurance are two distinct markets—a position that Justice Elena Kagan referred to as "cutting the baloney thin"[38]—and that the government was seeking to impose an insurance mandate precisely because some people are inactive in the insurance market.

In both the public debate and oral argument at the Supreme Court, the law's opponents said that if Congress could compel people to buy health insurance, it might be able to compel them to buy broccoli, cell phones, or other private goods. To respond to that objection, the government sought to identify a set of limiting principles that distinguish health care from other products whose required purchase might conceivably advance a public purpose. In health care, unlike other markets, people can go into the market and obtain services without the ability to pay, displacing the costs onto others and substantially raising the costs of insurance. Federal law requires hospitals to provide emergency care regardless of a patient's resources. In a revealing exchange with Justice Scalia, Solicitor General Verrilli observed that people without the ability to pay can obtain treatment because of "the social norms . . . to which we've obligated ourselves."

"Well, don't obligate yourself to that," Scalia responded.

Taken aback, Verrili responded, "Well, I can't imagine that that—that the Commerce Clause would—would forbid Congress from taking into account this deeply embedded social norm."

"You could do it," Scalia insisted.[39] In other words, we could leave the sick and injured without treatment if they couldn't pay for it. The exchange epitomized two diametrically opposed views of the constitutional relevance of widely recognized moral obligations.

In its defense of the mandate, besides citing the commerce clause, the government also invoked the taxing power of the federal government. To many observers, the taxing power seemed like the weaker of the two arguments because the Affordable Care Act used the word "penalty" rather than "tax" to describe the payments due for failing to comply with the mandate. Under the law, however, the failure to obtain minimum coverage had only one practical consequence: the individual would owe additional money to the Internal Revenue Service. Verrilli argued that the mandate should just be seen as establishing the condition—lack of insurance—triggering the tax. At oral argument, Chief Justice Roberts asked Verrilli why Congress didn't label it a tax, and Verrilli responded, "They might have thought, Your Honor, that calling it a penalty as they did would make it more effective in accomplishing its objectives." Smiling, Roberts said, "Well, that's the reason. They thought it might be more effective if they called it a penalty."[40] That exchange turned out to be more significant than many at the time realized.

Except for the chief justice, the Court split evenly on the constitutionality of the mandate. The four Democratic appointees held the mandate to be constitutional under both Congress's power to regulate commerce and its taxing power, while four conservatives, all Republican appointees, held that neither of those applied. Roberts cast the deciding vote, siding with his fellow conservatives on the commerce clause but with the liberals on the taxing power. Rather than regulating existing activity, Roberts wrote, the mandate "instead compels individuals to *become* active in commerce by purchasing a product, on the ground that their failure to do so affects interstate commerce"—and Congress's power did not extend that far. In a passage that recalled Kennedy's remarks during oral argument, Roberts wrote, "Accepting the government's theory [about the commerce clause] would give Congress the same license to regulate what we do not do, fundamentally changing the relation between the citizen and the federal government."[41] On the taxing power, however, Roberts ruled that the substance of the law, not its terminology, was dispositive in constitutional adjudication, and because the mandate had no significance other than triggering payments to the IRS that had all the relevant characteristics of a tax and did not exceed the Congress's taxing authority, the Court's duty was to uphold the mandate as constitutional. The Affordable Care Act would survive.

The Court's ruling on the Medicaid expansion may prove to be the more important part of the decision, though it received less attention at the time. Even the Republican state officials who initiated the Medicaid challenge had thought it was a long shot.[42] Although the Court had previously denied Congress the power to "commandeer" the states by imposing regulations on them, it had never declared a grant of funds to the states to be coercive. States have always had the right to decline to establish a Medicaid program; nine states refused to accept Medicaid funds until 1970 or later. In the original statute, Congress reserved the authority to change the program, and between 1965 and 2010 Congress amended it more than 50 times.[43] Like those previous revisions, the Affordable Care Act made a state's receipt of federal matching funds contingent on its compliance with the new rules. But this time the Court declared the threatened loss of all Medicaid funds to be unconstitutionally coercive. Roberts, joined by his four conservative brethren as well as Kagan and Stephen Breyer, held that the potential loss of funds for existing Medicaid beneficiaries was "a gun to the head" and therefore violated the states' sovereignty.[44] According to Roberts's opinion, Congress had so fundamentally changed Medicaid in the Affordable Care Act that there were, in effect, two separate Medicaid programs; consequently, it could not withhold funds for the old program if a state refused to undertake the new one. In her dissenting opinion, Justice Ruth Ginsberg insisted that the broadening of Medicaid coverage in the Affordable Care Act was no different from earlier extensions of eligibility. She noted that Congress could first have repealed the original Medicaid statute and then "enacted Medicaid II," combining all the eligible groups in one program. "By what right," she asked, "does a court stop Congress from building up without first tearing down?"[45]

In their joint dissent, the four right-wing justices said the entire Affordable Care Act was unconstitutional. Not content to strike down the individual mandate and related insurance-market reforms, the conservatives held that the subsidies, insurance exchanges, and employer requirements would also have to fall because they would not work as Congress intended. Rather than making the Medicaid expansion optional for the states, the conservatives would have annulled it altogether on the grounds that the Court should not introduce a "divisive dynamic" among the states in which some receive federal aid and others do not. After overturning all provisions related to the mandate and Medicaid, the conservatives declared that all unrelated provisions had to go because they were unrelated: "There is no reason to believe that Congress would have enacted them independently."[46]

The sheer radicalism of the dissent was breathtaking. "When a constitutional infirmity mars a statute," Justice Ginsberg wrote in her opinion, "the Court ordinarily removes the infirmity. It undertakes a salvage operation; it does not demolish the legislation."[47] The extremism of the Court's conservatives may have been the reason that Roberts refused to join them. A few days after the decision was announced, Jan Crawford of CBS reported that Roberts had initially sided with the conservatives but then switched sides and withstood a long effort led by Kennedy to bring him back into the fold.[48]

The long-term significance of the Court's decision was unclear. If strictly interpreted, the new limit on the scope of the commerce clause may not have far-reaching consequences. One of the Republicans who brought suit against the government, Florida's former attorney general Bill McCollum, unintentionally made this point when he said after the Court's decision, "Well, at least it's clear that they can't order you to buy broccoli," as if anyone was proposing to do that.[49] By arguing that the insurance mandate was unprecedented, Roberts appeared to concede that the ruling doesn't apply to any other existing legal requirement. In fact, the proposal most closely resembling the health insurance mandate has come from conservatives who want replace Social Security with a requirement to buy private annuities—an idea safe under Roberts's tax-power argument. Some observers suggested that Roberts was actually playing a "long" game, keeping his eye on long-term conservative goals.[50] The limit on the federal government's spending powers was a doctrinal victory with potentially enormous significance for federal-state relations. By making a seemingly nonpartisan decision about health care, Roberts may also have achieved more authority for the Court—and himself—on other controversial issues where his rulings are likely to be warmly received on the right.

The immediate result of the Court's decision, however, was to bolster the legitimacy of the Affordable Care Act. Polls showed more support for the law from Democrats (and less support for the Court from Republicans).[51] For other reasons as well, Democrats began to think that although health-care reform had given them trouble in the 2010 election, it could work in their favor in 2012.

Another Election, Another Survival Test

The achievement of large-scale social change, I suggested in the Introduction, often requires winning not one, but several elections. In July, after the Supreme Court made the Medicaid expansion optional for the states, the Congressional Budget Office projected that the Affordable Care Act would still increase the number of Americans with insurance coverage by 29 to 30 million.[52] Republican congressional leaders and their party's presidential candidate Mitt Romney were on record, however, as favoring not only the repeal of "Obamacare," but also the enactment of tax cuts and budget retrenchment that would require major reductions in Medicaid and other health programs. In addition, employment-based insurance was in the midst of a long-term decline that would likely continue under Republican policies. Depending on the outcome of the election, therefore, the uninsured population could either fall or rise substantially. Many other Americans would also be affected if provisions of the Affordable Care Act broadening their coverage were repealed by a new Congress and president. The voters had a choice between two different futures in health care, though many people did not realize what they had at stake.

Romney's stance on health-care reform in 2012 had changed since his first presidential campaign, when he lost the Republican nomination to

John McCain. In 2007 he touted the legislation he signed as governor: "If Massachusetts succeeds in implementing it, then that will be a model for the nation."[53] At one of the 2008 Republican primary debates, he declared, "I like mandates. The mandates work."[54] After Obama was elected, Romney urged him to follow the example of Massachusetts.[55] But Romney's role in bringing about the reforms that were the basis of "Obamacare" created an awkward problem for him as he sought to win over Republican primary voters in 2012. While refusing to repudiate his Massachusetts program, Romney distinguished it from the national legislation. Obama's plan was "a federal power grab," whereas his own plan was "a state solution to a state problem," he declared in May 2011, neglecting to mention that his plan depended on hundreds of millions of dollars in extra federal aid.[56] At a debate on June 12, a day after one of his Republican rivals coined the term "Obamneycare" for the Massachusetts and national laws, Romney tried to put the qualms of conservatives to rest: "If I'm elected president I will repeal Obamacare," he said, adding that on his first day in office he would "grant a waiver to all 50 states," a power that the law did not give the president.[57] In another era, a Republican who had been a moderate governor in a liberal state might have been proud of pioneering the middle-of-the-road approach to health-care reform adopted by a Democratic president. But to become his party's nominee in 2012, Romney could not be conciliatory; he had to be Obama's antithesis.

As the 2012 campaign began, Romney and Obama appeared to have had similar political experiences in reforming health care. Both had succeeded in enacting legislation and then failed to get much political credit for the accomplishment. But their experiences diverged during 2012. While Romney never derived any benefit from his Massachusetts program, Obama was able to turn the Affordable Care Act to political advantage. The Supreme Court decision contributed to that turnaround, but it wasn't the only factor. An unexpected political conflict early in the year helped lay the ground for a Democratic campaign emphasizing health issues of particular concern to women.

The unexpected battle concerned the coverage of contraceptives under the Affordable Care Act. In the original fight over the legislation, abortion monopolized the debate over reproductive issues; contraception never came up. In fact, hardly anyone registered the implications for contracep-tive coverage when a "women's health amendment" passed the Senate in December 2009; news reports at the time focused on a provision in the amendment that effectively retracted the controversial recommendations on mammography that the U.S. Preventive Services Task Force had re-cently published.[58] In August 2011, following guidance from the National Academy of Sciences, the Obama administration issued a preliminary rule on women's preventive services that made the contraception coverage ex-plicit. Just as insurance plans would have to cover certain other preventive services without deductibles or co-pays, so they would have to cover the full cost of contraceptives. The preliminary rule provided an exemption from this requirement to churches and houses of worship, but not to religiously affiliated institutions such as hospitals and universities. The latter could not exclude contraceptive coverage if they offered health insurance. Although the Catholic Church and conservatives objected to the rule and tried to per-suade the White House to reconsider, public reaction was still relatively muted. But when the administration issued a "final" rule on January 20, 2012, reaffirming the contraception mandate, Republicans denounced the decision as an attack on religious freedom, and all hell broke loose.

The conflict over the contraception mandate had its origins in a shift in thinking about insurance coverage of contraceptives that began in the 1990s. Traditionally, health insurance didn't cover contraceptives, and the extent of the government's role in relation to that coverage was summed up by the newspaper columnist Pauline Phillips ("Abigail van Buren") in a tart response to a reader's question:

> Dear Abby: Are birth control pills deductible?—Bertie
> Dear Bertie: Only if they don't work.[59]

In the mid-1990s, Planned Parenthood and other groups concerned with women's issues and public health began to challenge the insurance rules. After failing to pass national legislation requiring contraceptive coverage, they turned to the states, and beginning with Maryland in 1998, 28 states adopted contraception mandates.[60] One reason for the receptiveness to the mandates was the growing evidence that covering contraceptives did not raise the cost of insurance; indeed, by avoiding unwanted pregnancies—and attendant costs for prenatal care and deliveries—contraceptive coverage saves insurers money.[61] Some states that enacted mandates exempted churches but not religiously affiliated organizations, and when Catholic institutions sued for a broader exemption on grounds of religious freedom, the courts ruled against them. The Equal Employment Opportunity Commission, the federal agency charged with enforcing laws against discrimination in employment, ruled that employers were engaged in sex discrimination if they covered prescription drugs and preventive services but not contraceptives.

The Obama administration's decision to stand behind the contraception mandate in January 2012 came at a moment when social conservatives were at the center of the battle for the Republican presidential nomination. In the Iowa caucuses on January 3, the first voting of the election season, former Pennsylvania senator Rick Santorum had won a narrow victory over Romney and for a time commanded national attention. A conservative Catholic with support from evangelical Protestants, Santorum was personally opposed to contraception. "It's not O.K.," he had said, "because it's a license to do things in the sexual realm that is counter to how things are supposed to be."[62] A growing movement among social conservatives also equated some forms of contraception with abortion and regarded any government support for contraceptives as immoral. The social conservatives didn't approve of sex apart from marriage or of the government giving away things for free, and in their eyes the contraceptive policy epitomized both. But rather than attack the policy directly, they preferred to frame the issue as one of religious freedom. The Obama administration, in this view, wasn't guaranteeing rights to women; it was persecuting religious conservatives. Romney joined the attack, accusing Obama of infringing on religious freedom by requiring contraceptive coverage; he also supported efforts by Republicans to defund Planned Parenthood. In the Senate, Roy Blunt, a Missouri Republican, introduced a proposal to allow employers to deny their workers a health-insurance benefit—any benefit, not just contraceptives—if the employer objected to it on religious grounds. The proposal failed to pass, but every Republican senator except for Olympia Snowe, who had already announced her retirement, supported it. In the

House, Republicans held a hearing in February on the contraception issue, and they called five witnesses, all men, refusing to allow testimony by
a law student at Georgetown University, Sandra Fluke, who had been protesting the Jesuit institution's decision not to cover contraceptives. Instead
of giving formal testimony, Fluke spoke at an unofficial session organized
by House Democrats, where she noted that the cost of contraceptives came
to as much as $1,000 a year, and some women had to pay that cost out of
pocket even though they were prescribed contraceptives for a medical condition. In the following weeks, the right-wing radio host Rush Limbaugh
denounced Fluke as a "slut" and a "prostitute" because, he said, she was
asking to be paid for having sex. After Limbaugh singled her out more
than 20 times on his show, President Obama put in a call to Fluke thank-
ing her for standing up to the abuse.[63]

Some observers who suggested at the time that Obama would have to
bow to the demands of critics and exempt all religiously affiliated institutions misread the politics. Limbaugh and the Republicans were doing
the president a favor. Ever since the Affordable Care Act had passed,
Democrats had found it difficult to communicate the law's benefits to the
general public. No-cost contraceptives were literally a pocketbook issue of
considerable value, and outraged conservatives were helping to publicize
it. Polls showed that the contraceptive mandate was popular; there was
no split between Catholics and non-Catholics on the issue, and the religious conservatives who were upset were not going to vote for Obama anyway.[64] Covering contraceptives also had social consequences that some
conservatives might have appreciated. Studies have shown that eliminating the economic barriers to contraception, particularly the long-lasting
kind such as IUDs, sharply reduces the number of abortions. In a St. Louis
study, no-cost access to contraceptives for a group of low-income, uninsured women cut the rate of abortions to less than half the regional and
national rates; teen births in the study fell to 6.3 per 1,000 women, compared to a national rate of 34.3 per 1,000.[65] But it was the savings for insurers that proved to be the key to an initial compromise devised by the
Obama administration in the midst of the controversy. The employees of
religiously affiliated institutions would be guaranteed contraceptive coverage, but their employers would not have to pay for it. Instead, insurers

would be required to pay for contraceptives out of their own reserves, a requirement that was feasible because the employees' access to contraceptive would cut insurers' overall costs. The bishops rejected the compromise, but it satisfied some of the administration's Catholic critics, and though the battle went to the courts, it died down in the political arena. (A year later, on February 1, 2013, the administration extended the exemption from the mandate to any nonprofit that opposes contraception and "holds itself out as a religious organization," a concession that may have reflected an interest in strengthening the government's position in pending legal cases. The revised provision still guarantees contraceptive coverage to employees even when their employer does not provide it.)

It was in the wake of the public battle over contraception, in late March 2012, just before the Supreme Court took up the Affordable Care Act, that Obama decided to embrace the term "Obamacare," used originally only by the law's opponents as a pejorative. To the conservative base, Obama was a hated figure who wasn't a genuine American; right-wing media refused even to refer to the health-care law as the Affordable Care Act, as if use of the name represented an endorsement. Calling it "Obamacare" suggested that it was mainly for the benefit of minorities. But the president's political advisers concluded it was a mistake to run away from the name; Obama was firmly identified with the law, and he might as well make the most of it. "You want to call it Obamacare—that's okay, because I do care," Obama told an Atlanta audience. On Fox News, Obama adviser David Plouffe defiantly predicted that Republicans would eventually "regret turning this [into] 'Obamacare.' "[66]

The popularity of the benefits for women may have given Democrats more confidence to stand behind the legislation. Unlike the expansion of coverage to the uninsured, the contraception mandate and other regulations on women's preventive care went into effect before the election, on August 1, 2012. At the Democratic National Convention in early September, preventive health services for women received more attention than any other aspect of health-care reform. The Democrats' emphasis on the issue continued into the fall; during the second presidential debate on October 16, Obama mentioned Planned Parenthood five times. Republicans themselves raised the salience of reproductive issues. Responding to a question about exceptions for abortion in cases of rape, a Republican senate candidate in Missouri said that from what he understood, "If it's a legitimate rape, the female body has ways to try to shut that whole thing down." A Republican senate candidate in Indiana declared that a pregnancy resulting from rape is "something that God intended."[67] Whether or not God intended these statements, they were an answer to Democratic prayers.

In the fall, with the primaries behind him, Romney tried to move a bit back toward the center. "I'm not getting rid of all of health care reform," he said on September 8, identifying two provisions that he would keep: coverage of young adults under their parents' policies up to age 26 and guaranteed coverage of pre-existing conditions. But his campaign subsequently clarified that coverage of pre-existing conditions would be guaranteed only for people who maintained their coverage continuously, a protection already established under federal law.[68] Repeatedly, he attacked "Obamacare" for cutting Medicare, although the law cut no Medicare benefits and his running mate Paul Ryan had retained the lower payment rates to providers in the budget approved by House Republicans. In 2012 as in 2010, Republicans criticized Obama for cutting Medicare during the campaign and then demanded bigger cuts in Medicare as soon as the election was over.

After the election, one Republican was emphatic that the Democrats' "gifts" of health care to voters were a major factor in the outcome:

> Free contraceptives were very big with young college-aged women. And . . . Obamacare also made a difference for them, because as you know, anybody now 26 years of age and younger was now going to be part of their parents' plan, and that was a big gift to young people. They turned out in large numbers, a larger share in this election even than in 2008.

The president's health-care plan, this Republican added, had also been useful in mobilizing African-American and Hispanic voters:

> You can imagine for somebody making $25,000 or $30,000 or $35,000 a year, being told you're now going to get free health care, particularly if you don't have it, getting free health care worth, what, $10,000 per family, in perpetuity, I mean, this is huge. Likewise with Hispanic voters, free health care was a big plus.[69]

This Republican analyst was none other than Mitt Romney, explaining his own defeat. The promise of health insurance may not, however, have been as big a factor in the voting as Romney believed; according to a survey in the fall by Lake Research, 78 percent of the uninsured were unaware of the opportunities for coverage under the Affordable Care Act.[70] In a Kaiser tracking survey after the election, health care ranked only as a second-tier issue. But the Kaiser survey also found a shift toward support of the health-care legislation compared to earlier surveys; asked what they wanted to see happen with the law, 49 percent said they wanted it expanded, while 33 percent wanted it repealed.[71] When the 2012 campaign began, Republicans appeared to be more enthusiastic about voting than Democrats were, but in November, young and minority voters showed up at the polls in unexpected numbers. Health-care reform, notably the benefits for women, had been central in giving them a reason to turn out. The gender gap in voting approached record levels; women's votes were critical to Democrats' success in Senate contests, including the races in Missouri and Indiana that Republicans initially thought they would win.

The Democrats, however, did not enjoy a complete sweep. When all the voting in House races was added up, votes for Democrats exceeded votes for Republicans, but the Republicans nonetheless retained their majority, thanks in large part to aggressive gerrymandering after the 2010 census and the 2010 election. With their control of the House, Republicans are not in a position to repeal the Affordable Care Act, but they can prevent Democrats from making corrections and improvements to it.

In 2012 Republicans also consolidated gains they had made at the state level two years earlier. The number of states with one-party Republican control rose from 20 to 24, and as of early 2013 Republicans had a governor or a share in legislative power in another 14 states (Democrats had one-party control in just 12). Since the Medicaid expansion was now a state option, Republicans were therefore in position to block it in up to 38 states. They could also refuse to set up health insurance exchanges, leaving it to the federal government to establish them.

The Medicaid expansion poses a difficult choice for conservative state officials who regard it as ideologically abhorrent. States refusing to expand Medicaid eligibility not only prevent low-income people from obtaining health coverage; they also inflict damage on their local economies and health-care institutions. To be sure, the Medicaid expansion will cost the states money—but, according to the Congressional Budget Office, it will increase state Medicaid expenditures by less than 1 percent because the federal government pays nearly all the cost of newly eligible Medicaid beneficiaries (100 percent for the first three years, declining to 90 percent thereafter). As the number of uninsured drops, moreover, hospitals are relieved of much of their burden of uncompensated care and no longer need to transfer that cost to the privately insured. As a result, the Medicaid expansion also benefits the insured, who will no longer pay the indirect tax for uncompensated care that has long been hidden in their health-care and insurance bills. In addition, the influx of federal Medicaid dollars into a state has a multiplier effect on local economies as hospitals and other providers pay their suppliers and employees. These economic considerations may eventually persuade resisting red states to accept the Medicaid expansion, just as the states in the South and Southwest that refused to participate in Medicaid in 1965 eventually accepted the program.

States that reject the expansion of Medicaid will also put some of their own citizens in a worse position than low-income legal immigrants. Citizens with incomes below the poverty line are not eligible for subsidized private coverage in the insurance exchanges because Congress assumed Medicaid would cover them. But because the Affordable Care Act maintains a five-year waiting period for legal immigrants to qualify for Medicaid, it offers them the opportunity to buy insurance through the exchanges. As a result, in the Republican-controlled states that take advantage of the Supreme Court decision and refuse to expand Medicaid, a citizen may have just as low an income as an immigrant but be disqualified from the subsidized insurance that the immigrant is eligible to buy.[72]

Unwilling to have anything to do with "Obamacare," most Republican state officials have also refused to set up insurance exchanges. At least to begin with, only seventeen of the states are building their own exchanges, while seven others develop exchanges in partnership with the federal government and the rest leave the job entirely to Washington. A nationally operated exchange would have had many advantages if the law had envisioned it from the beginning; many states, especially the smaller ones, lack the necessary administrative capacities and computer systems. But after the states dithered for nearly three years over the decision, federal authorities found themselves at the end of 2012 with less than a year to organize the exchanges for the first open enrollment beginning October 1, 2013, for coverage starting the next January 1.

The difficulties in creating the new marketplaces look intimidating. Many of the uninsured do not know about the new opportunities for insurance, and there may not be adequate publicity to make them aware. The mandate that is supposed to induce the uninsured to buy coverage has especially weak penalties in the first year. Online systems that were supposed to provide one-stop service for Medicaid, CHIP, and the exchanges may not be ready. State decisions not to expand Medicaid eligibility will leave many of the poor confused and dismayed when they discover they have incomes too high to qualify for Medicaid in their state but too low to qualify for subsidies in the exchange. State officials may be unable or unwilling to enforce insurance regulations consistent with the new federal law and in line with the best interests of consumers using the exchanges. As a result, participation in the exchanges may be disappointingly low, and costs per insured discouragingly high. Under the most favorable circumstances, the rollout of so large and complex a program would be difficult. Its dependence on hostile state governments creates a much larger risk of poor performance and backlash. Shortly after the 2012 election, Henry Aaron, an economist at the Brookings Institution, said observers were correct in predicting that the fate of health-care reform depended on the election; only now, he suggested, the decisive election would come in 2016.[73]

The fate of reform will be uncertain as long as there is no political agreement about the obligation to provide health care for all, and one of the two major parties rejects that idea. According to Gallup surveys, the proportion of Republicans saying "it is the responsibility of the federal government to make sure all Americans have health coverage" fell from 38 percent in 2007 to 12 percent in 2012.[74] Perhaps some came to believe that the responsibility lies with state governments, though there is little sign of Republican-led states acting on that belief. Perhaps the rise of health care as a commercial enterprise in recent decades has simply changed how many Americans think about the subject. A commitment to care for all has traditionally been an important moral principle in medicine. "Well, don't obligate yourself to that," Justice Scalia said. If that is what his fellow conservatives believe, the United States is a long way from resolving the issue.

The Peculiar Struggle

The historian Arthur Schlesinger, Jr., once wrote that "in a democracy politics is about something more than the struggle for power or the manipulation of image. It is above all about the search for remedy."[75] The search for a remedy to America's problems in health care has turned into a peculiarly arduous struggle—peculiar in its duration, its rancor, and its salience and centrality in national politics. Other democracies long ago resolved whether they have an obligation to provide care for the sick and protection against medical costs. For a century the United States has been fighting over that issue, and instead of subsiding, the disagreements have intensified and at times shaken the political arena. In their euphoria immediately after the passage of the Affordable Care Act, its supporters believed they had achieved a historic breakthrough. But those who make history can never be sure of what history will make of them. If the opponents of the law ultimately succeed in unraveling it, the triumph of the Obama years will turn instead into another chapter in a story of triumphant reaction.

The American struggle over health care has also been peculiar because of the unusual lines on which it has been fought. If the "special interests" were arrayed on one side and the suffering masses on the other, the conflict would fit easily into a familiar populist picture of the world. But though the health insurers, drug companies, and other interests profit from the health system, they are not alone responsible for maintaining it. The bias against change also comes from members of the protected public. No other major democracy created a financing system that provides the biggest tax breaks to the people with the best private insurance; no other major democracy established a separate program for the elderly. A variety of other programs protect particular groups. These partial measures have become major obstacles to efforts to control costs and to extend protection to the uninsured. The resistance to reform didn't arise because Americans were such determined individualists that they rejected all government help; much of the resistance has come from members of an entitled majority with a privileged position in the public-subsidy system. The potency of these entitlements lies in the psychology of self-exemption they instill; the beneficiaries do not understand themselves as benefiting from government assistance or as sharing a common condition with the excluded. The tax subsidies for employment-based insurance are nearly invisible to those who receive them; Medicare invites seniors to believe that they have earned its benefits, whereas other claimants have not. Morally armed, they can reject helping others in need as a matter of high principle; after all, Americans shouldn't look to the government for help.

What is also peculiar about the American struggle over health care is that the problems do not just afflict the least powerful in the society. Many middle-class people who have the bad luck to get sick also get stuck without protection. Most of the uninsured are not the poorest of the poor, but working people in low-wage jobs—the kind of people who, as Bill Clinton used to say, "play by the rules." It's just that the rules of health insurance in America have been stacked against them. Americans are supposed to value work but apparently do not value it strongly enough to give workers a right to protection in ill health.

Several of those involved in passing the Affordable Care Act told me that they saw it as a last chance for health-care reform. After long careers fighting for universal health care, they doubted they would personally have another opportunity. But I also heard the view that as health costs rise, the chance of ever passing a universal program again may slip away for the country. The Affordable Care Act already represented a significant scaling back of liberal ambitions from Senator Kennedy's proposals in the 1970s or even what Clinton was calling for in the 1990s. In those debates, many Republicans had accepted the legitimacy of universal coverage as a national objective. That is no longer true; the earlier moral consensus has disappeared. The policies advocated by Republican leaders in Congress would raise the number of uninsured. Perhaps America will simply get used to the idea that although other countries can provide health care to all their people, the United States is too poor to afford it.

The difficulties in the search for remedy in health policy were not inevitable; at times alternatives were in reach that could have provided insurance protection to all and kept costs closer to the levels of other advanced nations. In 2010 Congress finally overcame the usual drumbeat of fear by the opponents of reform with moderate legislation that could help create a more just and efficient system. Two years later, the law survived efforts to overturn it in the Supreme Court and at the ballot box, but it continued to face deep resistance in states controlled by Republicans. Whether the reforms will achieve their objective remains uncertain; continuing increases in health costs could erode the commitment to health care for all. Giving up on that aim and rolling back the Affordable Care Act would not merely harm the people excluded from protection. It would be a confession of political helplessness in the face of a problem that has nagged at the national conscience for a century. The search for remedy would continue, but it would proceed under a shadow of uncertainty about whether Americans will ever be able to hold their fears in check and summon the elementary decency toward the sick that characterizes other democracies.

NOTES

Introduction: An Uneasy Victory

1. U.S. Bureau of the Census, "Uninsured Rose to 16.7% in 2009," September 17, 2010.
2. Congressional Budget Office, "How Many People Lack Health Insurance and for How Long?" 2003, at http://www.cbo.gov/ftpdocs/42xx/doc4210/05–12-Uninsured.pdf; U.S. Department of the Treasury, "The Risk of Losing Health Insurance over a Decade: New Findings from Longitudinal Data," 2009, at http://www.ustreas.gov/press/releases/docs/final-hc-report092009.pdf.
3. Organization for Economic Cooperation and Development (OECD), "Health at a Glance 2009: OECD Indicators," December 8, 2009, at http://www.oecd.org/health/healthataglance/. For the 1970 figures, see Kaiser Family Foundation, "Health Care Spending in the United States and OECD Countries," January 2007, at http://www.kff.org/insurance/snapshot/chcm010307oth.cfm. For the most recent U.S. figures, see U.S. Department of Health and Human Services, "National Health Expenditures: 2009 Highlights," at https://www.cms.gov/NationalHealthExpendData/downloads/highlights.pdf.
4. Uwe E. Reinhardt, Peter S. Hussey, and Gerard F. Anderson, "U.S. Health Care Spending in an International Context," *Health Affairs* (May/June 2004), 12.
5. McKinsey Global Institute, "Accounting for the Cost of Health Care in the United States" (McKinsey & Co, January 2007), at http://www.mckinsey.com/mgi/reports/pdfs/healthcare/MGI_US_HC_fullreport.pdf; ; Gerard F. Anderson et al., "It's the Prices, Stupid: Why the United States Is So Different from Other Countries," *Health Affairs* 22 (May–June 2003), 89–105; Gerard F. Anderson et al., "Health Spending in the United States and the Rest of the Industrialized World," *Health Affairs* 24 (July–August 2005), 903–914.
6. Commonwealth Fund, *Why Not the Best? Results from a National Scorecard on U.S. Health System Performance, 2008*, July 2008, chart pack, at http://www

.commonwealthfund.org/Content/Publications/Fund-Reports/2008/Jul/Why
-Not-the-Best—Results-from-the-National-Scorecard-on-U-S—Health-System
-Performance—2008.aspx. See also Commonwealth Fund, *Mirror, Mirror on the
Wall: How the Performance of the U.S. Health Care System Compares Internation-
ally, 2010 Update* (June 23, 2010), at http://www.commonwealthfund.org/Content/
Publications/Fund-Reports/2010/Jun/Mirror-Mirror-Update.aspx.

7. World Health Organization, *The World Health Report 2000,* Statistical Annex,
Table 10, 200, at http://www.who.int/whr/2000/en/annex10_en.pdf.

8. For the data on trust, see Tami Buh and Robert J. Blendon, "Trust in Government and Health Care Institutions," in Robert J. Blendon et al., *American Public
Opinion and Health Care* (Washington, DC: CQ Press, 2011), 15–38.

9. See Royce Carroll et al., "DW-NOMINATE Scores with Bootstrapped Standard
Errors," updated February 3, 2011, at http: //www.voteview.com/dwnominate
.asp. Thanks to Nolan McCarty for providing the data on individual senators for
2009. For background, see Nolan McCarty, Keith T. Poole, and Howard Rosen-
thal, *Polarized America: The Dance of Ideology and Unequal Riches* (Cambridge,
MA: MIT Press, 2008).

10. Kaiser Family Foundation and Health Research and Education Trust, *Employer
Health Benefits: 2006 Annual Survey,* Section 1, at http://www.kff.org/insurance/
7527/upload/7527.pdf.

11. Jared Bernstein and Elise Gould, "Income Picture, August 29, 2006," Economic Policy Institute, at http://www.epi.org/publications/entry/webfeatures_
econindicators_income20060829/.

12. July 2, 2008, at a meeting just after Tanden joined the Obama campaign. Interviews, Washington, DC, July 7 and July 21, 2010.

13. For my own proposal, which I presented to Rep. Henry Waxman and others, see
"Averting a Health-Care Backlash," *American Prospect* (December 8, 2009), available at http://www.prospect.org/cs/articles?article=averting_a_health_care_
backlash; and "A Health Insurance Mandate with a Choice," *New York Times,*
March 3, 2010.

14. Interview, Jonathan Gruber, Lexington, Massachusetts, August 20, 2010.

15. Harold Pollack, "The Cost of Delayed Reform," *American Prospect* (September
2010), A16–A17.

16. Noam N. Levey and Janet Hook, "Tough Debates Ahead as Senate Unveils
Health Plan," *Los Angeles Times,* November 19, 2009, available at http://articles
.latimes.com/2009/nov/19/nation/na-health-senate19.

Chapter 1. Evolution through Defeat

1. Although this chapter draws on previous work of mine, I have updated the
analysis to reflect recent scholarship. For my earlier treatment of the subject, see
The Social Transformation of American Medicine (New York: Basic Books, 1983).

2. Associated Press, "Health Talks in Overdrive with Obama Pushing," January 15,
2010.

3. See Lewis L. Gould, ed., *Bull Moose on the Stump: The 1912 Campaign Speeches of Theodore Roosevelt* (Lawrence: University Press of Kansas, 2008). For the one passing (and qualified) reference to health insurance I could find, see "Roosevelt's Creed Set Forth," *New York Times*, August 7, 1912.

4. For the AALL's "standard bill," see *American Labor Legislation Review* 6 (1916), 239–268. On the background of the AALL, see Irwin Yellowitz, *Labor and the Progressive Movement in New York State, 1897–1916* (Ithaca, NY: Cornell University Press, 1965), 55–59.

5. Roy Lubove, *The Struggle for Social Security* (Cambridge, MA: Harvard University Press, 1970), 45–51; Lawrence M. Friedman and Jack Ladinsky, "Social Change and the Law of Industrial Accidents," *Columbia Law Review* 67 (January 1967), 50–82.

6. Samuel Gompers, "Trade Union Health Insurance," *America Federationist* 23 (November 1916), 1072–1074, and "Compulsory Sickness Insurance," *National Civic Federation Review* 5 (April 1, 1920), 8; Philip Taft, *The A.F. of L. in the Time of Gompers* (New York: Harper and Row, 1957), 364–365.

7. Beatrix Hoffman, *The Wages of Sickness: The Politics of Health Insurance in Progressive America* (Chapel Hill: University of North Carolina Press, 2001), 137–162.

8. Ronald Numbers, *Almost Persuaded: American Physicians and Compulsory Health Insurance, 1912–1920* (Baltimore: John Hopkins University Press, 1978).

9. F. L. Hoffman, *Facts and Fallacies of Compulsory Health Insurance* (Newark, NJ: Prudential Press, 1917); Marquis James, *The Metropolitan Life: A Study in Business Growth* (New York: Viking Press, 1974), 73–93. B. S. Warren and Edgar Sydenstricker, "Health Insurance: Its Relation to Public Health," *Public Health Bulletin*, no. 76 (March 1916), 54.

10. Arthur Viseltear, "Compulsory Health Insurance in California, 1915–1918," *Journal of the History of Medicine and the Allied Sciences* 24 (April 1969), 151–182; Numbers, *Almost Persuaded*, 79–81.

11. Hoffman, *The Wages of Sickness*, 163–180.

12. Ohio Health and Old Age Insurance Commission, *Health, Health Insurance, Old Age Pensions* (Columbus, Ohio, 1919), 116.

13. I. S. Falk et al., *The Cost of Medical Care* (Chicago: University of Chicago Press, 1933), 89. The estimate was only for private expenditures; figuring in tax money spent on hospital care, the proportion of social costs for hospital care rose to 23 percent.

14. On the early development of Blue Cross, see C. Rufus Rorem, *Blue Cross Hospital Service Plans* (Chicago: Hospital Service Plan Commission, 1944); Michael M. Davis and C. Rufus Rorem, *The Crisis in Hospital Finance* (Chicago: University of Chicago Press, 1932); Louis S. Reed, *Blue Cross and Medical Service Plans* (Washington, DC: Federal Security Agency, 1949); and Robert Cunningham III and Robert Cunningham, Jr., *The Blues: A History of the Blue Cross and Blue Shield System* (DeKalb: Northern Illinois University Press, 1997).

15. Edwin Witte, *The Development of the Social Security Act* (Madison: University of Wisconsin Press, 1962), 174–175.

16. "A National Health Program: Report of the Technical Committee on Medical Care," in Interdepartmental Committee to Coordinate Health and Welfare Activities, *Proceedings of the National Health Conference,* July 18, 19, 20, 1938, Washington, DC (Washington, DC: U.S. Government Printing Office, 1938), 29–63; Robert F. Wagner, "The National Health Bill," *American Labor Legislation Review* 29 (1939), 13–44; Harvey Lebrun, "The Wagner-Murray-Dingell Bill: Big and Little Issues in It," American Association for Social Security, February 15, 1944.

17. Cass Sunstein, *The Second Bill of Rights: FDR's Unfinished Revolution and Why We Need It More Than Ever* (New York: Basic Books, 2004); David Blumenthal and James A. Morone, *The Heart of Power: Health and Politics in the Oval Office* (Berkeley: University of California Press, 2009), 52–53.

18. Blumenthal and Morone, *Heart of Power,* 56.

19. "A National Health Program: Message from the President," *Social Security Bulletin* 8 (December 1945), 8.

20. Richard Harris, *A Sacred Trust* (New York: New American Library, 1966); Monte Poen, *Harry S. Truman versus the Medical Lobby: The Genesis of Medicare* (Columbia: University of Missouri Press, 1979), 153–161; Blumenthal and Morone, *Heart of Power,* 87–90.

21. Starr, *Social Transformation of American Medicine,* 310–315. Some analysts argue that the entire employment-based insurance system was "accidental" because it was stimulated by World War II wage-and-price controls. But the efficiencies of using an employment base were far more important; the same system was emerging before the war and would have developed without it.

22. Jacob S. Hacker, *The Divided Welfare State: The Battle over Public and Private Social Benefits in the United States* (New York: Cambridge University Press, 2002), 239–241 (quotation from Marion Folsom, 241).

23. *Social Transformation of American Medicine,* 328–331.

24. Martha Derthick, *Policymaking for Social Security* (Washington, DC: Brookings Institution, 1979); Edward D. Berkowitz, *Mr. Social Security: The Life of Wilbur Cohen* (Lawrence: University Press of Kansas, 1995).

25. Derthick, *Policymaking for Social Security;* Theodore Marmor, *The Politics of Medicare* (Chicago: Aldine, 1973), 35–36.

26. The audio for Reagan's speech is available from the Ronald Reagan Presidential Library at http://www.youtube.com/watch?v=AYrlDlrLDSQ. For background on the campaign against Medicare, see Harris, *A Sacred Trust.*

27. For differing accounts of the Johnson-Mills telephone calls, see Blumenthal and Morone, *Heart of Power,* 164–165, 178–181, and Julian E. Zelizer, *Taxing America: Wilbur D. Mills, Congress, and the State, 1945–1975* (New York: Cambridge University Press, 1998), 225–229.

28. On the passage of Medicare, see Harris, *A Sacred Trust,* and Marmor, *The Politics of Medicare.*

29. See my "Health Care for the Poor: The Past Twenty Years," in Sheldon Danziger and Daniel Weinberg, eds., *Fighting Poverty: What Works and What Doesn't* (Cambridge, MA: Harvard University Press, 1986), 106–132.

30. Ibid.
31. Public Law No. 89–97, Sec 102A.
32. Derthick, *Policymaking for Social Security*, 336.
33. Blumenthal and Morone, *Heart of Power*, 192.
34. Robert Moffitt and Barbara Wolfe, "The Effect of the Medicaid Program on Welfare Participation and Labor Supply," *Review of Economics and Statistics* 74 (November 1992), 615–626.
35. In 1977 the first reliable, large-scale household survey to estimate the number of uninsured put that figure at 26.6 million people, or 12.6 percent of the population—a finding that was reported as a "surprise." (See "Many Found to Lack Medical Insurance," *New York Times*, October 22, 1980.) The proportion lacking coverage was probably lower in 1970 when unemployment was lower (3.9 percent in January 1970, compared with 7.5 percent in January 1977). In the early 1970s there was also broader eligibility for welfare and therefore Medicaid. The unemployment data are available at http://data.bls.gov/PDQ/servlet/SurveyOutputServlet. The 1977 health insurance findings are reported in J. A. Kasper et al., *Who Are the Uninsured?* (Hyattsville, MD: National Center for Health Services Research, 1980).

Chapter 2. Stumbling toward Comprehensive Reform

1. *New York Times*, July 11, 1969; Ronald Andersen, Joanna Kravits, and Odin W. Anderson, "The Public's View of the Crisis in Medical Care: An Impetus for Changing Delivery Systems?" *Economic and Business Bulletin* 24 (1974), 44–52. For a more extended discussion, see Paul Starr, *The Social Transformation of American Medicine* (New York: Basic Books, 1982), 379–398.
2. Karen Davis, *National Health Insurance: Benefits, Costs, and Consequences* (Washington, DC: Brookings, 1975), 109–110.
3. *Time*, June 7, 1971; David Blumenthal and James A. Morone, *The Heart of Power: Health and Politics in the Oval Office* (Berkeley: University of California Press, 2009), 232 (Nixon quoted).
4. Richard Nixon, "Special Message to Congress on Health Care," March 2, 1972, accessed at http://www.presidency.ucsb.edu/ws/index.php?pid=3757. For the 1971 poverty threshold, see Gordon M. Fisher, "The Development and History of the Poverty Thresholds," *Social Security Bulletin* 55 (1992), accessed at http://www.ssa.gov/history/fisheronpoverty.html.
5. Paul Starr, "The Undelivered Health System," *Public Interest*, no. 42 (Winter 1976), 66–85.
6. Starr, *Social Transformation of American Medicine*, 398–404.
7. F. J. Wainess, "The Ways and Means of National Health Care Reform, 1974 and Beyond," *Journal of Health Politics, Policy, and Law* 24 (1999), 305–333.
8. Blumenthal and Morone, *Heart of Power*, 240.
9. Wainess, "The Ways and Means of National Health Care Reform"; Theo Lippman, Jr., *Senator Ted Kennedy* (New York: Norton, 1976), 237–240 (Kennedy quotation, 240).

10. Davis, *National Health Insurance*, 85–89.

11. Wainess, "The Ways and Means of National Health Care Reform," 321; "Insuring the Nation's Health," *Newsweek* (June 3, 1974), 73–74.

12. Wainess, "The Ways and Means of National Health Care Reform," 322–328.

13. Victor R. Fuchs, *Who Shall Live?* (New York: Basic Books, 1974); Paul Starr, "The Politics of Therapeutic Nihilism," *Working Papers for a New Society* (Summer 1976), 48-55; Albert O. Hirschman, *The Rhetoric of Reaction: Perversity, Futility, Jeopardy* (Cambridge, MA: Belknap Press, 1991).

14. Peter Bourne quoted in Blumenthal and Morone, *Heart of Power*, 252–253.

15. Ibid., 272.

16. Edward M. Kennedy, *True Compass: A Memoir* (New York: Twelve, 2009), 359.

17. Office of Senator Edward M. Kennedy, "Detailed Explanation of Health Care for All Americans Act" (n.d., author's files); Paul Starr, "Kennedy's Conservative Health Plan," *New Republic* (June 9, 1979), 18–21.

18. Alain C. Enthoven, *Health Plan: The Only Practical Solution to the Soaring Cost of Medical Care* (Reading, MA: Addison-Wesley, 1980).

19. Starr, *Social Transformation of American Medicine*, 420–449.

20. On the history of prospective payment, I am generally indebted to Rick Mayes and Robert A. Berenson, *Medicare Prospective Payment and the Shaping of the U.S. Health Care* (Baltimore: Johns Hopkins University Press, 2006).

21. Ibid., 32.

22. Jon Gabel et al., "Withering on the Vine: The Decline of Indemnity Health Insurance," *Health Affairs* 19 (September–October 2000), 152–157.

23. Sara Rosenbaum et al., "EMTALA and Hospital 'Community Engagement': The Search for a Rational Policy," *Buffalo Law Review* 53 (2005), 499-535.

24. Richard Himelfarb, *Catastrophic Politics: The Rise and Fall of the Medicare Catastrophic Coverage Act of 1988* (University Park: Pennsylvania State University Press, 1995), 17–22.

25. Ibid., 33–42.

26. Ibid., 41, 55–72.

27. David G. Smith and Judith D. Moore, *Medicaid Politics and Policy, 1965–2007* (New Brunswick, NJ: Transaction, 2008), 145–183, 205–207.

28. Clinton quoted in Smith and Moore, *Medicaid Politics and Policy*, 182.

29. George J. Schieber et al., "Health System Performance in OECD Countries, 1980–1992," *Health Affairs* 13 (Fall 1994), 100–112.

30. T. R. Reid, *The Healing of America* (New York: Penguin Press, 2009), 162.

Chapter 3. The Shaping of the Clinton Health Plan, 1991–1993

1. For the argument at the time that changed conditions made health insurance a more potent issue for Democrats, see my "The Middle Class and National Health Reform," *American Prospect*, no. 6 (Summer 1991), 7–12. (This was the article, reprinted in *Harper's*, that James Carville read and led to his asking me to talk with Wofford.) For the background on Wofford's campaign and for evi-

dence on how media interpretations of Wofford's victory settled on his advocacy of a right to health care, see Jacob S. Hacker, *The Road to Nowhere: The Genesis of President Clinton's Plan for Health Security* (Princeton, NJ: Princeton University Press, 1997), 10–11, 16–19.

2. Philip F. Cooper and Barbara S. Shone, "More Offers, Fewer Takers for Employment-Based Health Insurance," *Health Affairs* (November–December 1997), 142–149.

3. U.S. Bureau of the Census, "Historical Health Insurance Tables," Table HI-1, "Health Insurance Coverage Status and Type of Coverage by Sex, Race and Hispanic Origin: 1987 to 2005," available at http://www.census.gov/hhes/www/hlthins/data/historical/orghihist1.html.

4. Robert J. Blendon et al., "Satisfaction with Health Systems in Ten Nations," *Health Affairs* 9 (Summer 1990), 185–192; Joel Cantor et al., "Business Leaders' Views on American Health Care," *Health Affairs* 10 (Spring 1991), 100.

5. George D. Lundberg, "National Health Care Reform: An Aura of Inevitability Is upon Us," *Journal of the American Medical Association* 265 (1991), 2566–2567.

6. This was the theme of much public opinion analysis at the time. See Robert J. Blendon and Karen Donelan, "The Public and the Emerging Debate over National Health Insurance," *New England Journal of Medicine* 323 (July 19, 1990), 208–212; John Immerwahr et al., *Faulty Diagnosis: Public Misconceptions about Health Care Reform* ([New York]: Public Agenda Foundation, 1992).

7. Among the accounts of this process, see Hacker, *The Road to Nowhere*, and Lawrence R. Jacobs and Robert Y. Shapiro, *Politicians Don't Pander* (Chicago: University of Chicago Press, 2000).

8. While the plan was being drafted, I wrote a record of the process for my files; that account is now available at http://www.princeton.edu/~starr/HealthReform/Starr_WritingofthePlan_6-20-93.pdf.

9. For the arguments at the time about Canada's lessons for the United States and the source of Canada's lower costs, see Theodore Marmor and Jerry L. Mashaw, "Canada's Health Insurance and Ours: The Real Lessons, the Big Choices," *American Prospect,* no. 3 (Fall 1990), 18–29; Steffie Woolhandler and David U. Himmelstein, "The Deteriorating Administrative Efficiency of the U.S. Health Care System," *New England Journal of Medicine* 324 (May 2, 1991), 1253–1258; and Robert G. Evans, "Canada: The Real Issues," *Journal of Health Policy, Politics, and Law* 17 (Winter 1992), 739–762.

10. "The President's Comprehensive Health Reform Program," February 6, 1992.

11. Alain Enthoven and Richard Kronick, "A Consumer-Choice Health Plan for the 1990s," *New England Journal of Medicine* 320 (January 5, 1989), 29–37; Paul M. Ellwood, Alain C. Enthoven, and Lynn Etheredge, "The Jackson Hole Initiatives for a Twenty-First Century American Health Care System," *Health Economics* 1 (1992): 149–168.

12. John Garamendi, "California Health Care in the 21st Century: A Vision for Reform," February 1992.

13. Starr, *Logic of Health-Care Reform*.

14. These papers were presented at a conference at Princeton University and published in a special issue of *Health Affairs* (January 1993); see also my "Healthy Compromise: Universal Coverage and Managed Competition under a Cap," *American Prospect*, no. 12 (Winter 1993), 44–52.

15. "Bill Clinton's American Health Care Plan" (Little Rock, AK, n.d.).

16. Bill Clinton, speech at Merck Pharmaceuticals, Rahway, New Jersey, September 24, 1992; Hacker, *Road to Nowhere, 112–115.*

17. Haynes Johnson and David S. Broder, *The System: The American Way of Politics at the Breaking Point* (Boston: Little Brown, 1996), 173; Bill Clinton, *My Life* (New York: Knopf, 2004), 547.

18. On the internal debate—which was misunderstood by many in the White House, then leaked and misreported in the press, finding its way into the work of historians and political scientists—see my record of the decision-making, "The Writing of the Plan," at http://www.princeton.edu/~starr/HealthReform/Starr_WritingofthePlan_6-20-93.pdf. On the final benefit package, see Congressional Budget Office, *An Analysis of the Administration's Health Proposal* (February 1994).

19. See "The Writing of the Plan."

20. I was unhappy about the turn toward stringent regulation. In a June 18, 1993, memo to Magaziner ("A Critique of Our Plan") uncovered years later in the archives by the conservative organization Judicial Watch, I wrote, "There is more regulation in this plan than I expected to see, and I worry about the wisdom of it. . . . I can think of parallels in wartime, but I have trouble coming up with a precedent in our peacetime history for such broad and centralized control over a sector of the economy." The memo is available at http://www.judicialwatch .org/files/2007/0108HRCHealthcareCritique_0.pdf .

21. On the plan's release, see Johnson and Broder, *The System*, 167–168.

Chapter 4. Getting to No, 1994

1. Quoted in Adam Clymer, "Any Additional Delay for Health Bill Means Death for Proposal This Year," *New York Times*, September 18, 1994.

2. Congressional Budget Office, "Estimates of Health Care Proposals from the 102nd Congress," July 1993, 21–28.

3. H.R. 5502; see Congressional Budget Office, "Estimates of Health Care Proposals from the 102nd Congress," July 1993, 29–38.

4. Congressional Budget Office, "An Analysis of the Managed Competition Act," April 1994.

5. Haynes Johnson and David S. Broder, *The System: The American Way of Politics at the Breaking Point* (Boston: Little Brown, 1996), 306–344.

6. Ibid., 127.

7. Mark V. Pauly et al., "A Plan for 'Responsible National Health Insurance,'" *Health Affairs* 10 (Spring 1991), 5–25.

8. Quoted in Jacob Heilbrun, "The Moynihan Enigma: Why the Senate's Intellectual Giant Is a Strangely Ineffective Lawmaker," *American Prospect* (July–August 1997), 18–29 (quotation, 22).

9. Johnson and Broder, *The System*, 353.

10. On the political consultants' advice, see Theda Skocpol, *Boomerang: Clinton's Health Security Effort and the Turn against Government in U.S. Politics* (New York: W. W. Norton, 1996), 118–125.

11. Bill Kristol, Project for the Republican Future, memo to "Republican Leaders," December 2, 1993; copy available at http://theplumline.whorunsgov.com/bill -kristols-1993-memo-calling-for-gop-to-block-health-care-reform/.

12. Elizabeth McCaughey, "No Exit," *The New Republic*. February 7, 1994, 21–25; James Fallows, "A Triumph of Misinformation," *Atlantic* (January 1995), at http:// www.theatlantic.com/politics/healthca/hcfallow.htm.

13. My discussion of the shifting position of business draws on the following: John B. Judis, "Abandoned Surgery: Business and the Failure of Health Reform," *American Prospect* (Spring 1995), 65–73; Cathy Jo Martin, "Mandating Social Change: The Business Struggle over National Health Reform," *Governance* 10 (1997), 397–428; and Peter Swenson and Scott Greer, "Foul Weather Friends: Big Business and Health Care Reform in the 1990s in Historical Perspective," *Journal of Health Politics, Policy, and Law* 27 (2002), 605–638.

14. Kathleen Hall Jamieson, "When Harry Met Louise," *Washington Post*, August 15, 1994.

15. Laura E. Tesler and Ruth E. Malone, " 'Our Reach Is Wide by Any Corporate Standard': How the Tobacco Industry Helped Defeat the Clinton Health Plan and Why It Matters Now," *American Journal of Public Health* 100 (July 2010), 1174–1188.

16. Alan Schick, "How a Bill Did Not Become a Law," in Thomas E. Mann and Norman Ornstein, eds., *Intensive Care: How Congress Shapes Health Policy* (Washington, DC: Brookings Institution, 1995), 227–272.

17. Johnson and Broder, *The System*, 363–366.

18. Bill Kristol, "Health: Congress Is Now More Dangerous Than Mr. Clinton," *Washington Times*, July 27, 1994.

19. Michael Beschloss, ed., *Reaching for Glory: Lyndon Johnson's Secret White House Tapes, 1964–1965* (New York: Simon & Schuster, 2001), 242. Johnson was quoting Sam Rayburn.

20. Hilary Stout, "Many Don't Realize It's the Clinton Plan They Like," *Wall Street Journal*, March 10, 1994, B1, B6.

21. See Lawrence R. Jacobs and Robert Y. Shapiro, "Don't Blame the Public for Failed Health Care Reform," *Journal of Health Politics, Policy, and Law* 20 (1995), 418.

22. Martin Gilens, "Inequality and Democratic Responsiveness," *Public Opinion Quarterly* 69 (2005), 778–796. Gilens' forthcoming book *Affluence and Influence* develops these findings in more detail.

23. See Ann E. Danelski et al., "The California Single-Payer Debate: The Defeat of Proposition 186," Kaiser Family Foundation, August 1995, available at

http://www.kff.org/statepolicy/loader.cfm?url=/commonspot/security/getfile.cfm&PageID=14427.

24. Skocpol, *Boomerang*, 182.

25. Gary C. Jacobson, "The 1994 House Elections in Perspective," *Political Science Quarterly* 111 (1996), 203–223 (quotation, 206). For Clinton's own analysis of the 1994 election, see Bill Clinton, *My Life* (New York: Knopf, 2004), 629–632.

Chapter 5. Comes the Counterrevolution, 1995–2006

1. Elizabeth Drew, *Showdown: The Struggle between the Gingrich Congress and the Clinton White House* (New York: Simon & Schuster, 1996), 276.

2. John F. Harris, *The Survivor: Bill Clinton in the White House* (New York: Random House, 2005), 215.

3. For a general discussion of health-care entitlements, see Timothy Stoltzfus Jost, *Disentitlement?* (New York: Oxford University Press, 2003), 23–62.

4. Alan S. Blinder and Janet L. Yellen, *The Fabulous Decade: Macroeconomic Lessons from the 1990s* (New York: Century Foundation Press, 2001), 15–24; Drew, *Showdown*, 71.

5. Jonathan Oberlander, *The Political Life of Medicare* (Chicago: University of Chicago Press, 2003), 164; Jost, *Disentitlement?* 138–161.

6. Oberlander, *The Political Life of Medicare*, 171–176; Drew, *Showdown*, 207, 242.

7. Oberlander, *The Political Life of Medicare*, 172.

8. Randall S. Brown et al., "Do Health Maintenance Organizations Work for Medicare?" *Health Care Financing Review* 15 (Fall 1993), 7–23.

9. Drew, *Showdown*, 206, 318 (Dole and Gingrich quoted).

10. Harris, *The Survivor*, 215. For Clinton's own account, see Bill Clinton, *My Life* (New York: Knopf, 2004), 681–683.

11. David G. Smith and Judith D. Moore, *Medicaid Politics and Policy, 1965–2007* (New Brunswick, NJ: Transaction, 2008), 227–243.

12. Ibid., 244–247; Bowen Garrett and John Holahan, "Health Insurance Coverage after Welfare," *Health Affairs* 19 (January–February 2000), 175–184.

13. Quoted in Smith and Moore, *Medicaid Politics and Policy*, 247.

14. Harris, *The Survivor*, 236 (Clinton quoted).

15. Len M. Nichols and Linda J. Blumberg, "A Different Kind of 'New Federalism'? The Health Insurance Portability and Accountability Act of 1996," *Health Affairs* 17 (May–June 1998), 25–42; Robert Kuttner, "The Kassebaum-Kennedy Bill—The Limits of Incrementalism," *New England Journal of Medicine* 337 (July 3, 1997), 64–68.

16. Robert Pear, "Insurers Fighting a Bipartisan Bill for Health Care," *New York Times*, February 2, 1996.

17. Kuttner, "The Kassebaum-Kennedy Bill—The Limits of Incrementalism"; Robert Pear, "Health Insurers Skirting New Law, Officials Report," *New York Times*, October 5, 1997; Robert Pear, "High Rates Hobble Law to Guarantee Health Insurance," *New York Times*, March 17, 1998.

18. Quoted in Robert Pear, "House Republicans Offer an Ambitious Plan to Expand Health Care Coverage," *New York Times,* March 9, 1996.

19. Kala Ladenheim, "Health Insurance in Transition: The Health Insurance Portability and Accountability Act of 1996," *Publius* 27 (Spring 1997), 33–51.

20. See Paul Starr, "An Emerging Democratic Majority," in Stanley B. Greenberg and Theda Skocpol, eds., *The New Majority* (New Haven: Yale University Press, 1997), 221–237.

21. The following discussion of SCHIP draws on Sara Rosenbaum et al., "The Children's Hour: The State Children's Health Insurance Program," *Health Affairs* (January–February 1998), 75–89; Sara Rosenbaum and Colleen Sonosky, "Medicaid Reforms and SCHIP: Health Care Coverage and the Changing Policy Environment," in Carol J. De Vita and Rachel Mosher-Williams, eds., *Who Speaks for America's Children?* (Washington, DC: Urban Institute Press, 2001), 81–104; Jonathan B. Oberlander and Barbara Lyons, "Beyond Incrementalism? SCHIP and the Politics of Health Reform," *Health Affairs* 28 (May–June 2009), w399–w410; and Jeanne Lambrew, *The State Children's Health Insurance Program: Past, Present, Future* (New York: Commonwealth Fund, 2007), at http://www.commonwealthfund .org/usr_doc/991_Lambrew_SCHIP_past_present_future.pd.

22. Lambrew, *The State Children's Health Insurance Program.*

23. Smith and Moore, *Medicaid Politics and Policy,* 251–258.

24. Marsha Gold, "Can Managed Care and Competition Control Medicare Costs?" *Health Affairs* (April 2, 2003), w176–w188.

25. Gail Jensen et al., "The New Dominance of Managed Care," *Health Affairs* 16 (January–February 1997), 125–136; Jon Gabel et al., "Withering on the Vine: The Decline of Indemnity Health Insurance," *Health Affairs* 19 (September–October 2000), 152–157.

26. Paul B. Ginsburg, "Competition in Health Care: Its Evolution over the Past Decade," *Health Affairs* 24 (November 2005), 1512–1522.

27. Blinder and Yellen, *The Fabulous Decade,* 73–79.

28. Joel Friedman and Isaac Shapiro, "Tax Returns: A Comprehensive Assessment of the Bush Administration's Record on Cutting Taxes" (Washington, DC: Center on Policy and Budget Priorities, April 23, 2004), available at http://www .cbpp.org/cms/index.cfm?fa=view&id=1811.

29. Katherine Q. Seelye, "Sensing Voter Interest, Gore Pushes Health Plan," *New York Times,* August 27, 2000.

30. Thomas R. Oliver, Phillip R. Lee, and Helene L. Lipton, "A Political History of Medicare and Prescription Drug Coverage," *Milbank Quarterly* 82 (2004), 283–354.

31. Karl Rove, *Courage and Consequence* (New York: Simon and Schuster, 2010), 373. For details on the later ethics investigations, see "Rove on Tactics Used to Pass Health Care Legislation: Do As I Say . . . ," Media Matters, March 22, 2010, at http://mediamatters.org/research/201003220078.

32. Oliver, Lee, and Lipton, "A Political History of Medicare and Prescription Drug Coverage."

33. MedPAC, *Report to the Congress: Medicare Payment Policy* (Washington, DC: MedPAC, March 2008).

34. Oliver, Lee, and Lipton, "A Political History of Medicare and Prescription Drug Coverage."

35. Alexandra Minicozzi, "Medical Savings Accounts: What Story Do the Data Tell?" *Health Affairs* 25 (January–February 2006), 256–267.

36. James C. Robinson and Paul B. Ginsburg, "Consumer-Driven Health Care: Promise and Performance," *Health Affairs* 28 (January 27, 2009), w272–w281.

37. Marc L. Berk and Alan C. Monheit, "The Concentration of Health Care Expenditures, Revisited," *Health Affairs* 20 (March–April 2001), 9–18.

38. For a comprehensive analysis and critique, see Timothy Stoltzfus Jost, *Health Care at Risk: A Critique of the Consumer-Driven Movement* (Durham, NC: Duke University Press, 2007).

39. Joseph P. Newhouse and the Insurance Experiment Group, *Free for All? Lessons from the Rand Health Insurance Experiment* (Cambridge, MA: Harvard University Press, 1993).

40. Dahlia K. Remler and Sherry A. Glied, "How Much More Cost Sharing Will Health Savings Accounts Bring?" *Health Affairs* 25 (July–August 2006), 1070–1078.

41. Jon B. Christianson, Paul B. Ginsburg, and Debra A. Draper, "The Transition from Managed Care to Consumerism: A Community-Level Status Report," *Health Affairs* 27 (September–October 2008): 1362–1370.

42. Elizabeth C. Hamel, Claudia Deane, and Mollyann Brodie, "Medicare and Medicaid," in Robert J. Blendon et al., *American Public Opinion and Health Care* (Washington, DC: CQ Press, 2011), 187.

43. Atul Gawande, "Getting There from Here," *The New Yorker,* January 26, 2009.

44. Robert J. Blendon and Drew E. Altman, "Voters and Health Care in the 2006 Election," *New England Journal of Medicine* 355 (November 2, 2006), 1928–1933; Hamel, Deane, and Brodie, "Medicare and Medicaid," 185.

45. Jared Bernstein and Elise Gould (Economic Policy Institute), "Income Picture, August 29, 2006," at http://www.epi.org/publications/entry/webfeatures_econindicators_income20060829/; Kaiser Family Foundation and Health Research and Education Trust, *Employer Health Benefits: 2006 Annual Survey,* Section 1, at http://www.kff.org/insurance/7527/upload/7527.pdf.

46. Kaiser Family Foundation and Health Research and Education Trust, *Employer Health Benefits,* 4; John Holahan and Allison Cook, "The U.S. Economy and Changes in Health Insurance Coverage, 2000–2006," *Health Affairs* 27 (February 20, 2008), w135–w144.

47. Peter J. Cunningham, "The Growing Financial Burden of Health Care: National and State Trends, 2001–2006," *Health Affairs* 29 (March 26, 2010), 1037–1044.

48. Cathy Schoen et al., "How Many Are Underinsured? Trends among U.S. Adults, 2003 and 2007," *Health Affairs* 27 (June 10, 2008), w298–w309.

49. Lambrew, *The State Children's Health Insurance Program: Past, Present, Future;* Rosenbaum and Sonosky, "Medicaid Reforms and SCHIP: Health Care Coverage and the Changing Policy Environment."

50. Mollyann Brodie et al., "Attitudes about Health Care Costs," in Blendon et al., *American Public Opinion and Health Care*, 77, 64.

51. See "Americans Spend More Out-of-Pocket on Health-Care Expenses, 2004," in "Health System Performance in Selected Nations: A Chartpack" (Commonwealth Fund, May 2007), 53, available at http://www.commonwealthfund.org/usr_doc/Shea_hltsysperformanceselectednations_chartpack.pdf; Jost, *Health Care at Risk*, 129.

Chapter 6. The Rise of a Reform Consensus, 2006–2008

1. Kate Kenski et al., *The Obama Victory: How Media, Money, and Message Shaped the 2008 Election* (New York: Oxford University Press, 2009).

2. Yu-Chu Shen and Stephen Zuckerman, "Why Is There State Variation in Employer-Sponsored Insurance?" *Health Affairs* 22 (January–February 2003), 241–251. On the impact of race on welfare policy in the states, see Matthew C. Fellowes and Gretchen Rowe, "Politics and the New American Welfare States," *American Journal of Political Science* 48 (2004), 362–373.

3. Robert S. Erikson et al., *Statehouse Democracy: Public Opinion and Policy in the American States* (New York: Cambridge University Press, 1993), esp. Ch. 4.

4. U.S. Bureau of the Census, "Number and Percentage of People without Health Insurance Coverage: by State Using 2- and 3-Year Averages: 2006–2007 and 2008–2009," at www.census.gov/hhes/www/hlthins/data/incpovhlth/2009/state.xls.

5. Deborah Stone, "Why the States Can't Solve the Health Care Crisis," *American Prospect*, no. 9 (Spring 1992), 51–60; Karen Pollitz and Eliza Bangit, *Federal Aid to State High-Risk Pools: Promoting Health Insurance Coverage or Providing Fiscal Relief?* (New York: Commonwealth Fund, 2005), available at http://www.commonwealthfund.org/Content/Publications/Issue-Briefs/2005/Nov/Federal-Aid-to-State-High-Risk-Pools—Promoting-Health-Insurance-Coverage-or-Providing-Fiscal-Relief.aspx.

6. M. A. Chirba-Martin and T. A. Brennan, "The Critical Role of ERISA in State Health Reform," *Health Affairs* 13 (March–April 1994), 142–156.

7. Richard A. Knox, "MASS. Enacts Health Bill; Care-For-All Act Is 1st in Nation," *Boston Globe*, April 14, 1988.

8. Interview, John McDonough, New York, September 15, 2010.

9. Interview, Andrew Dreyfus, Boston, February 23, 2011.

10. Interview, Tim Murphy, Boston, February 23, 2011.

11. Alice Dembner, "U.S. Threatens to Cut $600M in Medicaid," *Boston Globe*, November 11, 2004.

12. Interview, Jonathan Gruber, Lexington, Massachusetts, August 20, 2010.

13. Alice Dembner and Rick Klein, "Mass., US Reach Deal on Funding—Averts Major Cut In Medicaid Match," *Boston Globe*, January 15, 2005.

14. Scott S. Greenberger, "Romney Eyes Penalties for Those Lacking Insurance—Costs Are Key in Health Plan," *Boston Globe*, June 22, 2005.

15. Telephone interview, John Holahan, January 27, 2010.

16. Linda J. Blumberg et al., *Building the Roadmap to Coverage: Policy Choices and the Cost and Coverage Implications* (Blue Cross Blue Shield Foundation of Massachusetts, June 2005), available at http://www.agmconnect.org/doc/Building%20the%20roadmap%20to%20coverage%20Healthcare.pdf.

17. Scott S. Greenberger, "House Approves Healthcare Overhaul," *Boston Globe*, November 4, 2005.

18. Scott Greenberger, "State Senate Ok's Healthcare Plan," *Boston Globe*, November 10, 2005.

19. Scott Helman and Frank Phillips, "Hopes Fade on Reforms in Healthcare—Travaglini Shifts to Lesser Mass. Plan," *Boston Globe*, February 26, 2006.

20. Christopher Rowland, "Health Executives Emerge as State's New Power Players," *Boston Globe*, March 13, 2006.

21. Tara Sussman Oakman, Robert J. Blendon, and Tami Buhr, "The Massachusetts Health Reform Law: A Case Study," in Robert J. Blendon et al., *American Public Opinion and Health Care* (Washington, DC: CQ Press, 2011), 128–150.

22. For Romney's account, see Mitt Romney, "Health Care for Everyone? We Found a Way," *Wall Street Journal*, April 11, 2006.

23. Interview, Jon Kingsdale, Boston, April 30, 2010.

24. Jeffrey Krasner, "State OK's 7 Low-Cost Health Plans for Uninsured—Penalty for Failing to Get Coverage May Be Lifted for Some," *Boston Globe*, March 9, 2007.

25. Jon Kingsdale, "New Health Plans: Better Than What's Out There," *Boston Globe*, March 19, 2007.

26. Sharon K. Long, "On the Road to Universal Coverage: Impacts of Reform in Massachusetts at One Year," *Health Affairs* 27 (June 3, 2008), w270–w284; John E. McDonough et al., "Massachusetts Health Reform Implementation: Major Progress and Future Challenges," *Health Affairs* 27 (July–August 2008), w285–w297; Genevieve M. Kenney, Sharon K. Long, and Adela Luque, "Health Reform in Massachusetts Cuts the Uninsurance Rate Among Children in Half," *Health Affairs* 29, no. 6 (2010), 1242–1247.

27. Sharon K. Long and Karen Stockley, "Massachusetts Health Reform: Employer Coverage from Employees' Perspective," *Health Affairs* 28 (October 1, 2009), w1079–w1087.

28. For an account, see Martha Bebinger, "Mission Not Yet Accomplished? Massachusetts Contemplates Major Moves on Cost Containment," *Health Affairs* 28 (September 2009), 1373–1381.

29. Oakman, Blendon, and Buhr, "The Massachusetts Health Reform Law," 146.

30. Edmund Haislmaier, "The Significance of Massachusetts Health Reform," Heritage Foundation, April 11, 2006, at http://www.heritage.org/Research/Reports/2006/04/The-Significance-of-Massachusetts-Health-Reform.

31. Walter Zelman, *Swimming Upstream: The Hard Politics of Health Reform in California* (UCLA Center for Health Policy Research, June 2009), at http://www.statecoverage.org/files/California%20Reform%20Study%20FINAL.pdf; Peter Harbage, Leif Haase, and Len M. Nichols, *Lessons from California's Health Re-*

form Efforts for The National Debate (New America Foundation, March 7, 2008), at http://www.newamerica.net/publications/policy/lessons_californias_health _reform_efforts_national_debate. For a comparative analysis of the Massachusetts and California cases, see Anthony S. Chen and Margaret Weir, "The Long Shadow of the Past: Risk Pooling and the Political Development of Health Care Reform in the States," *Journal of Health Politics, Policy and Law* 34 (October 2009), 679–716.

32. Interview, Ron Pollack, Families USA, Washington, DC, May 19, 2010; Health Coverage Coalition for the Uninsured, "Expanding Health Care Coverage in the United States: A Historic Agreement," January 18, 2007, available at http://www .familiesusa.org/issues/uninsured/hccu/about-hccu.html.

33. Robert Pear, "Groups Offer Health Plan for Coverage of Uninsured," *New York Times*, January 19, 2007.

34. Telephone interview, Chris Jennings, September 9, 2010.

35. Robert Pear and Carl Hulse, "Congress Set for Veto Fight on Child Health Measure," *New York Times*, September 25, 2007; Jonathan B. Oberlander and Barbara Lyons, "Beyond Incrementalism? SCHIP and the Politics of Health Reform," *Health Affairs* 28 (May–June 2009), 399–410.

36. Telephone interview, Chris Jennings, September 9, 2010.

37. Jeanne M. Lambrew, John D. Podesta, and Teresa L. Shaw, "Change in Challenging Times: A Plan for Extending and Improving Health Coverage," *Health Affairs* (March 23, 2005), w5 119–w5 132.

38. These passages reflect a discussion with Wyden at the time he was working on the bill as well as a retrospective interview in his Senate office, December 9, 2010.

39. Jonathan Cohn, "What's the One Thing Big Business and the Left Have in Common," *New York Times*, April 1, 2007.

40. Andy Stern, "Horse-and-Buggy Health Coverage," *Wall Street Journal*, July 17, 2006.

41. Ylan Q. Mui and Dale Russakoff, "Wal-Mart, Union Join Forces on Health Care; Alliance's Goal Is to Improve Coverage," *Washington Post*, February 8, 2007.

42. Julie Hirschfeld Davis, "The Influence Game: Labor and Business, Joined in Health Care Cause, Now at Odds on Specifics," *Chicago Tribune*, February 16, 2009, at http://www.chicagotribune.com/news/nationworld/sns-ap-health-care -strange-bedfellows,0,6877237.story.

43. Ruth Marcus, "Universal Coverage's Mavericks; Harry and Louise, Meet Ron and Bob," *Washington Post*, February 27, 2008.

44. Interview, Rep. Jim Cooper, Washington, DC, July 1, 2010.

45. Ezra Klein, "Is the Healthy Americans Act a Basis for Compromise," *Washington Post*, June 24, 2009, at http://voices.washingtonpost.com/ezra-klein/2009/ 06/is_the_healthy_americans_act_a.html.

46. For the final version of AmeriCare, see H.R. 193, 11th Cong., 1st sess.

47. Jacob S. Hacker, "Health Care for America," Economic Policy Institute, January 11, 2007, at http://www.sharedprosperity.org/bp180.html.

48. Lewin Group, "Cost Impact Analysis for the 'Health Care for America' Proposal," February 2008, http://www.sharedprosperity.org/hcfa/lewin.pdf.

49. Roger Hickey, "Real Health Care Solutions," Campaign for America's Future, November 15, 2007, at http://www.ourfuture.org/blog-entry/real-health-care-solutions.

50. Mark Schmitt, "The History of the Public Option" Tapped, August 18, 2009, at http://www.prospect.org/csnc/blogs/tapped_archive?month=08&year=2009&base_name=the_history_of_the_public_opti.

51. Kaiser Family Foundation, "Kaiser Health Tracking Poll: Election 2008," Issue no. 6, March 2008, at http://www.kff.org/kaiserpolls/upload/7752.pdf.

52. Interview, Andy Stern, Washington, DC, May 6, 2010.

53. "Transcript: Senator Barack Obama," Center for American Progress Action Fund, http://www.americanprogressaction.org/events/healthforum/obama_transcript.html.

54. David Plouffe, *The Audacity to Win: The Inside Story and Lessons of Barack Obama's Historic Victory* (New York: Viking, 2009), 74.

55. John Heilemann and Mark Halperin, *Game Change* (New York: HarperCollins, 2010), 138.

56. *Meet the Press* transcript, February 4, 2007, http://www.msnbc.msn.com/id/16903253/ns/meet_the_press/.

57. For the video of his single-payer comments, see http://www.youtube.com/watch?v=fpAyan1fXCE.

58. Interview, Jonathan Gruber, Lexington, Massachusetts, August 20, 2010.

59. Obama '08, "Barack Obama's Plan for a Healthy America: Lowering Health Care Costs and Ensuring Affordable, High-Quality Health Care for All." (No longer available at BarackObama.com.)

60. Ezra Klein, "A Lack of Audacity," *American Prospect,* May 30, 2007, available at http://www.prospect.org/cs/articles?article=a_lack_of_audacity.

61. "Remarks of Senator Barack Obama," http://www.nytimes.com/2007/05/29/us/politics/28text-obama.html.

62. "Disease management programs," Obama's health policy advisers conceded, "vary in effectiveness, but *some programs do seem to save money.* A Rand study of health information technology estimated that prevention and disease management *could* lead to an additional $81 billion of savings." (emphasis added) David Blumenthal, David Cutler, and Jeffrey Liebman, "Obama Health Care Plan," http://www.nytimes.com/packages/pdf/politics/finalcostsmemo.pdf.

63. Telephone interview, David Cutler, September 1, 2010; Plouffe, *The Audacity to Win,* 75.

64. Interview, Neera Tanden, Washington, DC, July 7, 2010.

65. Hillary for President, "The American Health Choices Plan: Ensuring Quality, Affordable Health Care for All Americans," September 2007; Clinton specified the cap on premium costs later; see Kevin Sack, "Clinton Details Premium Cap in Health Plan," *New York Times,* March 28, 2008.

66. Patrick Healy and Robin Toner, "Public Policy with a Personal Message," *New York Times,* September 19, 2007. Shortly before her announcement, I had pub-

lished an article trying to clarify who made the decisions about the Clinton health plan in 1993. See my "The Hillarycare Mythology," *American Prospect* (October 2007), 12–18, and for my analysis of her 2007 proposal, "Hillary's Own Plan," *American Prospect* (September 24, 2007), at http://www.prospect.org/cs/articles?article=hillarys_own_plan.

67. "Democratic Presidential Candidates Participate in a Debate Sponsored by CNN," CQ Transcripts, January 31, 2008; see also Hillary Clinton's response to George Stephanopolous, ABC News, *This Week,* February 3, 2008, transcript at http://www.presidency.ucsb.edu/ws/index.php?pid=77316.

68. FactCheck.org, "Harry & Louise Again? Obama Mailer on Clinton Health Care Plan Lacks Context," February 4, 2008.

69. FactCheck.org, "Misleading Pennsylvania Voters," at http://www.factcheck.org/elections-2008/misleading_pennsylvania_voters.html.

70. Tom Daschle with David Nather, *Getting It Done* (New York: Thomas Dunne Books/St. Martin's Press, 2010), 83.

71. Interview, Neera Tanden, Washington, DC, July 7, 2010.

72. Robert Moffit and Nina Owcharenko, "The McCain Health Care Plan: More Power to Families," Heritage Foundation, Backgrounder #2198, at http://www.heritage.org/research/reports/2008/10/the-mccain-health-care-plan-more-power-to-families.

73. Transcript, Third Presidential Debate, October 15, 2008, at http://elections.ny-times.com/2008/president/debates/transcripts/third-presidential-debate.html.

74. Thomas Buchmueller, Sherry A. Glied, Anne Royalty, and Katherine Swartz, "Cost and Coverage: Implications of the McCain Plan to Restructure Health Insurance," *Health Affairs* 27, no. 6 (2008), w472–w481.

75. Ezra Klein, "Will This Man Fix American Health Care?" *American Prospect,* June 18, 2008, at http://www.prospect.org/cs/articles?article=will_this_man_fix_american_health_care.

76. Daschle, *Getting It Done,* 184–188.

77. Interview, Peter Orszag, New York City, September 16, 2010; Congressional Budget Office, *Budget Options,* vol. 1, *Health Care* (U.S. Congress, December 2008).

78. For the historical argument, see Beatrix Hoffman, "Health Care Reform and Social Movements in the United States," *American Journal of Public Health* 93 (January 2003), 75–85.

79. Interview with Jeff Blum and Ethan Rome, Washington, DC, May 21, 2010; Health Care for America Now, "Statement of Common Purpose," http://healthcareforamericanow.org/site/content/statement_of_common_purpose/. Richard Kirsch, *Fighting for Your Health* (forthcoming). Kirsch's book promises to be the definitive account of the progressive organizing underpinning the health-care campaign; I appreciate his willingness to share parts of the manuscript.

80. Interview with Gara LaMarche, New York, February 14, 2011; Ben Smith, "HCAN's Sponsor," Politico, at http://www.politico.com/blogs/bensmith/1110/HCANs_sponsor.html.

Chapter 7. Breaking Through, 2009–2010

1. James McGregor Burns, *Transforming Leadership* (New York: Grove Press, 2003).
2. Tom Daschle with David Narther, *Getting It Done* (New York: Thomas Dunne Books, 2010), 63.
3. Interview, Andy Stern, Washington, DC, May 6, 2010.
4. Max Baucus, "Reforming America's Health Care System: A Call to Action," Senate Finance Committee, November 12, 2008.
5. Harold Meyerson, "A Job for Henry Waxman," *Washington Post,* November 19, 2008; Paul Kane, "Rep. Dingell Loses Energy Post; Waxman to Head Key Panel; Change Is Blow to Automakers," *Washington Post,* November 21, 2008.
6. America's Health Insurance Plans, "We Believe Every American Should Have Access to Affordable Health Care Coverage: A Vision for Reform" (Washington, DC, 2008); Fran Lysiak, "Health Industry Proposes Coverage for All, Along with Individual Mandate," *Washington Post,* November 19, 2008.
7. David S. Broder, "Rising Hope for Fixing Health Care," *Washington Post,* November 23, 2008; "Health Reform's Moment," *Washington Post,* December 14, 2008.
8. Daschle, *Getting It Done,* 117.
9. "Transcript: Second Presidential Debate," October 7, 2008, at http://www.cbsnews.com/stories/2008/10/08/politics/2008debates/main4508405.shtml.
10. Matt Bai, "Taking the Hill," *New York Times Magazine,* June 7, 2009.
11. Paul Krugman, "Big Table Fantasies," *New York Times,* December 17, 2007.
12. White House, "Closing Remarks by the President at White House Forum on Health Reform, followed by Q&A, 3/5/09," at http://www.whitehouse.gov/the_press_office/Closing-Remarks-by-the-President-at-White-House-Forum-on-Health-Reform.
13. Letter to President Obama, May 11, 2009, at http://www.whitehouse.gov/assets/documents/05-11-09_Health_Costs_Letter_to_the_President.pdf.
14. For a detailed account of the PhRMA deal, see Paul Blumenthal, "The Legacy of Billy Tauzin: The White House-PhRMA Deal," Sunlight Foundation blog, February 12, 2010, at http://blog.sunlightfoundation.com/2010/02/12/the-legacy-of-billy-tauzin-thewhite-house-phrma-deal/; Jon Cohn, "How Big Pharma Extorted the White House," *New Republic,* August 25, 2009, at http://www.tnr.com/article/politics/drug-deal.
15. Rick Umbdenstock, Sister Carol Keehan, and Chip Kahn, "Statement about Agreement with White House and Senate Finance Committee on Health Reform," July 8, 2009, at http://www.aha.org/aha/press-release/2009/090708-jointst-covreform.pdf.
16. PolitiFact, "Negotiate Health Care Reform in Public Sessions Televised on C-SPAN," http://www.politifact.com/truth-o-meter/promises/obameter/promise/517/health-care-reform-public-sessions-C-SPAN/.
17. Letter to President Obama, April 20, 2009, at http://finance.senate.gov/newsroom/chairman/release/?id=9f070383-f76b-40fa-9c49-1769150af6eb.
18. Robert Pear, "45 Centrist Democrats Protest Secrecy of Health Care Talks," *New York Times,* May 12, 2009.

19. Robert Pear and David M. Herszenhorn, "Conservative Democrats Push Health Bill Changes," *New York Times,* July 22, 2009.

20. Matt Yglesias, "The Powers That Be," ThinkProgress, July 28, 2009, at http://yglesias.thinkprogress.org/2009/07/the-powers-that-be/.

21. Paul Kane and Shailagh Murray, "Lawmakers Cut Health Bills' Price Tag; Negotiators in House and Senate Move Toward Compromises on Reform Packages," *Washington Post,* July 30, 2009.

22. Senate Finance Committee, "Health Care Reform from Conception to Final Passage: Timeline of the Finance Committee's Work to Reform America's Health Care System," at http://finance.senate.gov/issue/?id=32be19bd-491e-4192–812f-f65215c1ba65.

23. Howard Baker, Tom Daschle, and Bob Dole, "Crossing Our Lines: Working Together to Reform the U.S. Health Care System," Bipartisan Policy Center, June 2009.

24. Richard Wolffe, *Revival: The Struggle for Survival inside the Obama White House* (New York: Crown, 2010), 70.

25. Dana Milbank, "At Breakfast, a Side of Political Sausage-Making," *Washington Post,* June 26, 2009.

26. Ben Smith, "Health Reform Foes Plan Obama's 'Waterloo,' " Politico, July 17, 2009, at http://www.politico.com/blogs/bensmith/0709/Health_reform_foes_plan_Obamas_Waterloo.html.

27. "McCaughey Claims End-of-Life Counseling Will Be Required for Medicare Patients," PolitiFact, July 23, 2009, at http://www.politifact.com/truth-o-meter/statements/2009/jul/23/betsy-mccaughey/mccaughey-claims-end-life-counseling-will-be-requi/.

28. For the Boehner and Fox quotations, see Angie Drobnic Holan, "PolitiFact's Lie of the Year: 'Death Panels,' " PolitiFact, December 18, 2009, at http://www.politifact.com/truth-o-meter/article/2009/dec/18/politifact-lie-year-death-panels/; Lee Fang, "Gohmert Trades Ideas with Conspiracy Theorist, Says Obama Health Plan Will 'Absolutely Kill Senior Citizens,' " ThinkProgress, July 27, 2009, at http://thinkprogress.org/2009/07/27/gohmert-conspiracies-alexjones/.

29. Holan, "PolitiFact's Lie of the Year: 'Death Panels.' "

30. Ezra Klein, "Is the Government Going to Euthanize Your Grandmother? An Interview with Sen. Johnny Isakson," *Washington Post,* August 10, 2009, at http://voices.washingtonpost.com/ezra-klein/2009/08/is_the_government_going_to_eut.html.

31. Frank I. Luntz, "The Language of Healthcare 2009," at http://wonkroom.thinkprogress.org/wp-content/uploads/2009/05/frank-luntz-the-language-of-healthcare-20091.pdf.

32. The video is at http://www.politico.com/news/stories/0309/19542.html.

33. Jonathan Martin, "Group Launches Health Care Offensive," Politico, March 3, 2009, http://www.politico.com/news/stories/0309/19542.html; Maggie Mahar, "Who Is Richard Scott—and Why Is He Saying These Things About Health Care Reform?" HealthBeat, March 3, 2009, at http://www.healthbeatblog.com/2009/

03/who-is-richard-scott-and-why-is-he-saying-these-things-about-healthcare-reform.html.

34. Jane Mayer, "Covert Operations: The Billionaire Brothers Who Are Waging a War Against Obama," *The New Yorker*, August 30, 2010, at http://www.newyorker.com/reporting/2010/08/30/100830fa_fact_mayer#ixzz1F1uGA8gN.

35. Tim Dickinson, "The Lie Machine," *Rolling Stone*, October 1, 2009.

36. "Rocking the Town Halls: Best Practices," http://thinkprogress.org/wp-content/uploads/2009/07/townhallactionmemo.pdf.

37. Adam C. Smith, "Protesters in Ybor City Drown Out Health Care Summit on Obama's Proposal," *St. Petersburg Times*, August 7, 2009, at http://www.tampabay.com/news/politics/article1025529.ece.

38. These details are culled from several accounts: Richard Kirsch, "The Guns of August," a chapter to appear in his *Fighting for Your Health* (forthcoming); Patricia Anstett and Kathleen Gray, "Tempers Flare over Health Plan," *Detroit Free Press*, August 7, 2009, at http://www.freep.com/article/20090807/NEWS06/908070387/Tempers-flare-over-health-care-plan; and "Insanity at Rep. John Dingell's Town Hall Meeting," DailyKos, August 6, 2009, at http://www.dailykos.com/story/2009/8/6/762891/-Insanity-at-Rep.-John-Dingells-Town-Hall-Meeting.

39. David D. Kirkpatrick, "White House Affirms Deal on Drug Costs," *New York Times*, August 5, 2009; Ryan Grim, "Internal Memo Confirms Big Giveaways in White House Deal with Big Pharma," Huffington Post, August 13, 2009, at http://www.huffingtonpost.com/2009/08/13/internal-memo-confirms-bi_n_258285.html.

40. Quoted in Karen Tumulty, "Why Grassley Turned on Health-Care Reform," *Time*, September 3, 2009, at www.time.com/time/politics/article/0,8599,1920209,00.html#ixzzotInk2Tkn.

41. Howard Kurtz, "Journalists, Left Out of the Debate: Few Americans Seem to Hear Health Care Facts," *Washington Post*, August 24, 2009.

42. Dickinson, "The Lie Machine."

43. Project for Excellence in Journalism, "Six Things to Know About Health Care Coverage: Opponents Win the Message Wars," June 21, 2010, at http://www.journalism.org/analysis_report/opponents_win_message_wars_0.

44. Pew Research Center for the People and the Press, "Health Care Reform Closely Followed, Much Discussed," conducted August 13–16, 2009, at http://people-press.org/reports/pdf/537.pdf; Kurtz, "Journalists, Left Out of the Debate."

45. Kirsch, "The Guns of August."

46. Mayer, "Covert Operations."

47. Drew Armstrong, "Insurers Gave U.S. Chamber $86 Million Used to Oppose Obama's Health Law," Bloomberg, November 17, 2010, at http://www.bloomberg.com/news/2010-11-17/insurers-gave-u-s-chamber-86-million-used-to-oppose-obama-s-health-law.html?cmpid=yhoo.

48. Interviews with Karen Ignagni, Washington, DC, June 15 and October 1, 2010.

49. "Transcript: Obama's Fifth News Conference," *New York Times,* July 22, 2009, at http://www.nytimes.com/2009/07/22/us/politics/22obama.transcript.html?_r=1&pagewanted=1.

50. Marc Ambinder, "Interview with AHIP's Karen Ignagni: We Won't Take Bait," *The Atlantic,* August 3, 2009, at http://www.theatlantic.com/politics/archive/2009/08/interview-with-ahips-karen-ignagni-we-wont-take-bait/22613/.

51. Brian Beutler, "Major Insurance Company Urges Employees to Attend Tea Parties," Talking Points Memo, August 19, 2009, at http://tpmdc.talkingpointsmemo.com/2009/08/major-health-insurance-company-urges-employees-to-attend-tea-parties.php.

52. Interview, Helen Darling, Washington, DC, July 7, 2010.

53. Kaiser Health Tracking Poll: August 2009, chartpack, at http://www.kff.org/kaiserpolls/upload/7965.pdf.

54. Jonathan Cohn, "How They Did It: The Inside Account of Health Care Reform's Triumph," *New Republic* (June 10, 2010), 14–25.

55. Project for Excellence in Journalism, "Six Things to Know About Health Care Coverage: Obama's Role in the Narrative," June 21, 2010, at http://www.journalism.org/analysis_report/obama%E2%80%99s_role_narrative.

56. In this section, I draw on my "Governing in the Age of Fox News," *The Atlantic* (January–February 2010), 95–98. For the evidence on the limits of presidential persuasion, see B. Dan Wood, *The Myth of Presidential Representation* (New York: Cambridge University Press, 2009), esp. Ch. 5.

57. Matthew A. Baum and Samuel Kernell, "Has Cable Ended the Golden Age of Presidential Television?" *American Political Science Review* 93 (March 1999), 99–114.

58. "24.7M Watch Obama's Prime Time Health Care Press Conference," Nielsen Wire, July 23, 2009, at http://blog.nielsen.com/nielsenwire/nielsen-news/obama-prime-time-health-care-press-conference.

59. "32.1 Million Watch President Obama's Health Care Address to Congress on TV," Nielsen Wire, September 10, 2009, at http://blog.nielsen.com/nielsenwire/media_entertainment/31-8-million-watch-president-obamas-health-care-address-to-congress-on-tv/.

60. For the text of Obama's speech, see http://www.nytimes.com/2009/09/10/us/politics/10obama.text.html.

61. Interview, Peter Orszag, New York, September 16, 2010. The $900 billon number came from Gruber's modeling. Interview, Nancy-Ann Min DeParle, Washington, DC, June 1, 2010.

62. Kaiser Health Tracking Poll: September 2009, at http://www.kff.org/kaiserpolls/posr092909pkg.cfm.

63. Ezra Klein, "Chuck Grassley Fundraises against Health-Care Reform," *Washington Post,* August 31, 2009, at http://voices.washingtonpost.com/ezra-klein/2009/08/chuck_grassley_fundraises_agai.html.

64. See Timothy Noah, "Don't Be Stupak: Abortion Foes Meddle with Private Health Insurance," *Slate,* November 4, 2009, at http://www.slate.com/id/2234602/.

65. Shailagh Murray and Lori Montgomery, "Prospects for Public Option Dim in Senate; Key Committee Rejects Proposals for Government Health Insurance," *Washington Post,* September 30, 2009.

66. Congressional Budget Office, Letter to Sen. Reid, November 18, 2009, page 9, at http://www.cbo.gov/ftpdocs/107xx/doc10731/Reid_letter_11_18_09.pdf.

67. "Dean on Health Care: 'Kill the Senate Bill,'" Vermont Public Radio, December 15, 2009, at http://www.vpr.net/news_detail/86681/; Huma Khan and Jonathan Karl, "Howard Dean: Health Care Bill 'Bigger Bailout for the Insurance Industry Than AIG'; Top Democrat Urges Lawmakers to Kill the Bill and Start Over," ABC News, December 16, 2009, at http://abcnews.go.com/GMA/HealthCare/howard-dean-health-care-bill-bigger-bailout-insurance/story?id=9349392.

68. Karl Rove, *Courage and Consequence* (New York: Simon and Schuster, 2010), 373.

69. David M. Herszenhorn, "In Health Vote, a New Vitriol," *New York Times,* December 24, 2009.

70. Dan Balz and Jon Cohen, "Poll Finds Mass. Vote Reflects Ongoing Trend; Anger Seen in GOP Wins in November Also Drove Party's Upset Tuesday," *Washington Post,* January 23, 2010.

71. David M. Herszenhorn, "Supported by Brown, Massachusetts Reform Was a Model for Democrats in Washington," *New York Times,* January 20, 2010, at http://prescriptions.blogs.nytimes.com/2010/01/20/supported-by-brown-mass-health-plan-was-a-model-for-democrats/.

72. Kaiser Health Tracking Poll: January 2010, at http://www.kff.org/kaiserpolls/upload/8042-C.pdf.

73. Fred Barnes: "Look, it is dead. It is dead in the House. It is dead in the Senate." Sean Hannity: "Prince Harry [Reid] has to accept the fact that his health care bill is dead." For these and other comments at the time, see "Flashback: Media Repeatedly Declared Health Care Reform 'Dead' after Brown's Senate Victory," Media Matters, March 22, 2010, at http://mediamatters.org/research/201003220039.

74. David M. Herszenhorn, "The Numbers Come Out Just Where Obama Wanted, with No Magic Involved," *New York Times,* March 19, 2010.

75. Barack Obama, victory speech, St. Paul, Minnesota, at http://www.youtube.com/watch?v=kbbIQFcEhcQ.

76. Eric Pooley, *The Climate War* (New York: Hyperion, 2010), 360–361.

77. Ryan Lizza, "As the World Burns," *The New Yorker,* October 11, 2010.

Chapter 8. The Affordable Care Act as Public Philosophy

1. Congressional Budget Office, Letter to Speaker Nancy Pelosi, March 20, 2010, at http://www.cbo.gov/ftpdocs/113xx/doc11379/AmendReconProp.pdf.

2. In this chapter, when I refer to the Affordable Care Act, I mean the act as revised by the Health Care and Education Reconciliation Act. For the texts, see H.R. 3590, 111th Cong., 2d sess., at http://www.gpo.gov/fdsys/pkg/BILLS-111hr3590enr/pdf/BILLS-111hr3590enr.pdf, and H.R. 4872, 111th Cong., 2d sess., at http://www.gpo.gov/fdsys/pkg/BILLS-111hr4872enr/pdf/BILLS-111hr4872enr.pdf. For a handy ref-

erence, see Kaiser Family Foundation, "Summary of New Health Care Reform Law," at http://www.kff.org/healthreform/upload/8061.pdf.

3. In earlier work I distinguished among four structures of inequality: mass exclusion, minority exclusion, multi-tier universal coverage, and broad-based universalism. The Affordable Care Act is an instance of multi-tier universal coverage, not broad-based universalism. For that earlier work, see Paul Starr, "The Politics of Health Care Inequalities," in David E. Rogers and Eli Ginzberg, eds., *Medical Care and the Health of the Poor* (Boulder, CO: Westview Press, 1993), 21–32.

4. Aaron Yellowitz, "ObamaCare: A Bad Deal for Young Adults," Cato Institute, October 9, 2009, at http://www.cato.org/pubs/bp/bp115.pdf.

5. U.S. Census Bureau, "Income, Poverty, and Health Insurance Coverage in the United States: 2009," Current Population Reports, September 2010, 26, at http://www.census.gov/prod/2010pubs/p60–238.pdf.

6. Sharon K. Long, Alshadye Yemane, and Karen Stockley, "Disentangling the Effects of Health Reform in Massachusetts: How Important Are the Special Provisions for Young Adults?" *American Economic Review: Papers & Proceedings* 100 (May 2010), 297–302.

7. Eli Y. Adashi, H. Jack Geiger, and Michael D. Fine, "Health Care Reform and Primary Care—The Growing Importance of the Community Health Center," *New England Journal of Medicine* 362 (April 28, 2010), 2047–2050, at http://healthpolicyandreform.nejm.org/?p=3377.

8. For my own view on immigration, see "Why Immigration Reform Matters," *American Prospect* (July–August 2007), 3; for more on how the Affordable Care Act affects immigrants, see Maria C. Abascal, "Reform's Mixed Impact on Immigrants," *American Prospect* (September 2010), A17–A18.

9. In this section, I draw on my *Freedom's Power: The History and Promise of Liberalism* (New York: Basic Books, 2008).

10. This formulation, which comes from *Freedom's Power,* owes a debt to Ronald Dworkin's thinking about principles of human dignity in *Sovereign Virtue: The Theory and Practice of Equality* (Cambridge, MA: Harvard University Press, 2000) and *Is Democracy Possible Here?* (Princeton, NJ: Princeton University Press, 2007); for more discussion, see my review of the latter in *New York Review of Books,* July 16, 2009.

11. Transcript, "The Second Presidential Debate," October 7, 2008, http://elections.nytimes.com/2008/president/debates/transcripts/second-presidential-debate.html.

12. If the employer offers inadequate insurance (a plan that covers less than 60 percent of allowable costs or for which any employee must pay more than 9.5 percent of income), the employer must pay a penalty of $3,000 for each subsidized employee up to a total no greater than $2,000 per total full-time employees after the first 30 employees.

13. Christine Eibner, Peter S. Hussey, and Federico Girosi, "The Effects of the Affordable Care Act on Workers' Health Insurance Coverage," *New England Journal of Medicine* 363 (October 7, 2010), 1393–1395.

14. Robert E. Moffitt. "Personal Freedom, Responsibility, and Mandates," *Health Affairs* 13 (Spring 1994), 101–104 (quotations, 101, 103).

15. See Mark Blumenthal, "Polling on the Individual Mandate," December 15, 2009, at http://www.pollster.com/blogs/polling_on_the_individual_mand.php ?nr=1. For an analysis based on 2008 data, see Tara Sussman, Robert J. Blendon, and Andrea Louise Campbell, "Will Americans Support the Individual Mandate?" *Health Affairs* (April 21, 2009), w501–w509. Support for the mandate went up when questions in polls suggested it would not apply if insurance was too expensive, or that it would be coupled with provisions to make it affordable.

16. Paul Starr, "Averting a Backlash," *American Prospect,* December 8, 2009, at http://prospect.org/cs/articles?article=averting_a_health_care_backlash; "A Health Insurance Mandate with a Choice," *New York Times,* March 3, 2010; and "The Opt-Out Compromise," *American Prospect,* March 9, 2010, at http://prospect.org/cs/articles?article=the_opt_out_compromise.

17. January Angeles, "Some Recent Reports Overstate the Effect on State Budgets of the Medicaid Expansions in the Health Reform Law," Center on Budget and Policy Priorities, October 21, 2010, 3, at http://www.cbpp.org/files/10–21–10health.pdf.

18. Stan Dorn and Matthew Buettgens, "Net Effects of the Affordable Care Act on State Budgets," Urban Institute, December 2010, at http://www.urban.org/UploadedPDF/1001480-Affordable-Care-Act.pdf.

19. See my "Troubled States," *American Prospect* (March 2011), 3.

20. The Basic Health Program option, introduced to meet concerns from the state of Washington's representatives, could turn out to be an important sleeper provision of the law. See Stan Dorn, "The Basic Health Program Option under Federal Health Reform: Issues for Consumers and States," AcademyHealth State Coverage Initiatives, March 2011, at http://www.rwjf.org/files/research/72024.pdf.

21. MedPAC, *Report to the Congress: Medicare Payment Policy* (Washington, DC: MedPAC, March 2008).

22. This section draws on my article, "The Preventive Turn in Health-Care Reform," *American Prospect* (September 2010), A19.

23. U.S. Preventive Services Task Force, "Screening for Breast Cancer," release date: October 2008; updated: November 2009, at http://www.uspreventiveservicestaskforce.org/uspstf/uspsbrca.htm.

24. Congressional Budget Office, *Key Issues in Analyzing Major Health Insurance Proposals* (December 2008), 60, at http://www.cbo.gov/ftpdocs/99xx/doc9924/12–18-KeyIssues.pdf.

25. Jonathan Oberlander and Joseph White, "Public Attitudes toward Health Care Spending Aren't the Problem; Prices Are," *Health Affairs* 28 (September–October, 2009), 1285–1293. I made the case for an American version of global budgeting in *The Logic of Health-Care Reform* ([Knoxville, TN]: Grand Rounds Press, 1992).

26. Robert A. Berenson, "Unleashing Restraint," *American Prospect* (September 2010), A20–A22.

27. Andrea M. Sisko et al., "National Health Spending Projections: The Estimated Impact of Reform through 2019," *Health Affairs* 29 (October 2010), 1–9.

28. David M. Cutler, Karen Davis, and Kristof Stremikis, "The Impact of Health Reform on Health System Spending," Commonwealth Fund, 2010, at http://www.commonwealthfund.org/~/media/Files/Publications/Issue%20Brief/2010/May/1405_Cutler_impact_hlt_reform_on_hlt_sys_spending_ib_v4.pdf.

29. Nancy-Ann DeParle, "New Report on National Health Expenditures" (White House blog), at http://www.whitehouse.gov/blog/2010/09/09/new-report-national-health-expenditures; Jonathan Gruber, "The Cost Implications of Health Care Reform," *New England Journal of Medicine* 362 (June 3, 2010), 2050–2051.

Chapter 9. Reform's Uncertain Fate

1. Some sections of this chapter draw on my "The Next Health-Reform Campaign," *American Prospect* (September 2010), A3–A7.

2. Interview, Nancy-Ann DeParle, Washington, June 1, 2010.

3. N. C. Aizenman and Robert Barnes, "Controversial Mini-Med Plans to Live on through Waivers," *Washington Post,* March 27, 2011.

4. Letter from Secretary Kathleen Sebelius to Karen Ignagni, September 24, 2010, at http://www.hhs.gov/ociio/regulations/children19/ignagni.pdf.

5. U.S. Department of Health and Human Services, "Uninsured Americans with Pre-existing Conditions Continue to Gain Coverage through Affordable Care Act," February 10, 2011, at http://www.hhs.gov/news/press/2011pres/02/20110210a.html; Harold Pollack, "The Cost of Delayed Reform," *American Prospect* (September 2010), A16–A17; "State by State Enrollment in the Pre-Existing Condition Insurance Plan," accessed December 14, 2012, at http://www.healthcare.gov/news/factsheets/2012/11/pcip11162012a.html.

6. Joanne Kenen, "National Reform Meets Politics in the States," *American Prospect* (September 2010), A11–A15.

7. Mollyann Brodie et al., "Liking the Pieces, Not the Package: Contradictions in Public Opinion during Health Reform," *Health Affairs* 29 (June 2010), 1125–1130.

8. Kaiser Health Tracking Poll: October 2010, at http://www.kff.org/kaiserpolls/upload/8115-F.pdf.

9. CNN Opinion Research Poll, December 27, 2010, at http://i2.cdn.turner.com/cnn/2010/images/12/27/rel17h.pdf. See Matt Yglesias, "The Median Voter Supports the Affordable Care Act," ThinkProgress, December 27, 2010, at http://yglesias.thinkprogress.org/2010/12/the-median-voter-supports-the-affordable-care-act/.

10. "The Associated Press 2010 Health Care Reform Survey by Stanford University with the Robert Wood Johnson Foundation Conducted by Knowledge Networks" (Menlo Park, CA: Knowledge Networks, n.d.).

11. See Morris P. Fiorina, with Samuel J. Abrams, and Jeremy C. Pope, *Culture War? The Myth of a Polarized America,* 2nd ed. (New York: Pearson Longman, 2006).

12. Brodie et al., "Liking the Pieces, Not the Package"; Kaiser Health Tracking Poll: November 2010, at http://www.kff.org/kaiserpolls/upload/8120-F.pdf. See,

more generally, Alan I. Abramowitz, *The Polarized Public? Why American Government Is So Dysfunctional* (Boston: Pearson, 2013), 10–11.

13. Kaiser Health Tracking Poll: October 2010.

14. Nate Silver, "Democrats Aren't Running from Health Care, but What Are They Running On?" Five Thirty Eight (*New York Times* blog), September 7, 2010, at http://fivethirtyeight.blogs.nytimes.com/2010/09/07/democrats-arent-running-from-health-care-but-what-are-they-running-on/.

15. Kaiser Health Tracking Poll: November 2010, at http://www.kff.org/kaiserpolls/upload/8120-F.pdf.

16. John Sides, "Political Science Forecasts for the 2010 Election," The Monkey Cage, September 7, 2010, at http://www.themonkeycage.org/2010/09/political_science_forecasts_fo.html.

17. Eric McGhee, Brendan Nyhan, and John Sides, "Midterm Postmortem," *Boston Review*, November 11, 2010, at http://bostonreview.net/BR35.6/sides.php.

18. See figure, "Margin of Victory (Defeat) for Democratic Incumbents Based on Health Care Vote," in Nate Silver, "Health Care and Bailout Votes May Have Hurt Democrats," Five Thirty Eight (*New York Times* blog), November 16, 2010, at http://fivethirtyeight.blogs.nytimes.com/2010/11/16/health-care-bailout-votes-may-have-hurt-democrats/; Ben Smith, "No Shelter in Health-Care Opposition," Politico, November 3, 2010, at http://www.politico.com/blogs/bensmith/1110/No_shelter_in_health_care_opposition_.html.

19. Kaiser Health Tracking Poll, November 2010.

20. Byron Tau, "Seniors Fled Democrats in Midterms," Politico, November 8, 2010, at http://www.politico.com/news/stories/1110/44802.html; Jonathan Chait, "The Age Gap," *New Republic*, November 8, 2010, at http://www.tnr.com/blog/jonathan-chait/78982/the-age-gap.

21. Lydia Saad, "Verdict on Healthcare Reform Bill Still Divided," Gallup, June 22, 2010, at http://www.gallup.com/poll/140981/verdict-healthcare-reform-bill-divided.aspx.

22. Drew Altman, "Seniors and Health Reform," Kaiser Health Foundation, July 28, 2010, at http://www.kff.org/pullingittogether/072710_altman.cfm. For the survey, see Kaiser Health Tracking Poll, July 2010, at http://www.kff.org/kaiserpolls/upload/8084-F.pdf.

23. "Elizabeth C. Hamel, Claudia Deane, and Mollyann Brodie, "Medicare and Medicaid," in Robert J. Blendon et al., *American Public Opinion and Health Care* (Washington, DC: CQ Press, 2011), 155.

24. Robert J. Blendon and John M. Benson, "Attitudes about the U.S. Health System and Priorities for Government Action," in Robert J. Blendon et al., *American Public Opinion and Health Care* (Washington, DC: CQ Press, 2011), 58.

25. "The Associated Press 2010 Health Care Reform Survey."

26. Edwin Park, "Ryan's Rx for Medicaid Means Millions More Uninsured or Underinsured Seniors, People with Disabilities, and Children," April 4, 2011, Center on Budget and Policy Priorities, at http://www.offthechartsblog.org/ryan

%E2%80%99s-rx-for-medicaid-means-millions-more-uninsured-or-underin sured-seniors-people-with-disabilities-and-children/#more-2812. For more, see Kaiser Commission on Medicaid and the Uninsured, "Implications of a Medic- aid Block Grant," April 2011, at http://www.kff.org/medicaid/upload/8173.pdf.

27. Congressional Budget Office. *Long-Term Analysis of a Budget Proposal by Chair- man Ryan.* April 5, 2011, 24; Paul N. Van de Water, "Ryan Budget Would Increase Health Care Spending for Medicare Beneficiaries," Center on Budget and Policy Priorities, April 8, 2011, at http://www.offthechartsblog.org/ryan-budget-would -increase-health-care-spending-for-medicare-beneficiaries/.

28. Ron Wyden, "So Much for Choice and Competition," *Huffington Post,* April 9, 2011, at http://www.huffingtonpost.com/sen-ron-wyden/so-much-for-choice -and-co_b_847080.html; John McDonough, "Holes in the ACA: A Damage As- sessment," Boston.com, January 14, 2013, at http://www.boston.com/lifestyle /health/health_stew/2013/01/holes_in_the_aca_a_damage_asse.html.

29. Tucker Reals, "Obama: GOP Tried to 'Sneak' Agenda into Budget," CBS News, April 15, 2011, at http://www.cbsnews.com/8301–503544_162–20054185–503544 .html.

30. "Transcript: Sens. Dodd, Grassley on 'FNS,' " Fox News, at http://www.foxnews .com/story/0,2933,526301,00.html.

31. *Wickard v. Filburn,* 317 U. S. 111 (1942).

32. *Gonzales v. Raich* 545 US 1 (2005).

33. Testimony of Charles Fried, Senate Judiciary Committee, February 2, 2011, at http://judiciary.senate.gov/pdf/11–02–02%20Fried%20Testimony.pdf; Bradford Plumer, "The Individual Mandate Is a 'No-Brainer,' " *New Republic,* February 2, 2011, at http://www.tnr.com/blog/jonathan-cohn/82678/charles-fried-the-indi vidual-mandate-no-brainer.

34. "In the Supreme Court of the United States, Department of Health and Human Services, et al., v. Florida, et al.," Washington, DC, March 27, 2012 [hereafter "official transcript"], 4–5.

35. Official transcript, 11.

36. See Einer Elhauge, "If Health Insurance Mandates Are Unconstitutional, Why Did the Founding Fathers Back Them?" *New Republic,* April 13, 2012; Elhauge, "A Response to Critics on the Founding Fathers and Health Insurance Mandates," ibid, April 19, 2012; and Elhauge, "A Further Response . . ." April 21, 2012. These and other articles by Elhauge have been an invaluable resource.

37. Official transcript, 24.

38. Ibid, 65.

39. Ibid, 20.

40. Ibid, 50.

41. *National Federation of Independent Business et al. v. Sebelius,* Opinion of C.J. Rob- erts, 20, 23–24.

42. Kevin Sack and Eric Linchtblau, "For Attorneys General, A Long Shot on Health Care Law Brings Payoffs," *New York Times,* July 1, 2012.

43. *National Federation of Independent Business et al. v. Sebelius*, Opinion of J. Ginsburg, 40.

44. Opinion of C.J. Roberts, 51.

45. Opinion of J. Ginsburg, 51.

46. Dissent of Scalia, Kennedy, Thomas, Alito, 63.

47. Opinion of J. Ginsburg, 40.

48. Jan Crawford, "Roberts Switched Views to Uphold Health Care Law," CBS News, July 1, 2012, at http://www.cbsnews.com/8301-3460_162-57464549/roberts-switched-views-to-uphold-health-care-law/

49. Sack and Linchtblau, "For Attorneys General, A Long Shot on Health Care Law Brings Payoffs."

50. Jeffrey Toobin, *The Oath: The Obama White House and the Supreme Court* (New York: Doubleday, 2012).

51. Andrea Campbell and Nathaniel Persily, "The Health Care Case in the Public Mind: How the Supreme Court Shapes Opinion about Itself and the Laws It Considers," in Nathaniel Persily, ed., *The Health Care Case: The Supreme Court's Decision and Its Implications* (forthcoming).

52. Congressional Budget Office, *Estimates for the Insurance Coverage Provisions of the Affordable Care Act Updated for the Recent Supreme Court Decision* (July 2012), 13.

53. Ryan Lizza, "Romney's Dilemma: How His Greatest Achievement Has Become His Biggest Liability," *The New Yorker*, June 6, 2011.

54. "Transcript: ABC News/Facebook/WMUR Republicans Debate," January 5, 2008, at http://abcnews.go.com/Politics/Vote2008/story?id=4091645&page=1&singlePage=true#.UGTA8RjuamH.

55. Mitt Romney, "Mr. President, What's the Rush?" *USA Today*, July 30, 2009, 7A.

56. "Romney: No Apologies for RomneyCare," *The Atlantic*, May 12, 2011, at http://www.theatlantic.com/politics/archive/2011/05/romney-no-apologies-for-romneycare/238826/.

57. For the video, see "Tim Pawlenty Walks Back 'Obamneycare,'" ABC News, June 13, 2011, at http://abcnews.go.com/Politics/video/tim-pawlenty-walks-back-obamneycare-13833453.

58. Robert Pear and David M. Herszenhorn, "Senate Backs Preventive Health Care for Women," *New York Times*, December 4, 2009.

59. Margalit Fox, "Pauline Phillips, Flinty Adviser to Millions as Dear Abby, Dies at 94," *New York Times*, January 17, 2013.

60. Neera Tanden, "The 1990s Roots of the Contraception Battle," *New Republic*, March 12, 2012, at http://www.tnr.com/article/politics/101567/neera-tanden-contraception?utm_source=The+New+Republic&utm_campaign=9b0824f4c8-TNR_Pol_031212&utm_medium=email#; Irin Carmon, "Whose Freedom on Contraception?" *Salon*, March 15, 2012, at http://www.salon.com/2012/03/15/whose_freedom_on_contraception/singleton/.

61. Testimony of Guttmacher Institute to the Committee on Preventive Services for Women, Institute of Medicine, January 12, 2011, http://www.guttmacher.org/pubs/CPSW-testimony.pdf.

62. "Check Point: Santorum on Financing for Family Planning Programs," *New York Times*, February 23, 2012.

63. Erik Wemple, "Rush Limbaugh's 'Personal Attack' on Sandra Fluke? More like 20 Attacks," *Washington Post*, March 5, 2012; Jonathan Weisman, "Obama Backs Student in Furor with Limbaugh on Birth Control," *New York Times*, March 2, 2012.

64. According to the February Kaiser tracking survey, 63 percent of the public supported the contraceptive requirement, http://www.kff.org/kaiserpolls/upload /8281-F.pdf. A majority of Catholics supported the requirement. Cathy Lynn Grossman, "New Surveys: Catholics Want Birth Control Coverage," *USA Today*, February 7, 2012, at http://content.usatoday.com/communities/Religion/post /2012/02/contraception-catholic-bishops-obama-hhs/1.

65. Jeffrey F. Peipert et al., "Preventing Unintended Pregnancies by Providing No-Cost Contraception," *Obstetrics & Gynecology* 120 (December 2012), 1291–1297.

66. Chris Cillizza and Aaron Blake, "President Obama Embraces 'Obamacare' Label. But Why?" *Washington Post*, March 26, 2012, at http://www.washingtonpost .com/blogs/the-fix/post/president-obama-embraces-obamacare-label-but-why /2012/03/25/gIQARJ5qaS_blog.html?wprss=rss_the-fix.

67. John Eligon and Michael Schwirtz, "In Rapes, Candidate Says, Body Can Block Pregnancy," *New York Times*, August 20, 2012; Jonathan Weisman, "Rape Comment Draws Attention in Indiana," *New York Times*, October 24, 2012.

68. Sahil Kapur, "Romney: Sorry, No Preexisting Conditions Guarantee Unless You're Already Insured," TPM, September 10, 2012, at http://2012.talkingpoints-memo.com/2012/09/mitt-romney-obamacare-preexisting-condition.php.

69. Ashley Parker, "Romney Blames Loss on Obama's 'Gifts' to Minorities and Young Voters," *New York Times*, November 14, 2012.

70. Sarah Kliff, "Millions Will Qualify for New Options under the Health Care Law. Most Have No Idea," *Washington Post*, November 21, 2012.

71. Kaiser tracking survey: November 2012, at http://www.kff.org/kaiserpolls/up load/8382-F.pdf.

72. This was a consideration in Arizona Governor Jan Brewer's decision to go ahead with the Medicaid expansion. Sarah Kliff, "Arizona Could Make the Medicaid Expansion an Immigration Fight," *Washington Post*, January 25, 2013.

73. Conference, "What's Next for Health Reform?" Princeton University, November 16, 2012.

74. Gallup, "In U.S., Majority Now Against Gov't Healthcare Guarantee," November 28, 2012, at http://www.gallup.com/poll/158966/majority-against-gov-healthcare -guarantee.aspx?utm_source=alert&utm_medium=email&utm_campaign =syndication&utm_content=morelink&utm_term=Politics—USA.

75. Arthur Schlesinger, Jr., "The Liberal Opportunity," *American Prospect* (Spring 1990), 10–18.

Stupak, Bart, 224–25, 234
Summers, Larry, 196
Supplemental Security Income, 55, 165
Supreme Court, 30, 278–86, 287
suspicion of government, 8, 11, 214–17
Sutton, Jeffrey, 179
Sweden, 5
Sweet, Thaddeus, 34

Tanden, Neera, 187–88
Tauzin, Billy, 204
tax credits: *2007–2008* proposals, 175, 177–78, 185, 188–89; and abortion coverage, 224–25; Affordable Care Act, 243; Bush proposal, 85; Earned Income Tax Credit, 137; in Massachusetts, 170; Obama/ Democratic plan, 22, 213; public opinion, 181; Republican proposals, 80, 83, 174, 202–3. *See also* tax exclusion
taxes: Bush cuts, 146–47, 183–84, 186, 197, 257; under the Clinton plan, 97–98; under the Garamendi plan, 88; high-cost insurance tax, 17, 230–31, 234, 258–59; HSAs' benefits, 151, 154; insurance tax deduction proposed, 188; Medicare taxes, 69, 107, 234, 257; Obama/ Democratic plan and, 210, 223, 230–31; under pay-or-play, 85; under single-payer plans, 84; tanning salons, 261; value-added tax, 178. *See also* tobacco tax
tax exclusion: Affordable Care Act and, 22, 258–59; Clinton plan and, 98; Cooper bill and, 106; costs and inequities, 42, 258; McCain proposal and, 188; origins, 4, 42; as subsidy, 19; unlimited, 132; widely misunderstood, 188–89; Wyden-Bennett bill and, 178. *See also* health savings accounts; tax credits

Tea Party groups, 214–16, 219, 234
Texas, 164
therapeutic nihilism, 59
Thomas, Bill, 145
tobacco industry, 116
tobacco tax: children's coverage funded, 142, 167, 177, 256; Clinton plan, 95, 116; "mainstream group" proposal, 121
town hall meetings, 214–16
treatment effectiveness, 263
Truman, Harry, 40–41, 73, 76, 103

underinsurance, 5, 156
unemployment insurance, 34, 37–38
unfunded mandates, 71, 164
uninsured people: *1970s*, 1, 5, 50, 287(n35); *1989–1995*, 79, 100; *1995–2010*, 1, 5, 156, 176; access to care, 242–43; Affordable Care Act's effect on, 240, 256–57; demographic factors, 163–64; highlighted by Obama, 222; in Massachusetts, 167, 168, 173; paid for by taxes and the insured, 242, 250; political power lacking, 7–8. *See also* history of health-care legislation; Medicaid
unions: and the *2007* coalition proposal, 176; health benefits won, 42; high-cost insurance tax opposed, 230–31; and Kennedy plans, 56, 60, 75; "mainstream group" proposal opposed, 122; and Progressive health insurance proposals, 31–32; social programs supported, 35. *See also specific organizations*
UnitedHealthcare, 145, 218, 219
universal coverage: British model, 18, 40 (*see also* British health care); Enthoven market model, 62, 85–86, 89–90; Medicare model, 18; Obama campaign plan short of, 185; reasons for American lack, 72–76; seniors opposed to, 275. *See also* history of